D1627177

Healing Practices: Alternative Therapies for Nursing

Karen Lee Fontaine

Professor
Purdue University Calumet
Hammond, Indiana

Prentice Hall
Upper Saddle River, NJ 07458

Library of Congress Cataloging-in-Publication Data

Fontaine, Karen Lee,
    Healing practices : alternative therapies for nursing / Karen Lee Fontaine.
    p.   cm.
    Includes bibliographical references and index.
    ISBN 0-8385-0385-3
    1. Nursing.   2. Alternative medicine.   I. Title.
    RT42 .F64 2000
    615.5—dc21   99-32976
                                                                            CIP

Publisher: *Julie Alexander*
Editor-in-Chief: *Cheryl Mehalik*
Acquisitions Editor: *Maura Connor*
Director of Manufacturing and Production: *Bruce Johnson*
Managing Production Editor: *Patrick Walsh*
Senior Production Manager: *Ilene Sanford*
Production Liaison: *Julie Boddorf*
Full Service Production/Formatting: *BookMasters, Inc.*
Creative Director: *Marianne Frasco*
Cover Design Coordinator: *Maria Guglielmo*
Cover Designer: *Bruce Kenselaar*
Marketing Manager: *Kristin Walton*
Printer/Binder: *R.R. Donnelley & Sons*
Editorial Consultant: Patricia L. Cleary, San Francisco, California

© 2000 by Prentice-Hall, Inc.
Upper Saddle River, New Jersey 07458

Disclaimer   The facts of this text have been drawn from scientific literature and are intended to be educational in nature. In no way, however, are any of the suggestions meant to take the place of advice given by licensed health care professionals. The information should not beconsidered prescriptive advice, but rather a set of possible options for people and their health care providers to consider.
    Consult your primary health care provider before instituting any medical treatment. As such, the author disclaims any liability arising directly or indirectly from information contained in this text.

Care has been taken to confirm the accuracy of information presented in this book. The authors, editors, and the publisher, however, cannot accept any responsibility for errors or omissions or for consequences from application of the information in this book and make no warranty, express or implied, with respect to its contents.
    The authors and publisher have exerted every effort to ensure that drug selections and dosages set forth in this text are in accord with current recommendations and practice at the time of publication. However, in view of ongoing research, changes in government regulations, and the constant flow of information relating to drug therapy and drug reactions, the reader is urged to check the package inserts of all drugs for any change in indications of dosage and for added warnings and precautions. This is particularly important when the recommended agent is a new and/or infrequently employed drug.

Printed in the United States of America

10 9 8 7 6 5 4

ISBN 0-8385-0385-3

Prentice-Hall International (UK) Limited, *London*
Prentice-Hall of Australia Pty. Limited, *Sydney*
Prentice-Hall Canada Inc., *Toronto*
Prentice-Hall Hispanoamericana, S.A., *Mexico*
Prentice-Hall of India Private Limited, *New Delhi*
Prentice-Hall of Japan, Inc., *Tokyo*
Prentice-Hall Singapore Pte. Ltd.
Editora Prentice-Hall do Brasil, Ltda., *Rio de Janeiro*

This book is dedicated to
my mother, Vera J. Lee, thank you for giving me so much
and
Patti Cleary for her unending support, sense of humor,
and incredible mastery of the English language

Contents

Try This

Preface

As nursing moves into the twenty-first century, it is advancing beyond the Western biomedical model to incorporate many healing tools used by our Asian, Latino, Native American, African, and European ancestors. We are rapidly rediscovering that these ancient principles and practices have significant therapeutic value. Some see this movement as a "return to our roots." Others believe it is a response to runaway health care costs, growing dissatisfaction with high-tech medicine, and increasing concern over the adverse effects and misuse of medications. The growth of consumer empowerment also fuels this movement.

As nurses, how do we begin to assimilate thousands of years of healing knowledge? How do we begin this journey of integrating healing practices into our own lives? In our professional practice, how do we model healthful living? How do we help consumers choose their own healing journeys? How do we break down the barriers between conventional and alternative medicine? Learning about healing practices, like anything else, is a slow process involving a steady accumulation of bits of information and skills that eventually form a coherent pattern called knowledge. While it is possible to learn a great deal about healing practices from reading, thinking, and asking questions, you must in the long run learn about healing through participation. Without hands-on experience, you can be a good student but you can never be a great nursing practitioner of the healing arts. I trust this text will be one step in a lifelong exploration and experience of healing practices.

Consumers do not wish to abandon conventional medicine but they do want to have a range of options available to them including herbs, nutrition, manual healing methods, mind-body techniques, and spiritual approaches. Some healing practices, such as exercise, nutrition, meditation, and massage, promote health and prevent disease. Others, such as herbs or homeopathic remedies, address specific illnesses. Many other healing practices do both. The rise of chronic disease rates in Western society has motivated consumers to increasingly consider self-care approaches. As recently as the 1950s, we lived in a world of curable disease, largely infectious, where medical interventions were both appropriate and effective and only 30 percent of all disease was chronic. Now, 80 percent of all disease is chronic. Western medicine, with its focus on acute disorders, trauma, and surgery, is considered to be the best high-tech medical care in the world. Unfortunately, it cannot respond adequately to the current epidemic of chronic illnesses.

Ethnocentrism, the assumption that one's own cultural or ethnic group is superior to others, has often prevented Western health care practitioners from learning "new" ways to promote health and prevent chronic illness. With consumer demand for a broader range of options, we must open our minds to the idea that other cultures and countries have valid ways of preventing and curing diseases that could be good for Western societies. Although the information may be new to us, many of these traditions are hundreds or even thousands of years old and have long been part of the medical mainstream in other cultures.

I have titled this book *Healing Practices: Alternative Therapies for Nursing* because I believe we need a merger of alternative approaches with our Western-based nursing practices. I have tried to provide enough information about alternative therapies to help guide your practice decisions. This text, as an overview and practical guide for nurses, does not pretend to be an exhaustive collection of all the facts and related research in the area of alternative medicine, nor does it offer meticulous documentation for all claims made by the various therapies. The goal of the text is to motivate you, the reader, to explore alternative approaches, increase your knowledge about factors that contribute to health and illness, and expand your professional practice appropriately.

It is possible to classify alternative practices in any number of ways. I have chosen to present more than 40 approaches categorized into seven units. In Unit One, I introduce the philosophical approaches to both Western biomedicine and alternative or complementary medicine. Concepts common to many approaches are defined and discussed such as energy, breath, spirituality, and healing. Unit Two presents a number of health care practices that have been systematized throughout the centuries and throughout the world. These typically include an entire set of values, attitudes, and beliefs that generate a philosophy of life, not simply a group of remedies. Unit Three is comprised of chapters relating to botanical healings used by 80 percent of the world's population. Chapter discussions cover herbs and nutritional supplements, naturopathy, homeopathy, and aromatherapy. Unit Four presents manual healing methods, some from ancient times and some developed in the latter half of the twentieth century. The chapters are chiropractic, massage, pressure point therapies, hand-mediated biofield therapies, and physical and biofield therapies.

The chapters in Unit Five are types of mind-body techniques for healing and include yoga, meditation, hypnotherapy and guided imagery, dreams, biofeedback, and movement-oriented therapies. Unit Six presents two spiritual approaches to therapeutic intervention: working with shamans and the use of faith and prayer. Unit Seven includes three chapters on miscellaneous practices: bioelectromagnetics, detoxifying therapies, and animal-assisted therapy.

The appendix provides specific information on alternative therapies for common health problems. It is meant to provide education for the management of the types of problems that respond well to alternative therapies and lifestyle modification.

This book does not recommend treatments but rather describes alternative practices, their backgrounds and claims, preparation of practitioners, concepts, diagnostic methods, treatments, and evidence of research studies. Integrated nursing practice is an important section of every chapter. This section is designed to help you, the nurse, expand your practice by providing you with specific information and suggestions. A consistent feature is TRY THIS to give you an example of how these practices can be integrated into your own life, as well as giving you ideas for client education. A list of resources is also included in the chapters.

Nursing is in a unique position to take a leadership role in integrating alternative healing methods into Western health care systems. We have historically used our hands, heart, and head in more natural and traditional healing interactions. As nurses, by virtue of our education and relationships with clients, we can help consumers assert their right to choose their own healing journey and the quality of their life and death experiences.

Karen Lee Fontaine

UNIT I
HEALING PRACTICES: COMPLEMENTARY/ALTERNATIVE THERAPIES FOR NURSES

But why, when all is said and done, does integration in health care matter? I believe it matters because we cannot afford to overlook or waste any knowledge, experience, or wisdom from different traditions that could be brought to bear in the cause of helping those who suffer.

Charles, Prince of Wales, at Buckingham Palace,
October 21, 1997

1 Integrative Healing

It is part of the cure to wish to be cured.

Seneca

Not everything that can be counted
counts, and not everything that counts
can be counted.

Albert Einstein

Most of nursing education in the United States, Canada, the United Kingdom, Europe, and Australia, often referred to as Western countries, has been under the umbrella of biomedicine, and thus Western nurses are familiar and comfortable with its beliefs, theories, practices, strengths, and limitations. Fewer nurses have studied alternative medical theories and practices and as a result may lack information or even harbor misinformation about these healing practices. Unlike the medical profession in general, the profession of nursing has traditionally embraced the concepts of holism and humanism, commonly embodied in alternative therapies, in its approach with clients. Nurses have long believed that healing and caring must be approached holistically and that biological, psychological, emotional, and spiritual aspects of health and illness are equally important. Our humanistic perspective includes propositions such as the mind and body are indivisible, people have the power to solve their own problems, people are responsible for the patterns of their lives, and well-being is a combination of personal satisfaction and contributions to the larger community. This theoretical basis gives us a solid foot in each camp and places us, as nurses, in the unique position to help create a bridge between biomedicine and alternative medicine (Lamont, 1967; Leininger, 1997; Peplau, 1952; Rogers, 1970; Roy, 1976).

BACKGROUND

Many interesting exchanges around the world have debated the appropriate terminology of various healing practices. Some people become vested in the use of particular terms and have difficulty getting past the language limitations. For example, many people view the term *alternative medicine* as being too narrow or misleading and are concerned that the term lacks a full understanding of traditional healing practices. It would be more helpful for a common language to be developed without people being captive to it. As language evolves, the terms used today may be quite different from those used 20 years from now. For consistency purposes, the terms chosen for this text are *conventional medicine* or *biomedicine* to describe Western medical practices and the terms *alternative medicine* or *complementary medicine* to describe other healing practices. There are no universally accepted terms. For example, the term *alternative medicine* is used more in the United States while *complementary medicine* is used in Europe. The following list presents commonly used words and their counterparts:

Mainstream	Complementary/alternative
Modern	Ancient
Western	Eastern
Allopathic	Homeopathic
Conventional	Unconventional
Orthodox	Traditional
Biomedicine	Natural medicine
Scientific	Indigenous healing methods

The line between conventional and alternative medicine is imprecise and frequently changing. For example, is the use of megavitamins or diet regimes to treat disease considered medicine, a lifestyle change, or both? Can having one's pain lessened by massage be considered a medical therapy? How should spiritual healing and prayer—some of the oldest, most widely used, and least studied traditional approaches—be classified (*Alternative Medicine*, 1994)? Although the terms *alternative* or *complementary* are frequently used, in some instances they represent the primary treatment modality for an individual. Thus, conventional medicine sometimes assumes a secondary role and actually becomes a complement to the primary treatment modality.

Conventional Medicine

Biomedical or Western medicine is only about 200 years old. It is founded on the philosophical beliefs of René Descartes (1596–1650), that the mind and body are separate, and on Sir Isaac Newton's (1642–1727) principles of physics, that the universe is like a large mechanical clock where everything operates in a linear, sequential form. This mechanistic perspective of medicine views the human body as a series of body parts. It is a reductionistic approach in which the person is converted into increasingly smaller components: systems, organs, cells, and biochemicals. People are reduced to patients, patients are reduced to bodies, and bodies are reduced to machines. Health is viewed as the absence of disease or in other words, nothing being broken at the present time. The focus of sick care is on the symptoms of dysfunction. Doctors are trained to fix or repair broken parts through the use of drugs, radiation, surgery, or replacement of body parts. The approach is aggressive and militant with physicians being in a war against disease, with a take-no-prisoners attitude. Both consumers and practitioners of biomedicine believe it is better to:

- do something rather than wait and see whether the body's natural processes resolve the problem.
- attack the disease directly by medication or surgery rather than try to build up the person's resistance and ability to overcome the disease.

Biomedicine views the person primarily as a physical body, with the mind and spirit being separate and secondary, or at times, even irrelevant. It is powerful medicine in that it has virtually eliminated some infectious diseases such as small pox and polio. As a "rescue" medicine, the biomedical approach is wonderful. It is highly effective in emergencies, traumatic injuries, bacterial infections, and some highly sophisticated surgeries. In these cases, treatment is fast, aggressive, and goal-oriented, with the responsibility for cure falling on the practitioner. The priority of intervention is on opposing and suppressing the symptoms of illness. This approach is evidenced in many medications with prefixes such as "an" or "anti" as in analgesics, anesthetics, anti-inflamatories, and antipyretics. Because conventional medicine is preoccupied with parts and symptoms and not with whole working systems of matter, energy, thoughts, and feelings, it does not do well with long-term systemic illnesses such as arthritis, heart disease, and hypertension (Cantor and Rosenzweig, 1997; Fries, 1993; Seaward, 1994).

Alternative Medicine

Alternative medicine is an umbrella term for hundreds of therapies drawn from all over the world. Many forms have been handed down over thousands of years, both orally and as written records. They are based on the medical systems of ancient peoples, including Egyptians, Chinese, Asian Indians, Greeks, and Native Americans. Others, such as osteopathy and naturopathy, evolved in the United States over the past two centuries. Still others, such as some of the mind-body and bioelectromagnetic approaches, are on the frontier of scientific knowledge and understanding.

Although they represent diverse approaches, alternative therapies share certain attributes.They are based on the paradigm of whole systems and the belief that people are more than physical bodies with fixable and replaceable parts. Mental, emotional, and spiritual components of well-being are considered to play a crucial and equal role in a person's state of health. Since body, mind, and spirit are one unified reality, all illness is considered to be somatopsychic or psychosomatic, "somatic" meaning physiologic and "psychic" meaning psychologic. Even Hippocrates, the father of Western medicine, espoused a holistic orientation when he taught doctors to observe their patients' life circumstances and emotional states. Socrates agreed, declaring, "Curing the soul; that is the first thing." In alternative medicine, symptoms are believed to be an expression of the body's wisdom as it reacts to cure its own imbalance or disease. Other threads or concepts common to most forms of alternative medicine include the following:

- An internal self-healing process exists within each person.
- People are responsible for making their own decisions regarding their health care.
- Nature, time, and patience are the great healers.

When Albert Einstein (1879–1955) introduced his theory of relativity in 1905, the way of viewing the universe changed dramatically. Einstein said that all matter is energy, energy and matter are interchangeable, and all matter is connected at the subatomic level. No single entity could be affected without all connecting parts being affected. In this view, the universe is not a giant clock, but a living web. The human body is animated by an integrated energy called the *life force*. The life force sustains the physical body but is also a spiritual entity that is linked to a higher being or infinite source of energy. When the life force flows freely throughout the body, a person experiences optimal health and vitality. When the life force is blocked or weakened, organs, tissues, and cells are deprived of the energy they need to function at their full potential, and illness or disease results.

The value of alternative medicine is especially effective for people with chronic, debilitating illnesses for which conventional medicine has few, if any, answers. It has much to offer in the arena of health promotion and disease prevention. As costs of conventional medicine grow and people continue to suffer from chronic illnesses and degenerative diseases, the place of alternative medicine is moving closer to the mainstream. Box 1.1 provides an overview of the paradigms of conventional and alternative medicine.

ASSUMPTIONS

In understanding conventional and alternative medicine, it is helpful to study the assumptions basic to their theories, practices, and research. These assumptions include the origin of disease, the meaning of health, the curative process, and health promotion.

	Conventional Medicine	Alternative Medicine
Box 1.1: Paradigms of Medicine		
View		
Mind/body/spirit	are separate	are one
The body is	a machine	a living microcosm of universe
Disease results when	parts break	energy/life force becomes unbalanced
Role of medicine	to combat disease	to restore mind/body/spirit harmony
Approach	treat and suppress symptoms	search for patterns of disharmony or imbalance
Focuses on	parts/matter	whole/energy
Treatments	attempt to "fix" broken parts	support self-healing
Primary interventions	drugs, surgery, radiation	diet, exercise, herbs, stress management, social support
System	sick care	health care

Origin of Disease

Biomedicine and alternative medicine have widely divergent assumptions regarding the origin of disease. Biomedicine was shaped by the observations that bacteria were responsible for producing disease and pathologic damage and that antitoxins and vaccines could improve a person's ability to ward off the effects of pathogens. Armed with this knowledge, physicians began to conquer a large number of devastating infectious diseases. As the science developed, physicians came to believe that germs and genes caused disease and once the offending pathogen, metabolic error, or chemical imbalance was found all diseases would eventually yield to the appropriate vaccine, antibiotic, or chemical compound. Conventional medicine has also been influenced by Darwin's concept of survival of the fittest, which says that all life is a constant struggle and that only the most successful competitors survive. When this concept is applied to medicine it is translated that we live under constant attack by the thousands of microorganisms that, in the Western view, cause most diseases. People must defend themselves and counterattack with treatments that kill the enemy (*Alternative Medicine,* 1994; Castleman, 1996). Based on this assumption, symptoms are regarded as harmful manifestations and should be suppressed. For example, a headache is an annoyance that should be eliminated and a fever should be reduced with the use of medications.

Alternative medicine is based on the belief of a life force or energy that flows through each person and sustains life. Balance refers to harmony among organs in the body and among body systems, and in relationships to other individuals, society, and the environment. A balanced organism presents a strong defense against external insults such as bacteria, viruses, and trauma. When the life force or energy is blocked or weakened, the vitality of organs and tissues is reduced, oxygen is diminished, waste products accumulate, and organs and tissues degenerate. Symptoms are the body's way of communicating that the life force has been blocked or weakened resulting in a compromised immune system. Disease is not necessarily a surprise encounter with a bacteria or virus, since these surround us constantly, but rather the end result of a series of events that began with a disruption of the life force (Monte, 1997). Based on this assumption, symptoms are not suppressed unless they endanger life such as a headache from an aneurysm or a fever above 105°F. Rather, symptoms are cooperated with because they express the body's wisdom as it reacts to cure its own disease. For example, a headache is a signal that one's whole system needs realignment, and a fever may be the result of the breakdown of bacterial proteins or toxins. When symptoms are suppressed, they are not resolved but merely held off, gathering energy for renewed expression as soon as the outside, counteractive force is removed.

Meaning of Health

If you were to ask a healer from the Chinese, Indian, or Native American traditions about the meaning of health, you would hear answers very different from those that would be given by a Western physician. The biomedical view of health, in the past, was often described as the absence of disease or other abnormal conditions. That definition expanded to include the view that health is not a static condition; the body undergoes constant change and adaptation to both internal and external environmental challenges. The majority of conventional medical practitioners would define health as a state of well-being. They may disagree, however, about who determines well-being—the health professional or the individual.

Those practicing alternative medicine describe health as a condition of wholeness, balance, and harmony of the body, mind, emotions, and spirit. Health is not a concrete goal to be achieved; rather, it is a lifelong process that represents growth toward potential, an inner feeling of aliveness. Physical aspects include optimal functioning of all body systems. Emotional aspects include the ability to feel and express the entire range of human emotions. Mental aspects include feelings of self-worth, a positive identity, a sense of accomplishment, and the ability to appreciate and create. Spiritual aspects involve self, others, and society. Self components are the development of moral values and finding a meaningful purpose in life. Spiritual factors relating to others include the search for meaning through relationships and the feeling of connectedness with others and with an external power often identified as God or the divine source. Societal aspects of spiritual health can be understood as a common humanity and a belief in the fundamental sacredness and unity of all life. These beliefs motivate people toward truth and a sense of fairness and justice to all members of society. The World Health Organization (WHO) states that "the existing definition of health should include the spiritual aspect and that health care should be in the hands of those who are fully aware of and sympathetic to the spiritual dimension."

Curative Process

The curative process is another example of divergent viewpoints. Conventional medicine promotes the view that external treatments—drugs, surgery, radiation—cure people, and practitioners are trained to fix or repair broken parts. The focus is on the disease process or abnormal condition. Alternative practitioners look at conditions that block the life force and keep it from flowing freely through the body. Healing occurs when balance and harmony are restored. The focus is on the health potential of the person rather than the disease problem. The cure model and the healing model are presented with greater detail in chapter 2.

Health Promotion

Conventional and alternative medical systems have somewhat different foci on promotion of health. The thrust by conventional medicine is toward disease prevention. Consumers are taught how to decrease their risk of cancer, cardiac disorders, and other life-threatening diseases that kill most people prematurely in Western society. As important as these behaviors are, however, disease prevention is only one piece of health promotion. Health promotion, from the alternative perspective, is a lifelong process that focuses on optimal development of our physical, emotional, mental, and spiritual selves. An individual's world views, values, lifestyles, and health beliefs are considered to be of critical importance. Consumers are encouraged to adopt healthier lifestyles, to accept increased responsibility for their own well-being, and through greater self-reliance, to learn how to handle common health problems on their own.

RESEARCH

Scientific beliefs rest not just on facts but on paradigms (broad views of how these facts are related and organized). Differences in views among groups of nursing and medical researchers are a reflection of the different scientific paradigms in which each group believes. This understanding may provide some insight into the ongoing conflict between quantitative and qualitative researchers, nursing and medical researchers, Western and Eastern researchers, and conventional and alternative medical researchers. A common yet seemingly almost invisible presumption is that "experts" of conventional medicine are entitled and qualified to pass judgment on the scientific and therapeutic merits of alternative therapies. Since the paradigm is quite different, they are not qualified (*Alternative Medicine,* 1994).

Particulate-deterministic, or quantitative, research represents the principles of Western scientific method, which include formulating and testing hypotheses and then rejecting or not rejecting the hypotheses. Every question is reduced to the smallest possible part. Results can be replicated and generalized. Outcomes can be predicted and controlled. Particulate-deterministic research is said to be objective in that the observer is separate from that which is being observed. Another part of this objective paradigm is that all information can be derived from physically measurable data. This type of research has been extremely effective for isolating causative factors of disease and developing cures. On the other hand, it cannot explain the whole person as an integrated unit (Guzzetta, 1989; Micozzi, 1996; Newman et al., 1991).

Interactive-integrative research studies the context and meaning of interactive variables as these variables form patterns reflective of the whole. Researchers observe, document, analyze, and qualify the interactive relationship of variables. In the science of physics, it is believed that objectivity is ultimately not possible. The Heisenberg uncertainty principle states that the act of observing phenomena necessarily influences the behavior of the phenomena being observed. Another part of the paradigm relates to the belief that interactions between living organisms and environments are transactional, multidirectional, and synergistic in ways that cannot be reduced. This holistic approach (the whole is greater than the parts) is basic to the interactive-integrative paradigm (Guzzetta, 1989; Micozzi, 1996; Newman et al., 1991).

The unitary-transformative approach to research represents a significant paradigm shift. A phenomenon is viewed as an integral, self-organizing unit embedded in a larger, self-organizing unit. Change is nonlinear and unpredictable as systems move through organization and disorganization. Knowledge is a function of both the observer and the phenomenon being studied and involves pattern recognition. Knowledge is personal in that it includes thoughts, values, feelings, choices, and purpose (Newman et al., 1991).

Just as conventional and alternative medicine complement one another, so do multiple perspectives of research. Some research explores patterns about which little is known (interactive-interpretative) while other research validates new knowledge and predicts outcomes of interventions (particulate-deterministic). Yet other research may help us understand such aspects as the mutuality of nurse-client encounters (unitary-transformative). All paradigms are needed to further scientific knowledge.

Jean Watson's article on caring knowledge (1990) included a wonderful metaphor from Margaret Mead's book, *Blackberry Winter* (pp. 289–290), which Watson believes is relevant to nursing science. Mead is discussing the theoretical physicist Oppenheimer (1904–1967) and his well-chosen metaphor of science as a house:

> I would like to see us build a NEW room in that vast and rambling structure [of a house called "science"]. This room, like the others, would have no door and over the entrance would be the words, THOUGHT, REFLECTION, CONTEM-PLATION. It would have no tables with instruments, no whirring machinery. There would be no sound except the soft murmur of words carrying the thought of men [and women] in the room. It would be a Commons Room to which men [and women] would drift in from those rooms marked geology, anthropology, taxonomy, technology, biology, paleontology, logic, mathematics, psychology, linguistics, and many others. Indeed, from without the walls of the House would come poets and artists. All these would drop in and linger. This room would have great windows; the vistas our studies have opened. Men [and women] singly or together would from time to time walk to those windows to gaze out on the land-scape beyond. This landscape in all its beauty, sometimes gentle, sometimes ter-rible, cannot be seen fully by any one of the occupants of the room. Indeed, it cannot be known fully by a whole generation of men [and women]. Explorers of each generation travel into its unknown recesses and, with luck, return to share their discoveries with us. So the life of the NEW room would go on—thought, reflection, contemplation—as the explorers bring back their discoveries to share with the room's occupants. This landscape that we gaze on and try to understand is an epic portion of the human experience.

Those who limit themselves to Western scientific research have virtually ignored anything that cannot be perceived by the five senses and repeatedly measured or quantified. It is dismissed as superstitious and invalid if it cannot be scientifically explained by cause and effect. Many continue to cling with an almost religious fervor to this cultural paradigm about the power of science. Nonwestern, scientific paradigms are considered to be inferior at best and in-accurate at worst. And yet, biomedical research cannot explain many of the phenomena that concern alternative practitioners regarding caring-healing processes. When therapies such as acupuncture or homeopathy are observed to result in a physiologic or clinical response that cannot be explained by the biomedical model, many have tried to deny the results rather than modify the scientific model (Micozzi, 1996; Watson, 1995). In contrast to the biomedical perspective, Buckminster Fuller, an American architect and inventor, said, "Eighty percent of reality cannot be perceived or detected through the five senses." If people limit themselves to the five senses, they will never come to understand human energy fields, electromagnetic fields, thoughts as a form of energy, or the healing power of prayer.

Conventional medicine believes that procedures and substances must pass the double-blind study to be proven effective. As a testing method, the double-blind study examines a single procedure or substance in isolated, controlled conditions and measures results against an inactive procedure or substance (called a placebo). This approach is based on the assumption that single factors cause and reverse illness, and that these factors can be studied alone and out of context. Alternative medicine, however, believes that no single factor causes anything nor can a magic substance single-handedly reverse illness. Multiple factors contribute to illness, and multiple interventions work together to promote healing. The double-blind method is incapable of reconciling this degree of complexity and variation.

Although major alternative medical systems may not have a great deal of quantitative research, they are generally *not* experimental. They rely on well-developed clinical observational skills and experience that is guided by their explanatory models. Likewise, 70 to 85 percent of biomedical practices are guided by observation and experience and have *not* been tested quantitatively. New medicines must have rigorous proof of efficacy and safety before clinical use. The use of tests, procedures, and treatments, however, are not similarly constrained (Grimes, 1993). A tiny fraction of new devices undergoes formal review by the Food and Drug Administration before marketing approval. Western physicians, like alternative practitioners, use the same well-developed clinical observational skills and experience guided by their explanatory biomedical model. Thus, the argument really becomes one of cultural turf rather than scientific method (Cassidy, 1996).

This text does not offer meticulous documentation for all claims which are made by the various therapies. The Office of Alternative Medicine (OAM) at the National Institutes of Health has been mandated to facilitate the evaluation of alternative medical treatments and to provide the public with this information. There may be a wait for new knowledge from quantum physics and psychoneuroimmunology before alternative medicine can be understood in terms of the biomedical model. Successful alternative therapies, however, should not be withheld from the public while research is being debated. Box 1.2 lists the institution-affiliated centers for research on alternative medicine.

Box 1.2: Institution-Affiliated Centers of Research on Alternative Medicine

Institution	Specialty of Center
Bastyr University Bethel, WA	HIV/AIDS
Columbia University New York, NY	Women's health issues
Harvard Medical School Boston	General medical conditions
Kessler Institute for Rehabilitation West Orange, NJ	Stroke and neurological conditions
Palmer Center for Chiropractic Research Davenport, IA	Chiropractic
Stanford University Palo Alto, CA	Aging
University of Arizona Health Science Center Tucson	Pediatric conditions
University of California Davis	Asthma, allergy, and immunology
University of Maryland School of Medicine Baltimore	Pain
University of Michigan Ann Arbor	Cardiovascular diseases
University of Minnesota Medical School Minneapolis	Addictions

Box 1.2: Institution-Affiliated Centers of Research on Alternative Medicine (*continued*)

Institution	Specialty of Center
University of Texas Health Science Center Houston	Cancer
University of Virginia Charlottesville	Pain

Source: Medical News & Perspective, November 11, 1998. *JAMA.* 280(18): 1553.

CONSUMERS

Many Americans are looking outside of conventional medicine for relief of illness and improvement of health. According to a random survey in 1997, 32–54 percent of adults (83 million people) in the United States used one or more types of alternative medicine in the past year, often to treat a chronic medical condition as listed in Box 1.3. Sixty percent of these consumers did not discuss the use of alternative therapies with their primary conventional practitioner, even though the vast majority used both approaches simultaneously. In total, they made 629 million visits to alternative healers, which was nearly 243 million more visits than to all U.S. primary care physicians. They spent approximately $27 billion out-of-pocket on alternative therapies (Eisenberg et al., 1998). Another study of consumers of family practice medicine found that 50 percent had used at least one form of alternative medicine and 53 percent of these did not discuss the use with their primary practitioner (Elder et al., 1997). Studies thus far have demonstrated that consumers of alternative medicine tend to be better educated and have a higher socioeconomic status than the general population. The use of alternative medicine is most likely underestimated since the studies have focused on English-speaking individuals, often in small numbers, and have omitted prayer and other religious/spiritual resources from the studies (Eisenberg et al., 1998).

Burg (1998) and associates surveyed the use of alternative therapies by conventional health care professionals. In this study more than half of the respondents reported that they had used one or more types of alternative therapies, the most frequent being massage, relaxation techniques, dietary supplements, and chiropractic. The highest overall use was reported by allied health

Box 1.3: Thirteen Most Frequently Reported Conditions of Those Seeking Alternative Therapies

Problem	Percentage of Sufferers
Neck problems	57
Back problems	48
Anxiety	43
Depression	41
Headaches	32
Arthritis	27
GI problems	27
Fatigue	27
Insomnia	26
Sprain/strains	24
Allergies	17
Lung problems	13
Hypertension	12

Source: Eisenberg et al., 1998. Trends in Alternative Medicine Use in the United States, 1990–1997. *JAMA*. 280(18): 1569–1576.

professionals followed by nursing, dentistry, pharmacy, veterinary medicine, and medicine. Alternative medicine use appears to be similar to rates of use in the general population.

The mainstream medical community can no longer ignore alternative therapies. The public interest is extensive and growing. One has only to look at the proliferation of popular health books, health food stores, and clinics offering healing therapies to realize that this interest cannot be dismissed. Americans spent an estimated $32.7 billion on alternative therapies in 1997, of which more than $19 billion was out-of-pocket. In other words, Americans want something more than biomedicine, and they are willing to pay for it (Eisenberg et al., 1998).

What are consumers seeking from alternative medicine? Some have the same goal for both types of medicine, such as the use of pain medications and acupuncture to control chronic pain. Other consumers may have a different expectation for each approach, such as seeing a conventional practitioner for antibiotics to eradicate an infection and using an alternative practitioner to improve natural immunity through a healthy lifestyle. A person receiving chemotherapy may use meditation and visualization to control the side effects of the chemotherapeutic agents. People who combine conventional and alternative therapies are making therapeutic choices on their own and assuming responsibility for their own health (Lazar, and O'Connor, 1997).

It is important for nurses to understand the reasons consumers choose alternative practitioners. Some utilize alternative healers because of financial, geographic, and cultural barriers to biomedical care. Many turn to alternative healers for a sense of hope, control, personal attention, physical contact, and regard for the whole person that seems to be overlooked in conventional medicine. Some of the common reasons for seeking alternative practitioners are listed in Box 1.4.

Because alternative therapists are rushing to meet the demand, it is increasingly difficult for consumers to figure out how and where to get the best health care. It may be problematic to find reliable information to help separate the healers from those who pretend to have medical knowledge. Consumers should beware of healers who (Tiedje, 1998):

- say they have all the answers
- maintain that theirs is the only effective therapy
- promise overnight success
- refuse to include other practitioners as part of the healing team
- seem more interested in money than in people's well-being

Box 1.4: Reasons for Choosing Alternative Therapies

Pursue therapeutic benefit
Seek a degree of wellness not supported in biomedicine
Attend to quality of life issues
Prefer high personal involvement in decision making
Believe conventional medicine treats symptoms not underlying cause
Find conventional medical treatments to be lacking or ineffective
Avoid toxicities and/or invasiveness of conventional interventions
Decrease use of prescribed or OTC medications
Identify with a particular healing system as a part of cultural background

---

Sources: Dunn and Perry, 1997. Primary Care: Clinics in Office Practice, 24(4): 715–721; Lazar and O'Connor, 1997. Primary Care: Clinics in Office Practice, 24(4): 699–714.

Some alternative specialties are more regulated and licensed than others, but none come with guarantees any more than conventional medicine comes with guarantees. Most consumers locate alternative therapists through friends, family, an exercise instructor, health food stores, and referral lines at local hospitals. Nurses must initiate discussion with clients regarding alternative medicine. The most frequent reason clients give for not discussing their use of alternative medicine is the fear of ridicule or censure on the part of the conventional health care provider. In light of this fear, nurses must create a safe climate in which clients can openly discuss these issues. Nurses must remain nonjudgmental and supportive if they are to help people achieve their health care goals.

INTEGRATED NURSING PRACTICE

In the past 20 years, nursing has been moving away from a biomedical orientation that has largely defined and directed it toward a nursing-caring-healing model. Watson (1997) describes it as a shift from *nursing qua medicine* paradigm (nurses helping doctors practice medicine) to a *nursing qua nursing* paradigm (practicing the distinct art and science of nursing). This movement has reconnected us with the finest tradition of Florence Nightingale in using our hands, heart, and head in creating healing environments. The modern nurse-healer draws upon biomedical and caring/healing models by utilizing technology and focusing on caring relationships and healing processes. Dossey, Keegan, Lolkmeier, and Guzzetta (1989) have described the modern nurse-healer as a hybrid of scientific skills and spiritual commitment. We need scientific principles, methods, and skills, but we also need to teach people ways to become more self-reliant as we shift in the role from caregiver to healer.

In 1979, Watson published her text *Nursing: The Philosophy and Science of Caring,* which evolved from her experiences of nursing within the limitations of traditional biomedical models. She sought to bring new meaning to the nursing paradigm of caring-healing and health. Her ten carative factors, listed in Box 1.5, became a philosophical and conceptual guide toward a model of nursing that is well known throughout the world. Reading this list, it becomes obvious how nursing as a caring profession embraces philosophical perspectives similar to those of many alternative healing systems and therapies.

The art of nursing is in being there, with another person or persons, in a context of caring. It is the capacity of the nurse "to receive another human being's expression of feelings and to experience those feelings for oneself" (Chinn and Watson, 1994, p. xvi). Caring involves compassion and sensitivity to each person within the context of her or his entire life. In the past, the biomedical model urged us not to care too much or get too involved. Caring, successful nurses, however, do get involved with clients as they practice

---

Box 1.5: Watson's Ten Carative Factors

1. Forming a humanistic-altruistic system of values.
2. Enabling and sustaining faith-hope.
3. Being sensitive to self and others.
4. Developing a helping-trusting, caring relationship (seeking transpersonal connection).
5. Promoting and accepting the expression of positive and negative feelings and emotions.
6. Engaging in creative, individualized, problem-solving, caring processes.
7. Promoting transpersonal teaching-learning.
8. Attending to supportive, protective, and/or corrective mental, physical, societal, and spiritual environments.
9. Assisting with gratification of basic human needs while preserving human dignity and wholeness.
10. Allowing for, and being open to, existential-phenomenological, and spiritual dimensions of caring and healing that cannot be fully explained scientifically through modern Western medicine.

Source: Watson, in *Blueprint for Use of Nursing Models* (New York: NLN Press, 1996), 141–184.

---

nursing as an art instead of nursing as just a day-to-day job. Caring is a philosophy or context wherein we practice nursing. What makes our practice caring are not the tools we use but the attitude or perspective we bring. It is possible, of course, to use the tools of alternative therapies in the same reductionistic way of biomedicine. For example, if one knows the pressure point for headaches and simply uses this pressure point for pain relief without any further assessment, it could hardly be considered holistic or healing. The symptom of headache has been addressed, but the meaning of the headache and the person's experience of the pain has been totally ignored.

Before nurses can care for clients, they must first learn to value and care for themselves. One of your goals in reading this text might be discovering how to care for yourself more effectively because it is only when we can care first for ourselves that we have the energy to care for our patients. Caring for yourself means reducing unnecessary stress, managing conflict more effectively, communicating with family and friends more clearly, and taking time out for yourself. Caring for yourself includes developing a daily routine in practices such as relaxation, meditation, prayer, yoga, communion with nature, and other such forms of contemplation. In Watson's words, "If one is to work from a caring-healing paradigm, one must live it out in daily life" (1997, p. 51). The following guidelines will help you maintain your self-care practices (Jahnke, 1997):

- Choose self-care activities that appeal to you and fit into your lifestyle.
- Do one or more of these practices every day. Consider them as important as you do rest and daily hygiene activities.
- Seek guidance and support from teachers/practitioners if appropriate.
- Find a good spot for your practice that is physically and mentally comfortable.
- Build up your practice slowly. Success is not gained by aggressive or compulsive practice.
- Look for opportunities to practice with others.
- Focus on relaxing. The foundation of all self-healing, health enhancement, stress mastery, and personal empowerment is deep relaxation.

Much data is currently being gathered relating to the concept of the nurse as healer. The principles that have thus far been identified are listed in Box 1.6. Read these principles closely. You will see the same precepts appearing again and again in the various healing practices described in this text.

The plurality of the sick-care, health-care systems may be one of its greatest strengths. It enables us to meet the diverse needs of diverse populations. The

---

Box 1.6: Principles of Nurse Healers' Practice

1. There is a unity and interdependence within the mind, body, and spirit.
2. Health is a process that may include dis-ease.
3. One's attitudes and beliefs toward life (mental-emotional energy fields or consciousness) is a major etiological factor in health and disease.
4. One's health and disease are manifested in one's lifestyle, habits, and conscious awareness, as well as the body's physical being and energy.
5. The self is empowered with the ability to create or maintain health/disease.
6. Changes in health can occur through experiential learning, which is defined as a change in behavior that occurs as a result of living through an activity, event, or situation.
7. Experiential learning is essential to changing one's lifestyle for high-level wellness.
8. Human beings are energy fields.

Box 1.6: Principles of Nurse Healers' Practice (*continued*)

9. Healing involves a transformational change that encompasses the whole person; it requires the involvement of the spiritual, emotional, and intellectual domains, as well as the physical body.

10. Energy fields can become unbalanced as a response to stress in any one of the three domains of body, mind, and spirit.

11. The client-practitioner relationship is one of partnership—equal with differing responsibilities.

12. Any modality or health system that supports healing should be valued.

13. Each health system should be respected for the resources and the tools that it offers while being challenged to prove its credibility.

14. Each person is an open system with the environment without separating boundaries.

15. Energy fields are constantly interacting.

Source: Keegan, *The Nurse as Healer* (Albany, NY: Delmar, 1994).

question is, how can we combine the best ideas of conventional nursing practice and alternative healing practices? First, we must have education. At the basic level, our nursing curricula must include courses in caring and alternative medicine. All nurses could learn Therapeutic Touch, healthy dietary plans, the use of basic herbs, as well as the use of visualization and prayer in the healing process. We must also participate in continuing education courses to expand our knowledge beyond the basic level. With additional education, we can learn such things as basic massage and reflexology, meditation, and yoga. Some nurses will choose to continue their education by completing formal programs in alternative medicine such as naturopathy, ayurveda, homeopathy, chiropractic medicine, or hypnotherapy. Nurses should also participate in research on the effectiveness of alternative therapies.

Next, we must provide community education. We must provide people with information, tools, skills, and support to enable them to make healthy decisions about life and negotiate their way through the health care systems. We must also attempt to keep ourselves healthy most of the time. We should exemplify good health, since teaching by example is a powerful influence. We can teach wherever our practice is located: acute care, long-term care, community nurse-managed centers, and in areas of advanced practice nursing. And, finally, we must document our findings, utilize and participate in nursing research, and design new studies to measure the effectiveness of various healing practices.

REFERENCES

Alternative Medicine: Expanding Medical Horizons. 1994. A report to the National Institutes of Health on Alternative Medical Systems and Practices in the United States. U.S. Government Printing Office. Washington, DC.

BURG, M. A. et al. 1998. Personal use of alternative medicine therapies by health science center faculty. *JAMA.* 280(18): 1563.

CANTOR, I. S., and S. ROSENZWEIG. 1997. Anthroposophic perspectives in primary care. Complementary and Alternative Therapies in Primary Care. *Primary Care: Clinics in Office Practice.* 24(4): 867–885.

CASSIDY, C. M. 1996. Cultural context of complementary and alternative medical systems. In M. S. MICOZZI, ed. *Fundamentals of Complementary and Alternative Medicine.* New York: Churchill Livingstone, 9–34.

CASTLEMAN, M. 1996. *Nature's Cures.* Emmaus, PA: Rodale Press.

CHINN, P. and J. WATSON, eds. 1994. *Art and Aesthetics in Nursing.* New York: NLN Press.

Department of Health and Human Services (DHHS). 1991. *Healthy People 200.* Washington, DC; Publication number (PHS) 91-50213.

DOSSEY, B. M., L. KEEGAN, L. G., LOLKMEIER, and C. E. GUZZETTA, eds. 1989. *Holistic Health Promotion: A Guide for Practice.* Rockville, MD: Aspen.

DUNN, L. and B. L. PERRY. 1997. Where your patients are. Complementary and Alternative Therapies in Primary Care. *Primary Care: Clinics in Office Practice.* 24(4): 715–721.

EISENBERG, D. M. et al. 1998. Trends in alternative medicine use in the United States, 1990–1997. *JAMA.* 280(18): 1569–1576.

ELDER, N. C., A. GILLCRIST, and R. MINZ. 1997. Use of alternative health care by family practice patients. *Arch Fam Med.* 6: 181–184.

FRIES, J. F., et al. July 29, 1993. Reducing health care costs by reducing the need and demand for medical services. *N Eng J Med.* 329(5): 321–325.

GRIMES, D. A. June 16, 1993. Technology follies. The uncritical acceptance of medical innovation. *JAMA.* 269(23): 3030–3033.

GUZZETTA, C. E. Research and holistic implications. 1989. In B. M. DOSSEY, L. KEEGAN, L. G. LOLKMEIER, and C. E. GUZZETTA, eds. *Holistic Health Promotion: A Guide for Practice.* Rockville, MD: Aspen, 85–92.

JAHNKE, R. 1997. *The Healer Within.* San Francisco: Harper.

KEEGAN, L. 1994. *The Nurse as Healer.* Albany, NY: Delmar.

LAMONT, C. 1967. *The Philsosophy of Humanism.* New York: Frederick Ungar Pub.

LAZAR, J. S. and B. B. O'CONNOR. 1997. Talking with patients about their use of alternative therapies. Complementary and Alternative Therapies in Primary Care. *Primary Care: Clinics in Office Practice.* 24(4): 699–714.

LEININGER, M. 1997. Alternative to what? Generic vs. professional caring, treatments, and healing modes. *J Transcultural Nrsg.* 9(1): 37.

MEAD, M. 1972. *Blackberry Winter.* New York: William Morrow.

MICOZZI, M. S. 1996. Characteristics of complementary and alternative medicine. In M. S. MICOZZI, ed. *Fundamentals of Complementary and Alternative Medicine.* New York: Churchill Livingstone, 3–8.

MONTE, T. 1997. *The Complete Guide to Natural Healing.* New York: Perigee.

NEWMAN, M. A., A. M. SIME, S. A. CORCORAN-PERRY. 1991. The focus of the discipline of nursing. *Adv Nurs Sci.* 14(1): 1–6.

PEPLAU, H. E. 1952. *Interpersonal Relations in Nursing.* New York: Putnam.

ROGERS, M. E. 1970. *The Theoretical Basis of Nursing.* Philadelphia: F. A. Davis.

ROY, C. 1976. *Introduction to Nursing: An Adaptation Model.* Englewood Cliffs, NJ: Prentice-Hall.

SEAWARD, B. L. 1994. Alternative medicine complements standard. *Health Progress.* 15(9): 52–57.

TIEDJE, L. B. 1998. Alternative health care: An overview. *JOGNN.* 27(5): 557–562.

WATSON, J. 1997. The theory of human caring: Retrospective and Prospective. *Nurs Sci Quart.* 10(1): 49–52.

WATSON, J. 1996. Watson's theory of transpersonal caring. In P. H. WALKER, and B. NEWMAN, eds. *Blueprint for Use of Nursing Models: Education, Research, Practice, and Administration.* New York: NLN Press, 141–184.

WATSON, J. 1995. Nursing's caring-healing paradigm as exemplar for alternative medicine? *Alternative Therapies.* 1(3): 64–69.

WATSON, J. 1990. Caring knowledge and informed moral passion. *Adv Nurs Sci.* 13(1): 15–24.

2 Basic Concepts Guiding Alternative Therapies

Wounds don't disappear, they heal. Our wounds are part of who we are. We need them because they bear witness to the pain we have endured and the damage that has been done to us. They are precious to us because they help us tell our story to ourselves and to those we love.

William H. Thomas,
Open Hearts, Open Minds

Serious illness doesn't bother me for long because I am too inhospitable a host.

Albert Schweitzer

In this book, separate chapters are devoted to each of the most widely used methods in alternative medicine. Since there is a sharing of principles, overlap occurs in the various types of alternative practices. While practices are grouped in units, many of the practices could be placed in several units. Thus, before reading specifics on each practice, it may be helpful to introduce several concepts common to most healing practices. These are balance, spirituality, energy, and breath.

BALANCE

An expression in the Native American culture, "walking in balance" describes the philosophy of a peaceful coexistence and harmony with all aspects of life. This concept of balance is found in all cultures throughout time. In terms of optimal wellness, the concept of balance consists of mental, physical, emotional, and spiritual components. Not only does each component in and of itself have to be balanced, equilibrium is needed among the components. Physical aspects include optimal functioning of all body systems. Emotional aspects include the ability to feel and express the entire range of human emotions. Mental aspects include feelings of self-worth, a positive identity, a sense of accomplishment, and the ability to appreciate and create. Spiritual aspects involve moral values, a meaningful purpose in life, and a feeling of connectedness to others and a divine source. Walking in balance is a learned skill and one that must be practiced regularly to engage in the process of healthful living. This concept of balance appears again and again throughout the various alternative healing practices (Seaward, 1997).

Circadian Rhythms

Universal rhythmic cycles are observed in plants, animals, and people referred to as circadian rhythms. The word *circadian* derives from the Latin, *circa diem,* which means "about a day." Circadian rhythms are regular fluctuations of activity and rest of a variety of physiologic processes that occur every 23–27 hours. Most familiar is the 24-hour temperature and sleep patterns. Less well known is the fact that immunity to viruses and infection is not equal at all hours of the day since gamma globulin, which contains the most antibodies, is lower in the early hours of the morning, when most people are usually sleeping. Interestingly, blood clots at a faster rate in mid to late day than in the early hours of the morning. Taking this factor into consideration, hospitals might schedule elective surgeries later in the day rather than the typical morning schedule (Luce, 1997).

The constant rhythmic processes bring about a dynamic, healthy balance in our bodies. Systole and diastole of the cardiovascular system regulate blood pressure. The inspiration and expiration of the respiratory system allow for gas exchange. The nervous system has a number of processes including depolarization and repolarization, excitation and recovery, and arousal and sleep. Attention to the rhythmic nature of one's own being reveals an intimate relationship with the rhythms of the surrounding natural world.

Musical Rhythms

Health is about balance or harmony of body, mind, and spirit. In a state of optimal health, all frequencies are in harmony, like a finely tuned piano. In fact, music is often used in healing from the ancient sounds of the drum, rattle, bone flute, and other primitive instruments to the current use of music as a prescription for health. The Chinese are producing musical recordings with some curious titles. *Obesity, Constipation,* and *Liver, Heart, and Lungs* are three examples. Most of the recordings use traditional Chinese instruments and are meant to be "taken" as an individual would take an herbal medicine, to help cope with the problems or strengthen the organs described in the titles. For headaches and migraines, the Japanese suggest Mendelssohn's "Spring Song," Dvorak's "Humoresque," or even a dose of George Gershwin's "An American in Paris." At hospitals throughout India, traditional Indian music is used medicinally to balance the rhythms of the body. Western researchers have lately established the healing and creative powers of sound and music in general and in particular Mozart's music, which seems to have a special ability to improve learning and healing. It is thought that his music facilitates certain complex neuronal patterns in the cerebral cortex, increasing left-brain activities such as logical thinking as well as strengthening the creative right-brain processes. Vibrating sounds create energy fields of resonance and movement in the surrounding space. These energies are absorbed and subtly alter one's internal rhythms (Campbell, 1998; Chopra, 1991). See Box 2.1 for other findings related to the use of music as therapy.

SPIRITUALITY

Spiritual healing techniques and spiritually based health care systems are among the most ancient healing practices. Spirit is the liveliness, richness, and beauty of one's life. Spirituality is the drive to become all that one can be, and it is bound to intuition, creativity, and motivation. It is the dimension that involves relationship with oneself, with others, and with a higher power. It involves finding significant meaning in the entirety of life, including illness and death (Wright, 1998).

The materialism of North American culture of the 1980s has given way to a period of reflectiveness. People are searching for a wholeness in their lives and a way to allow their innermost selves to grow and expand. Spiritual healing practices guide people to places within themselves they did not know existed through techniques as ancient as prayer, contemplation, meditation, drumming, storytelling, and mythology. In consciously awakening the energies of the spirit, people are able to move toward healing places and sacred moments in their lives.

During periods of stress, illness, or crisis, people search for meaning and purpose in their pain and suffering. They ask questions such as "Why am I sick?" or "Why did this bad thing happen?" This spiritual quest for meaning can lead to insight and healing or to fear and isolation. In the words of Ken Wilber,

> A person who is beginning to sense the suffering of life, is, at the same time, beginning to awaken to deeper realities, truer realities. For suffering smashes to pieces the complacency of our normal fictions about reality, and forces us to become alive in a special sense—to see carefully, to feel deeply, to touch ourselves and our world in ways we have heretofore avoided. It has been said, and truly I think, that suffering is the first grace (Borysenko and Borysenko, 1994, p. 191).

Box 2.1: Healthful Music

- A study on the effects of music on nearly 97,000 people before, during, and after surgery found that 97% reported that listening to slow baroque or classical music helped them relax and reduced their postoperative disorientation.
- Twenty-seven people with rheumatoid arthritis used Guided Imagery and Music (GIM) for 18 weeks and reported a reduction in both pain and psychological distress as well as improvement in walking.
- Children with attention deficit disorder (ADD) who listened to Mozart were able to improve their attention, have better control over their moods, lessen their impulsivity, and improve their social skills.
- At the Ireland Cancer Center at the University Hospital of Cleveland, 19 children demonstrated a significant increase in salivary immunoglobulin A (IgA) after a single half-hour music therapy session. IgA, an antibody in saliva, is a principle marker in enhanced resistance to disease.
- In a study of 20 developmentally disabled children, most of whom had cerebral palsy, 75% demonstrated improved attention, reduced hypersensitivity, and improved coordination after listening to baroque compositions by Vivaldi and Bach.
- Cathie E. Guzzetta, R.N., Ph.D., the director of Holistic Nursing Consultants in Dallas, Texas, found that relaxation and music therapy are effective in lowering mean heart rate from 100 to 82 beats per minute and systolic blood pressure from 150 to 130 mm/Hg. Phyllis Updike, R.N., D.N.S., found that music therapy significantly reduced both systolic and diastolic blood pressure, mean arterial pressure, and heart rate. Clients also reported a decrease in anxiety and pain.

Source: Campbell, The Riddle of the Mozart Effect, *Natural Health* (January–February 1998), 114–119.

Spirituality is not religion. Spirituality, however, is the search for wholeness and purpose that underlies the world's religions. Remove the dogma, the politics, and cultural influence from any of the world's religions, and you find the same questions, the same seeking, and the same answers. The concept of spirituality does not undermine any religion but rather enhances all religions by illuminating their commonalities and the commonality between all people. It makes us far more similar to each other than it makes us different.

Many traditions also speak of spiritual guides. Some of us think of them as guardian angels, others as Beings of Light who guide people through near-death experiences. Buddhists think of them as *devas*. Cherokees call them *Adawees,* the great protectors of the Four Directions. *Malakh,* or messenger, is the Hebrew word for angel. There are the cherubim and the seraphim and the four great archangels: Uriel, Raphael, Michael, and Gabriel. The Iranian angel Vohu Manah is believed to have revealed the message of God to Zoroaster some 2,500 years ago. Similarly, the Archangel Gabriel is credited for revealing the Koran to Mohammed a thousand years later. Gabriel, honored by Jews, Christians, and Muslims, has a special role as a mediator between human consciousness and the higher realms from which spirit descends into the body. Although no Western scientific evidence supports the existence of angels, one can find phenomenological evidence. Many first-person accounts of near-death occurrences involve angels and similar experiences from people of different ages, from diverse cultures, with different personal and religious beliefs (Borysenko and Borysenko, 1994; Moss, 1996). A number of books provide more information about angels including *Angels, an Endangered Species* by Malcolm Godwin, *A Book of Angels* by Sophy Burnham, and *Many Lives, Many Masters* by Brian Weiss.

ENERGY

The concept of energy has been recognized for centuries, and in most cultures. Many ancient and current cultures have great respect for the subtle and unseen forces in life. Most spiritual traditions share the belief that energy is the bridge between spirit and physical being. Meditation and prayer are believed to be subtle energy phenomena that represent contact with the spiritual dimension.

Chinese Taoist scholars believed that energy, not matter, was the basic building material of the universe. Albert Einstein and other physicists proved that matter and energy are the same and that energy is not only the raw material of the cosmos but the glue that holds it together. Modern scientists now look at the universe in terms of forces instead of tiny particles of matter. Their experimental findings are similar to the intuitive observations of China's ancient scholars. Everything in the world—animate and inanimate—is made of energy. People are beings of energy, living in a universe composed of energy (Collinge, 1998).

Although Western scientists agree that energy comprises all things, when this notion is applied to the human body, they do not yet fully agree that a distinct energy system exists within the physical body. In order for energy to be "real," it must be measurable by scientific instruments. By this logic, of course, brain waves did not exist prior to the invention of EEG equipment! Since technology is not yet capable of measuring all the energy fields in the body, references to energy are conspicuously absent in conventional medicine (Collinge, 1998). Chin (1995, p. viii) believes that in the not-too-distant future, Western scientists will begin to agree that humans are a "matrix of interacting multidimensional energy fields."

For more than 2,000 years, various practitioners around the world have insisted that a person is more than the physical body. According to these healers, a "life force" of subtle energy surrounds and permeates every person. Energy is viewed as the force which integrates the body, mind, and spirit; it is that which connects everything. The Japanese call this energy *ki* (pronounced key), the Tibetans refer to it as *lung* (pronounced loong), the Polynesians call it *mana,* Native Americans call it *oki, orenda,* or *ton,* Americans call it subtle energy, the Greeks call it *pneuma,* and the Hindus give it the name *prana.* Prana is sometimes translated from the Sanskrit as "primary energy," "breath," or "vital force." The Chinese refer to this energy as *qi* or *chi* (pronounced chee) and believe that it takes the form of two opposite but complementary phases, yin and yang. Yin is the earth, moon, night, fall and winter, cold, wetness, darkness, the feet, the left side, the female gender, and passivity. Yin is involved in tissue growth. Yang is the sun, day, spring and summer, heat, dryness, light, the head, the right side, the male gender, and aggressiveness. Yang is involved in tissue breakdown. It is believed that each person is a unique combination of the complementary energies of yin and yang. Wholeness is comprised of this union of opposites. See Figure 2.1 for the T'ai Chi symbol, which illustrates the yin and yang of Chinese thought. The white dot on the black portion of the symbol and the black dot on the white section are reminders that each quality contains some of its opposite. Further descriptions of yin and yang are found in chapter 3.

It is believed that qi creates qi. In other words, physical activities such as eating, work, and rest, as well as nonphysical aspects of life such as will, motivation, feelings, desires, and a sense of purpose in life, are all made possible by qi. Those same activities and aspects also create more qi. Most

Yang   Yin

Figure 2.1:   T'ai Chi Symbol

schools of thought basically agree on the following points regarding energy (Collinge, 1998):

- Energy comes from one universal source.
- Movement of energy is the basis of all life.
- Matter is an expression of energy, and vice versa.
- All things are manifestations of energy.
- The entire earth has energetic and metabolic qualities.
- People are composed of multiple, interacting energy fields that extend out into the environment.
- People's relationships with one another are shaped by the interactions of their energies.

Qi, kei, or prana have no exact counterpart in conventional medicine, though the concept of "bioenergy" is beginning to emerge in Western vocabulary.

Chakras

The Hindu concept of chakras (a Sanskrit word for "spinning wheel") describes seven major energy centers within the physical body. Chakras have been described by most eastern cultures and several South American cultures (such as Mayan) for thousands of years. Chakras are major centers of both electromagnetic activity and circulation of vital energy. They are usually thought of as funnels of perpetually rotating energy and are considered the gateways through which energy enters and leaves the body. Each chakra in the body is recognized as a focal point of life force relating to physical, emotional, mental, and spiritual aspects of people and are the network through which the body, mind, and spirit interact as one holistic system. Figure 2.2 illustrates the sites of the chakras in the body.

The concept of chakras may be foreign to the Western scientific mind, but they are not completely unknown to those familiar with Judeo-Christian culture, particularly in the artwork and sculptures passed down through the ages. For centuries, the crown chakra, which signifies a conscious awareness of the divine, has been painted as a halo over those who are consciously aware of a divine presence in their lives (Seaward, 1997).

The seven main chakras are vertically aligned up the center of the body from the base of the pelvis to the top of the head. Each has its own individual characteristics and functions and each has a corresponding relationship to various organs and structures of the body, to one of the endocrine glands, as well

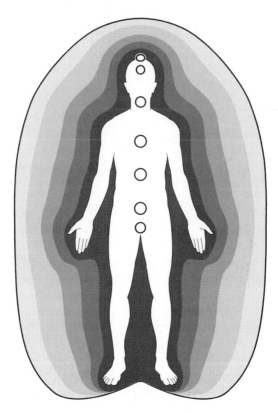

Figure 2.2:   The Chakras and the Auric Field

as to one of the seven colors of the rainbow spectrum. The characteristics of the seven major chakras are described in Box 2.2. Of the many smaller chakras throughout the body, the most significant are in the palms of the hands. The hand chakras are considered extensions of the heart chakra and, as such, radiate healing and soothing energies. Spiritual healers who practice the laying on of hands concentrate energy in their hand chakras. All the chakras have purpose, function, and frequency. These are:

- to regulate the human energy system and maintain an equilibrium of health (purpose).
- to link body, mind, and spirit and exchange energy (function).
- each operates at its own optimum frequency; generally the lower the chakra on the body, the lower its frequency; if one is out of sync, all others will be also (frequency).

Box 2.2: The Chakras

1. Root Chakra

Location: base of the spine
Center of: physical vitality, urge to survive
Gland: adrenal glands
Organs/structures: kidneys, bladder, spine
Color: red

2. Sexual or Navel Chakra

Location: slightly below the navel, in front of the sacrum
Center of: sexual energy, ego, extrasensory perception
Gland: gonads
Organs/structures: reproductive organs, legs
Color: orange

3. Solar Plexus Chakra

Location: slightly above the navel
Center of: unrefined emotions, urge for power
Gland: pancreas
Organs/structures: stomach, liver, gall-bladder
Color: yellow

4. Heart Chakra

Location: middle of the chest at the height of the heart
Center of: unconditional affection, compassion, devotion, love, spiritual growth
Gland: thymus
Organs/structures: heart, liver, lungs, circulatory system
Color: emerald

5. Throat Chakra

Location: throat area
Center of: communication, self-expression, creativity
Gland: thyroid
Organs/structures: throat, upper lungs, digestive tract, arms
Color: blue

Box 2.2: The Chakras (*continued*)

6. Third Eye Chakra

Location: middle of the forehead, a little higher than the eyebrows

Center of: the will, intellect, spirit, spiritual awakening, visualization

Gland: pituitary

Organs/structures: spine, lower brain, left eye, nose

Color: purple

7. Crown Chakra

Location: at the top of the head at the fontenal

Center of: highest level of consciousness or enlightenment, intuition, direct spiritual vision

Gland: pineal

Organs/structures: upper brain, right eye

Color: golden-white

The main purpose in working with and understanding the chakras is to create integration and wholeness within people. The chakras are the "doorways" through which the energy from within and without is distributed to cells, tissues, and organs. If chakras stop functioning properly, the intake of energy will be disturbed and the body organs served by that chakra will not get their needed supply of energy. Eventually organ functioning will be disrupted, leading to weakened organs with a diminished immune defense. If this process continues, the end result will be dysfunction and disease (Dale, 1997). Dr. Dean Ornish, well-known for his program to reverse blocked coronary arteries through diet, exercise, support groups, and meditation without surgery or drugs, believes that a closed heart chakra (unresolved anger and fear) is related to the closed coronary arteries. Consequently, the meditation technique he incorporates into his program involves opening the heart chakra. His holistic approach has now become a recognized program practiced nationwide (Seaward, 1997).

Aura

Closely related to the chakras is the concept of aura. The aura is the energy field surrounding each person as far as the outstretched arms and from head to toe. This energy field is both an information center and a highly sensitive perceptual system that transmits and receives messages from the internal and external environment. Each of the seven layers of the auric field is associated with a chakra; the first layer is related to the first chakra, and so on. Each layer has physical, mental, emotional, and spiritual dimensions and purposes and the layers function together through the transmission of energy. See Box 2.3 for the characteristics of the auric field and Figure 2.2 for a diagrammatic view of the auric field. Virtually every alternative healing therapy has a way of interpreting the body's subtle energy, which will be discussed throughout this text. For further information on energy and spirituality, see Caroline Myss's book *Anatomy of the Spirit* and Richard Gerber's text *Vibrational Medicine.*

Meridians

A person's vital energy is not simply radiated outward but has patterns of circulation within the body, referred to as the meridian system. Meridians are a network of energy circuits or lines of force that run vertically through the body connecting all parts. Meridians may be understood more clearly if they are compared to a major city's highway system with entrance and exit ramps, merging roads, and connecting surface streets. If a flood blocks an exit ramp, the streets served by this ramp are inaccessible, which, in turn, affects the people who live and work on those streets. Also, the traffic may be backed up on the highway waiting for the ramp to reopen, creating a traffic jam. Meridians operate this way in a person's body. If some kind of blockage affects one's hip, for example, the pathways of energy leading to that hip get "backed up." Pain or discomfort restrict the motion of the hip, which puts a different strain on the foot, and the foot in a different position creates a strain on other sets of muscles. These changes in the body's general posture affect the positions of the internal organs, which, in turn, restricts the nutrition to the organs, alters organ function, and thereby changes the body's balance. As the body and mind are affected, the person will think and feel differently, leading to more tension and more changes (Schwartz, 1996).

Each meridian passes close to the skin's surface at places called *hsueh,* which means cave or hollow and is translated as point or acupuncture point. Since each meridian is associated with an internal organ, the acupuncture points offer surface access to the internal organ systems. The flow of qi can be strengthened or weakened by manipulating specific points. Keeping the flow of energy open and regular contributes to a state of balance and health.

The California Institute for Human Science is the American center for research on a machine called the AMI, an acronym for "apparatus for meridian identification." The AMI measures the flow of ions through the body and in ten minutes can give a complete evaluation of the condition of a person's

Box 2.3: Seven Layers of the Auric Field

Level 1. Etheric body

Location: 1/4 inch to 2 inches beyond the physical body

Center of: physical functioning and physical sensation

Color: light blue to gray

Level 2. Emotional body

Location: 1 to 3 inches beyond the physical body; roughly follows the outline of the physical body

Center of: emotional aspects of person

Color: all colors of the rainbow

Level 3. Mental body

Location: 3 to 8 inches beyond the physical body

Center of: instinct, intellect, intuition

Color: bright yellow with additional colors superimposed

Level 4. Astral body

Location: 6 to 16 inches beyond the physical body

Center of: love

Color: same colors as in level 3 but infused with the rose light of love

Level 5. Etheric template body

Location: 18 inches to 24 inches beyond the physical body

Center of: higher will connected with divine will, speaking, listening, work, taking responsibility for our actions.

Color: clear lines on cobalt blue background

Level 6. Celestial body

Location: 24 inches to 33 inches beyond the physical body

Center of: celestial love, spiritual ecstasy, protection and nurturance of all life

Color: shimmering pastel colors

Box 2.3: Seven Layers of the Auric Field (*continued*)

Level 7. Causal body

Location: 30 inches to 42 inches, forming an egg shape around body

Center of: higher mind; integration of spiritual and physical body

Color: shimmering gold threads

---

meridian system and the corresponding internal organs related to those meridians. This stream of ions is not vital energy or qi itself. Rather, it is a secondary electromagnetic effect of qi—in a sense, its imprint in the physical domain. The AMI is now becoming available for wide distribution as a diagnostic tool in medicine (Collinge, 1998).

Energy Concentration

People's mind's energy, or willpower, can be developed to control their body's energy system to an extraordinary degree. Healers can concentrate and manipulate energy in remarkable ways. Dr. Green at the Menninger Clinic compared average people to healers by measuring the electrical field on their hands. Ordinary people varied from 0 to 50 millivolts of energy in their hands. (A millivolt is 1/1,000 of a volt.) When he measured the electrical energy of the hands of people who worked as traditional healers, he found that they all produced at least 4 volts of energy, more than 80 times more energy than the average person. One Chinese qi gong master produced 200 volts, the equivalent of 4,000 times more energy. Dr. Green also attempted to trace the source of the healers' electricity. It seemed to come from the central body in the area between the solar plexus and the lower abdomen. The Chinese refer to this spot as the *tan dien* or the home of qi, and the Hindu refer to it as the solar plexus chakra or the seat of prana (Castleman, 1996).

Grounding and Centering

Two terms common in various healing practices and related to energy and balance are *grounding* and *centering*. Grounding, as its name suggests, relates to one's connection with the ground and, in a broader sense, to one's whole contact with reality. Being grounded suggests stability, security, independence, having a solid foundation, and living in the present rather than escaping into dreams. It means having a mature sense of responsibility for oneself. Much of the sense of grounding comes from identification with the lower half of one's body—the parts of being that are less conscious and have more instinctive functions of movement. Learning to breathe into the belly, for example, is vital for grounding, for if the breath is shallow, contact with feelings and reality is limited. Many of the practices in this text, such as biofield therapies, mind-body techniques, and spiritual therapies, help to increase one's groundedness.

Centering refers to the process of bringing oneself to the center or middle. When people are centered, they are fully connected to the part of their bodies where all their energies meet. Centering is the process of focusing one's mind on the center of energy, usually in the navel or solar plexus chakra. All movement in the body originates from this center, providing the meeting point for body and mind. It is commonly considered the "earth" center, for it gathers energy from the earth rising up through the legs. Centering can be done through movement, as in T'ai Chi, or can be found in stillness, as in meditation. Being centered allows one to operate intuitively, with awareness, and to channel energy throughout the body.

BREATH

Breath is at the center of all spiritual and religious traditions. In many languages the words for *spirit* and *breath* are one and the same—Sanskrit *prana,* Hebrew *ruach,* Greek *pneuma,* and Latin *spiritus.* In Christianity, the Holy Spirit is referred to as "the breath of life." To inspire, or take in spirit, not only means to inhale but to encourage, motivate, and give hope. To expire, or lose spirit, not only means to exhale but to die, cease to exist, to end or be destroyed.

In Eastern cultures, when air is inhaled, so is vital energy, which flows into the body to nourish and enliven. In Traditional Chinese Medicine, the exhalation is considered the yin part of the breath, and the inhalation is yang. It is impossible to only breathe in without breathing out or to breathe out without breathing in. It is the continuous dynamic balance of yin and yang that contributes to health and well-being. Most of the healing traditions worldwide believe breath is the most important function of life and that restrictions in breathing lead to dysfunction and disease.

In Western culture, the breath has been considered simply a mechanical, metabolic function of the body. Scientists are now beginning to recognize that breath can be used for healing, improving the body's self-repair processes, and reducing vulnerability to illness. Oxygen is toxic to viruses, bacteria, yeasts, and parasites in the body. Cancer cells find it more difficult to survive in an oxygen-rich environment. Cullen (1983), in a 13-year study of longevity, found that respiratory capacity was actually more significant than tobacco use, insulin metabolism, or cholesterol levels in determining the length of people's lives. People with cancer and other illnesses involved in breath therapy groups demonstrate an average 46 percent increase in the levels of immunoglobulin A (IgA) immediately after the breathing sessions. IgA, an antibody in saliva, is the body's first line of defense against germs entering through the mouth and nose that produce respiratory tract infections. It is, of course, only one component of the immune system, but the results demonstrate that breathing techniques can enhance immunity (Collinge, 1998). Andrew Weil (1995a, p. 86) believes that "breath is the master key to health and wellness, a function we can learn to regulate and develop in order to improve our physical, mental, and spiritual well-being."

The breath is constantly adapting to accommodate the needs of the situation at hand. When people eat heavy meals or exercise rapidly, when their noses are congested or dry, or when their environment is filled with pleasant or unpleasant smells, their breathing changes. Every change in posture has an effect on the combination of muscles used to breathe. Breath does not feel the same standing or sitting as when one is lying down. Breathing also changes under stress. For example, anxious people take shallow "chest" breaths, using only their chest muscles to inhale rather than their diaphragms. As a result, only the top part of their lungs fills with air, depriving the body of the optimal amount of oxygen.

Many people, even when feeling relaxed, breathe in a shallow way that keeps them in a constant state of underoxygenation which contributes to a decreased level of energy and increased vulnerability to illness. The typical shallow chest breath moves about half a pint of air, while a full abdominal breath can move eight to ten times that amount. Forming healthy breathing habits can produce dramatic results. Probably no other single step that people can take will so profoundly and positively affect body, mind, and spirit. Deep breathing can counter stress. Just three deep, full belly breaths can move individuals from panic to calmness by increasing their oxygen intake. Much of perceived stress is worrying about the future or the past, and deep breathing is a great way to return people to the present. Twenty minutes of deep breathing exercises a day can lower blood pressure by increasing oxygen intake, which decreases work load on the cardiovascular system (Collinge, 1998).

INTEGRATED NURSING PRACTICE

In alternative medicine, the focus of restoring health is within each person and cannot be "given" to a client by any health care practitioner. Drugs, herbs, procedures, surgeries, or mind-body techniques may be helpful or necessary, but by themselves do not cure disease. People must, and do, rebalance and repair themselves. The profession of nursing was founded on this philosophy and view of life as noted by Florence Nightingale's basic premise that healing is a function of nature that comes from within the individual. She saw the role of the nurse as putting the "patient in the best condition for nature to act on him" (1969).

In contrast, biomedicine has taught people to listen to external authorities and to view themselves as helpless victims of disease. Conventional medicine is based on the idea of cure, which usually refers to the elimination of the signs and symptoms of disease. "Curing," however, is only effective for about 15–20 percent of the sick population. In 80–85 percent of acute disruptions of health, one of three things happens with or without medical intervention: the person gets well, develops a chronic disorder for which there is no cure, or dies. When the focus is on cure, death is seen as a failure. Certainly, the curative aspects of Western medicine have allowed many people to live healthy, productive lives. But for many others, fixing the body is not enough. As they search for meaning in their illness and their lives, as well as a sense of connectedness with others, they begin the healing process. Box 2.4 compares the philosophy and beliefs of the healing-nursing model with the curing medical model.

The concept of the "placebo effect" comes directly out of biomedicine's denial of the power of self-healing. In Western research studies, the placebo is a sham biomedical treatment with no inherent medical value. Most researchers dislike the placebo response because it complicates their experiments. In study after study, the placebo is effective in at least 30–35 percent of the cases. In fact, the rate is as high as 70 percent; typically 40 percent of individuals report excellent results and another 30 percent report good results (Benson, 1997; Roberts, 1995). Norman Cousins, author of *Anatomy of an Illness* and *The Healing Heart,* describes the placebo as the "doctor who resides within." In fact, this so-called placebo response in Western scientific literature demonstrates the unity of mind-body and provides great evidence of our self-curing capacity. Janet Quinn (1989, p. 554), an outstanding nursing leader, believes that since the site of all curing is within the individual, "there are no longer any 'real' or 'placebo' treatments and effects. There are only stimuli for healing processes." Andrew Weil (1995b, p. 52) regards the placebo response as a "pure example of healing elicited by the mind; far from being a nuisance, it is, potentially, the greatest therapeutic ally doctors can find in their efforts to mitigate disease."

Beliefs can also work against people. The "nocebo" is the placebo's negative counterpart. It is destructive thinking that contributes to sickness and even death. Our bodies are good at healing, but at times we inhibit this process by worrying or doubting our ability to overcome the illness. As nurses, we must routinely assess clients' beliefs and expectations for health and use them sys-

---

Box 2.4: The Cure Versus Heal Models

Cure-Medical Model	Heal-Nursing Model
Diseases are cured	People are healed
Focus on diagnosis	Focus on meaning
Patient is dependent	Person is autonomous
Effective for 15–20% of population; cure may or may not be possible	Effective for everyone; healing is always possible
Body is viewed as a machine; disease results when parts break	Body is a living microcosm of universe; disease results through unbalance
Role of medicine is to combat disease; practitioners are soliders in a war	Role of medicine is to restore harmony; practitioners are the peace corps, fostering learning and growth
Body is passive recipient of treatments to fix it	Body is capable of self-healing
Primary treatments are drugs, surgery, radiation	Primary treatments are diet, herbs, stress management, social support
Focus on pain	Focus on the human experience of pain, which is suffering
Caring is seen as a means to an end	Caring is the end in itself

Sources: Castleman, Nature's Cures (Emmaus, PA: Rodale Press, 1996); Quinn, 1997, Healing: A Model for an Integrative Health Care System, *Advanced Practical Nursing Quarterly* 3(1): 1–7; Shames, *The Nightingale Conspiracy* (Montclair, NJ: Enlightenment Press, 1993).

---

tematically in the healing process. The goal is not to deny reality, but to help people project healthy images. When a person acts "as if" the preferred reality were true, the body responds and improved health can emerge (Benson, 1997).

The word *heal* comes from the Greek word *halos* and the Anglo-Saxon word *haelan,* which mean "to be or to become whole." (Interestingly, the word *holy* is derived from the same source.) Thus "healing" means "making whole"—that is, restoring balance and harmony. It is movement toward a sense of wholeness and completion. Healing comes from surrendering to life as it is, including all feelings from anger and despair through joy and peacefulness. The irony is that in the process of accepting life as it is, most people feel more alive and live more fully, even when facing death. When the focus is on healing, success does not depend on whether the person lives. Healing can take place even as the body weakens. Through healing, people allow themselves to be everything they already are and move toward a greater sense of the meaning of their experiences. Even when nothing can be done physically to alter the course of disease, still much can be done in a caring sense, to make the human experience more meaningful and understandable (Quinn, 1997; Shames, 1993).

Nursing has always focused on creating healing environments for those who have been entrusted to our care. We create healing environments when we use our hands, heart, and mind to provide holistic nursing care. We create healing environments when we empower others by providing the knowledge, skills, and support that allow them to tap into their inner wisdom and make healthy decisions for themselves. Healing environments are a synthesis of the biomedical-curing approach and nursing-healing approach. We need a healthy balance between technology and compassion. We create healing environments when we take the time to be with clients in deeply caring ways. It is when we stop, become still, and enter the other's subjective world that we are able to be wholly present for that person. This moment of spiritual connection is uplifting to both client and nurse. Karilee Shames (1993, p. 131) described sacred healing moments that occurred when her "goal became to inspire, to share tenderness, and to help instill a will to live, or to surrender to the call of death peacefully, if that was most appropriate. In my highest vision, this is what nursing was all about."

We must also create healing environments for ourselves. Working with people can be draining work. As nurses, we need to learn how to restore our energy and replenish ourselves. You might compare your ability to care for others to a well of fresh, healing water. If the well is never dipped into, the water becomes stagnant and brackish. If the water is constantly drawn out and given away, with no source of replenishment, the well will soon run dry. What happens to nurses who don't sincerely care for others or take the time to replenish themselves? It soon becomes obvious by their behavior that they are stagnant or depleted; they are less patient, less tolerant, more irritable, and unhappy. Their state of "burnout" contaminates all aspects of their professional and personal lives.

When you care for others, care for yourself, and allow others to care for you; your well of healing is constantly being replenished. You will find many techniques in this book which you can incorporate into your daily life. It is important that you take time for yourself, even if for only ten minutes a day. Learning to take care of ourselves means letting go of self-defeating behaviors and attitudes. We must teach ourselves to relax without feeling guilty or selfish for taking time out. Self-renewal is a continuous process. To be there for others and care for them in their times of need, we must first look after our own well-being. It is only when we walk in balance that we can help others learn how to balance their lives.

TRY THIS: *Focused Breathing*

Breathing Clouds

Gently close your eyes and focus all your attention on the flow of air as you breathe in and exhale. After three to five breaths, visualize the air that you breathe into your lungs as a cloud of clean, pure, energized air. Tell yourself that the clean, fresh air that you breathe in through your nose has the power to clear your mind of distracting thoughts, as well as to cleanse and heal your body. As you slowly inhale this clean, pure air, feel the air enter your nose and travel up through the sinus cavity toward the top of your head. Visualize the air traveling down your spinal column and circulating throughout your abdominal area.

Now, as you exhale slowly and deeply, visualize that the air leaving your body is a dark, dirty cloud. This dark cloud of exhaled air symbolizes all your stressors, frustrations, and toxins. With each breath you take, allow the clean fresh air to enter and circulate and rejuvenate your body, while the exhalation of dark cloudy air helps to rid your body of its stress and tension. Repeat this breathing cycle for 5–10 minutes. As you continue this cycle of breathing clouds, visualize that as the body becomes more relaxed through the release of stress and tension, the color of the breath exhaled begins to change from dark to gray, perhaps even an off-white, a message from your mind that it is cleansed and refreshed.

Source: Seaward, *Stand Like Mountain Flow Like Water* (Deerfield Beach, FL: Health Communications, 1997), 114–115.

Breathing Energy

From a point beneath your feet, bring energy up through the chakras to a place above your head. Then spiral it around you and down back to where you started. You can fill the spiral with light or color, whatever feels best for you. If you encounter someone around whom you tend to become drained, run the energy quickly up and down.

Source: Rutherford, *Principles of Shamanism* (San Francisco: Thorsons, 1996).

REFERENCES

BENSON, H. 1997. *Timeless Healing.* New York: Fireside Book.

BORYSENKO, J. and M. BORYSENKO. 1994. *The Power of the Mind to Heal.* Carlsbad, CA: Hay House.

CAMPBELL, D. January–February 1998. The riddle of the Mozart Effect. *Natural Health.* 114–119.

CASTLEMAN, M. 1996. *Nature's Cures.* Emmaus, PA: Rodale Press.

CHIN, R. M. 1995. *The Energy Within.* New York: Marlowe & Co.

CHOPRA, D. 1991. *Perfect Health.* New York: Harmony Books.

COLLINGE, W. 1998. *Subtle Energy.* New York: Warner Books.

CULLEN, K. et al. 1983. Multiple regression analysis of risk factors for cardiovascular disease and cancer mortality in Busselton, West Australia: A thirteen-year study. *J Chronic Diseases.* 36: 371–377.

DALE, C. 1997. *New Chakra Healing.* St. Paul, MN: Llewellyn Pub.

IVKER, R. 1997. *Thriving.* New York: Crown.

LUCE, G. G. 1997. Biological rhythm in health and disease. In: D. S. SOBEL, ed. *Ways of Health: Holistic Approaches to Ancient and Contemporary Medicine.* New York: Harcourt Brace Jovanovich, 397–411.

NIGHTINGALE, F. 1969. *Notes on Nursing.* New York: Dover Press.

MOSS, R. 1996. *Conscious Dreaming.* New York: Crown Trade Paperbacks.

MYSS, C. 1996. *Anatomy of the Spirit.* New York: Three Rivers Press.

QUINN, J. F. 1989. On healing, wholeness, and the haelan effect. *Nurs and Health Care.* 10(10): 553–556.

QUINN, J. F. 1997. Healing: A model for an integrative health care system. *Adv Prac Nurs Q.* 3(1): 1–7.

ROBERTS, A. 1995. The powerful placebo revisited. *Body/Mind J.* 1(1): 35–45.

RUTHERFORD, L. 1996. *Principles of Shamanism.* San Francisco: Thorsons.

SCHWARTZ, C. 1996. *Four Paws, Five Directions.* Berkeley, CA: Celestial Arts.

SEAWARD, B. L. 1997. *Stand Like Mountain Flow Like Water.* Deerfield Beach, FL: Health Communications.

SHAMES, K. H. 1993. *The Nightingale Conspiracy.* Montclair, NJ: Enlightenment Press.

WEIL, A. 1995a. *Natural Health, Natural Medicine.* Boston: Houghton Mifflin.

WEIL, A. 1995b. *Spontaneous Healing.* New York: Knopf.

WRIGHT, K. B. 1998. Professional, ethical, and legal implications for spiritual care in nursing. *Image.* 30(1): 81–83.

UNIT II
SYSTEMATIZED HEALTH CARE PRACTICES

Our ideas must be as broad as Nature if they are to interpret Nature.

Sir Arthur Conan Doyle, Study in Scarlet

3 Traditional Chinese Medicine

Worms will not eat living wood where the vital sap is flowing; rust will not hinder the opening of a gate when the hinges are used each day. Movement gives health and life. Stagnation brings disease and death.

Ancient proverb in Traditional Chinese Medicine

The superior physician helps before the early budding of the disease. . . . The inferior physician begins to help when [the disease] has already set in.

The Yellow Emperor's Classic of Internal Medicine

Traditional Chinese Medicine (TCM) originated in Chinese culture more than 3,000 years ago and has spread, with variations, throughout other Asian countries, particularly Japan, Korea, Tibet, and Vietnam. As a comprehensive health system, it has a range of applications from preventive health care and maintenance to diagnosis and treatment of acute and chronic disorders.

BACKGROUND

TCM has a long and extensive history. Shen Nong, the Fire Emperor, said to have lived from 2698 to 2598 B.C., is considered the founder of herbal medicine in China. The written history itself is more than 2,500 years old, starting with the text on internal medicine of Huang Di, the Yellow Emperor. Written long before the birth of Hippocrates, the father of Western medicine, *Yellow Emperor's Inner Classic* covers such principles as yin and yang, the five phases, the effects of the season, and treatments such as acupuncture and moxibustion.

TCM is associated with early Taoists and Buddhists who observed energy within themselves, in plants and animals, and throughout the cosmos. Based on a belief in the natural order of the universe and the direct correlation between the human body and the cosmos, this philosophy stresses the constant search for harmony and balance in an environment of constant change. By the close of the Han era (A.D. 220), the Chinese had a clear grasp of pathology, preventive medicine, first aid, and dietetics, and had devised breathing practices to promote longevity. During the fourth and fifth centuries A.D., China's influence spread throughout Asia, and both Taoism and Buddhism had a marked impact on ideas about health. Sun Si Mian (A.D. 581–682), a famous physician, established himself as China's first medical ethicist. He advocated the need for rigorous scholarship, compassion toward patients, and high moral standards in physicians. In the eleventh century, TCM began to focus more on social phenomena, especially human relations and ethical behavior. Initially this orientation resulted in increased scientific medical study and publications. As TCM developed further, people began to take for granted that a breakthrough in one realm of knowledge would eventually solve all problems of human existence. (As in the West, some assume that advances in technology will solve all problems.) Eventually, sociological methods were used to solve medical problems, and clinical and empirical research reached a low point. Fortunately, the core of the scientific system was never obliterated, and this century has seen a worldwide revival of TCM (*Alternative Medicine,* 1994; Ergil, 1996; Porkert, 1979).

In China today, TCM is practiced in hospitals along with Western medicine. Physicians not only study principles of anatomy, histology, biochemistry, bacteriology, and surgery but also acupuncture, acupressure, and herbal medicine. Patients can choose TCM or Western approaches or a combination for their particular problem. Inpatient and outpatient care is provided in large, well-equipped hospitals, as well as private clinics and pharmacies.

CONCEPTS

A basic understanding of TCM requires recognition of its long-lived tradition, multiple philosophies, and varied practices. It is impossible to separate the individual concepts and the specific treatment approaches from the context of a complete theoretical system. Prevention, diagnosis, and treatment of diseases are based on the concepts of qi, yin and yang, the five phases, the five seasons, and the three treasures. Often only isolated fragments of TCM emerge in the West.

Qi

The concept most central to TCM is qi or chi (pronounced chee), which is translated as energy. Qi represents an invisible flow of energy that circulates through plants, animals, and people as well as the earth and sky. It is what maintains physiologic functions and the health and well-being of the individual. In TCM theory, energy is distributed throughout the body along a network of energy circuits or meridians, connecting all parts of the body. The many different types of qi in the body are described according to their source, location, and function. *Yin qi* supports and nourishes the body, *wei qi* protects and warms the body, *jing qi* flows in the meridians, *zang qi* flows in the organs, and *zong qi* is responsible for respiration and circulation. Obstructed qi flow in the human body can cause problems ranging from social difficulties to illness. Its effects are very individual—a person gets sick, has problems at work, or fights with family—and depend on each individual's unique qi. Certain TCM treatments such as meditation, exercise, and acupuncture are ways of enhancing or correcting the flow of qi (Ergil, 1996; Lagatree, 1996).

Yin and Yang

In the Taoist philosophy, wholeness is comprised of the union of opposites—dark and light, soft and hard, female and male, slow and fast, etc. These opposite but complementary aspects are called yin and yang. Originally the terms designated geographical aspects such as the shady and sunny side of a mountain or the southern and northern bank of a river. In modern terms they are used to characterize the polar opposites that exist in everything and make up the physical world.

From the health perspective, the basis of well-being is the appropriate balance of yin and yang as they interact in the body. Imbalance of yin and yang is considered to be the cause of illness. Yin is the general category for passivity and is like water with a tendency to be cold and heavy. Yin uses fluids to moisten and cool our bodies. It provides for restfulness as we slow down and sleep. Yin is associated more with substance than with energy. Things that are close to the ground are yin or more earthy. Yin is associated with the symptoms of coldness, paleness, low blood pressure, and chronic conditions. People with excess yin tend to catch colds easily, and are sedentary and sleepy. Yang is the general category for activity and aggressiveness. It is like fire with its heating and circulating characteristics. Associated with things higher up or more heavenly, yang is the energy that directs movement and supports its substance. Symptoms such as redness in the face, fever, high blood pressure, and acute conditions are associated with yang. People with excess yang tend to be nervous and agitated and cannot tolerate much heat (Monte, 1997; Schwartz, 1996).

It must be understood that yin and yang cannot exist independently of each other. Nothing is either all yin or all yang. They are complementary and depend on each other for their very existence—without night there can be no day, without moisture there can be no dryness, and without cold there can be no heat. It is the interaction of yin and yang that creates the changes that keep the world in motion; summer leads to winter, night becomes day. Yin and yang are used in both the diagnosis and treatment of illness. For example, if a person is experiencing too much stress, usually understood as an excess of yang, more yin activities, such as meditation and relaxation, are the appropriate treatment.

Five Phases

As they studied the world around them, the Chinese perceived connections between major forces in nature and particular internal organ systems. Seeing similarities between natural elements and the body, early practitioners developed a concept of health care that encompassed both natural elements and body organs. This theory is known as the Five Phases Theory (wu-hsing). Five elements—fire, earth, metal, water, wood—represent movement or energies that succeed one another in a dynamic relationship and in a continuous cycle of birth, life, and death. These elements do not represent static objects, since even mountains and rivers change constantly with time. In the Five Phases Theory, it is not the substances themselves that are important, but rather how they interact together to make up the essential life force or qi (Schwartz, 1996).

The rhythm of events resembles a circle known as the Creation Cycle. In this cycle, burning wood feeds fire; from its ashes, fire produces earth; earth in turn gives up its ore, creating metal; from condensation on its surface, metal brings forth water; and water nourishes and creates plants and trees, creating wood. Each element is related to a pair of internal organs. The yin organ is solid and dense, like the liver, while its yang partner is hollow or forms a pocket, like the gall bladder. The proper interaction of the organ partners influences how well the entire body functions. Fire is linked to the circulation of blood, hormones, and food. Its partner organs are the heart (yin) and small intestine (yang). Earth is linked to digestion and is comprised of the spleen/pancreas (yin) and the stomach (yang). Metal is linked to respiration and elimination and is made up of the lungs (yin) and large intestine (yang). Water is linked to elimination and is comprised of the kidneys (yin) and urinary bladder (yang). Wood is linked to toxic processing and is made up of the liver (yin) and gall bladder (yang). In addition, each organ is related to a time of day of optimal functioning. If a problem occurs during those hours when an organ is most vulnerable, the timing may alert a TCM practitioner to an imbalance in that organ system. Figure 3.1 illustrates the Five Phases of the Creation Cycle and their related yin and yang organs (Lagatree, 1996; Schwartz, 1996).

Five Seasons

The four cardinal compass directions—south, west, north, and east—are affiliated with four of the five elements: fire, metal, water, and wood. The fifth ele-

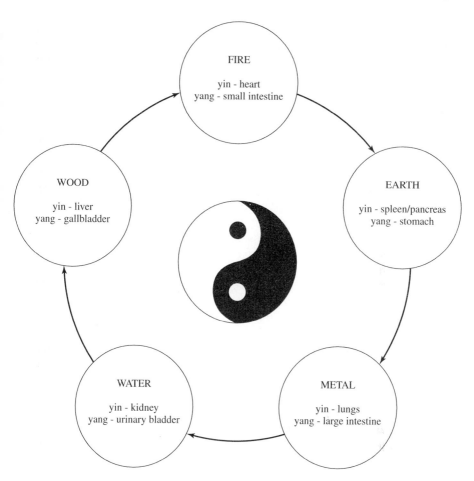

Figure 3.1:   Creation Cycle: Five Phases and Related Organ Systems

ment, earth, is depicted in the center. The Chinese place so much importance on the direction south, that they put it at the top of their maps and navigate from it in the same way that Westerners use north. Just as south rules the top of the compass, it also represents summer, the "high noon" of the year and is linked to fire. West, the direction of the setting sun, is associated with autumn and metal, which is used to make tools for harvesting. North is linked to winter and water, the opposite of the element of fire and is seen as a period of dormancy. East, the direction of the rising sun, is associated with spring and with wood, which represents all growing things. The fifth and central element, earth, is related to the late summer season and a time of maturity. Figure 3.2 illustrates the five directions as they correlate to the five seasons and the five elements.

SOUTH

Summer
Fire
Peak

EAST   CENTER   WEST

Spring   Late summer   Autumn
Wood   Earth   Metal
Growth   Maturity   Tools

NORTH

Winter
Water
Dormancy

Figure 3.2:   Five Directions/
Seasons/Elements

The etiology of disease in TCM is linked to the five phases, five seasons, and five directions. It is believed that if one component is overbearing and excessive, then another becomes weak and debilitated. It is a complex system of checks and balances that is often not easily grasped by those with a Western perspective. Diagnosis and treatment of illness depends on understanding the five elements, seasons, and directions and how they interact.

Three Treasures

The Chinese believe that a combination of life force elements make up the substance and functions of the body, mind, and spirit and that these three are all one and the same. One way to understand this connection is to think of water with its wet, fluid nature. Compare that to ice, which not only appears different but feels hard and cold. And then consider steam with its hot gaseous nature. Despite the differences in appearance, it is the same substance in three different forms. In the same way, body, mind, and spirit can be seen as different expressions of the same individual (Longo and Newhouse, 1984).

The Taoists call body, mind, and spirit, the three "vital treasures." They are *jing,* meaning basic essence, *qi* meaning energy or life force, and *shen* meaning spirit and mind. The balance of their abundance or deficiency influences the state of health. Jing is the essence with which people are born. It is similar to Western concepts of genes, DNA, and heredity. Essence is the gift of one's parents; it is the basic material in each cell that allows that cell to function. It is the bodily reserves that support life and must be restored by food and rest.

There are several types of qi. The hereditary qi, which is from the jing, the nutritive qi derived from food, and the cosmic qi from the air that is breathed. Wei qi is a specialized qi associated with the immune system. Wei qi circulates near the surface of the body and is the first level of protection when a bacteria or virus tries to enter the body. If the circulating wei qi is weak, it can allow a pathogen to enter the body and illness ensues.

The vital treasure known as shen is the gift of heaven and represents spiritual and mental aspects of life. Shen comprises one's emotional well-being, thoughts, and beliefs. It is the radiance, or inner glow, that can be perceived by others. In order for people to be healthy, their physical, emotional, mental, and spiritual aspects must be balanced (Schwartz, 1996).

VIEW OF HEALTH/ILLNESS

The Chinese regard the body as a system that requires a balance of yin and yang energy to enjoy good health. Each part of the body is also thought of as an individual system that requires its own balance of yin and yang to function properly. TCM assumes that a balanced body has a natural ability to resist or cope with agents of disease. Symptoms are caused by an imbalance of yin and yang in some part of the body, and illness can develop if the balance is disturbed for any length of time. Therefore, health is maintained by recognizing an imbalance before it becomes a disease. It is believed that everything needed to restore health already exists in nature and it is up to the individual, with or without the aid of a health practitioner, to free up energy and restore balance using diet, herbs, acupuncture, and other yin/yang treatments (Wensel, 1984).

The Chinese believe that all living things—people, the earth, the universe—are connected by cosmic energy. Thus the balance of qi in an individual is connected to the balance in the environment; the forces active within the world are the same forces active within the individual body. Simply put, nothing happens without consequence to something else. The concern for balance and harmony is not only reflected in the TCM approach to the individual but also in the view that the balance and well-being of the resources of the natural world and society are vital to the overall health of all who live on the earth. Practitioners never lose sight of the multifaceted relationship between individuals, communities, societies, and nature (AAOM, 1991).

Since the human body is a microcosm of the universe, extremes of climate in the body can create problems, just as extreme environmental conditions can wreak havoc on the environment. Sometimes people experience a "cold" or yin illness caused by too much coldness in the body. For example, the symptoms of a "cold" influenza include a low-grade fever, no sweating, headache, muscle aches, stuffy nose, and a cough with clear white phlegm. Some influenzas are "hot" or yang influenzas caused by too much heat in the body. Symptoms include high fever, sweating, headache, dry or sore throat, thirst, and nasal congestion with sticky or yellow mucus. Too much cold in the body requires "warming" remedies and too much heat in the body requires "cooling" remedies (Zhang, 1998).

DIAGNOSTIC METHODS

The TCM practitioner has four diagnostic methods (szu-chen): inspection, auscultation/olfaction, inquiry, and palpation. These methods gather information about the five phases and their related body systems. The practitioner examines how the person eats, sleeps, thinks, works, relaxes, dreams, and imagines. No part of the self is considered a neutral bystander when the body is in a state of imbalance.

Inspection

Inspection (wang), refers to the visual assessment of the spirit and physical body of patients. Spirit inspection or observation is an assessment of the person's overall appearance, especially the eyes, the complexion, and the quality of voice. Good spirit, even in the presence of serious illness, indicates a more positive prognosis. Tongue diagnosis is a highly developed system of inspection of the physical body. The tongue is considered to be the visual gateway to the interior of the body. The whole body "lives" on the tongue, rather like a hologram. Different areas of the tongue correspond to the five phases and related organ systems as seen in Figure 3.3. The central area of the tongue is related to the spleen/pancreas and stomach. The very back of the tongue reflects the kidneys and urinary bladder. The sides of the tongue are related to the liver and gall bladder. The very tip of the tongue corresponds to the heart and surrounding the heart are the lungs in the front one-third of the tongue.The practitioner inspects the color, shape, markings, and coating of the tongue to gather information about the state of balance in the person's body. For example, a moist tongue with a thin white coating may signal the presence of a "cold" or yin illness whereas a dry, yellow or dark tongue may signal a "hot" or yang illness (Ergil, 1996; Schwartz, 1996).

Auscultation/Olfaction

The second part of diagnosis, auscultation/olfaction (wen), refers to listening to the quality of speech, breath, and other sounds, as well as being aware of the

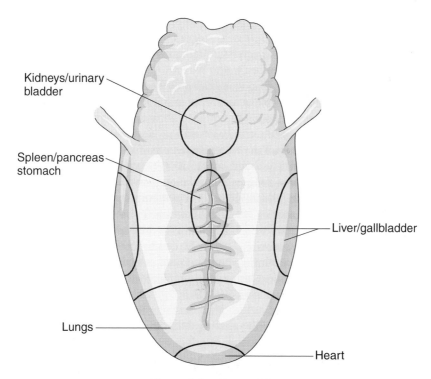

Kidneys/urinary bladder

Spleen/pancreas stomach

Liver/gallbladder

Lungs

Heart

Figure 3.3:   Tongue Map

odors of breath, body, and excreta. Types of sound are associated with the five phases and organ systems. How the person is breathing is a good indication of the status of the organs. Phases and organ systems are associated with specific odors such as sickly sweet, rotten, putrid, rancid, and scorched. Odors can arise from the skin itself or from the ears, nose, genitals, urine, stool, or bodily discharges. The breath may also have a distinctive odor. Usually the stronger the odor, the more serious the imbalance has become.

Inquiry

The third part of diagnosis, inquiry (wen), is the process of taking a comprehensive health, social, emotional, and spiritual history. The practitioner questions the person not only about the presenting complaint but about many other factors, including sensations of hot and cold, perspiration, excreta, hearing, thirst, sleep, digestion, emotions, sexual drive, and energy level.

Palpation

Palpation (qie) is the fourth diagnostic method and includes pulse examination, general palpation of the body, and palpation of the acupuncture points. Reading the pulses, or pulse diagnosis, can provide key information about the person's condition. For example, a fast pulse might indicate a problem with an overactive heart or liver; a slow pulse might indicate a sluggish digestive system; pulses described as wide, flat, and soft may indicate a spleen problem; and narrow, forceful pulses might indicate a liver dysfunction. The radial pulse is felt in three positions and two layers on both the right and left arm. The more superficial, or surface layer, belongs to the yang organs, while the deeper layer belongs to the yin organs. The locations of major points used in pulse diagnosis are illustrated in Figure 3.4. The pulse allows the practitioner to feel the quality of qi and blood at the different locations in the body. Twenty-nine pulse qualities are described according to size, rate, depth, force, and volume (Ergil, 1996; Schwartz, 1996). Examples of qualities are surging, scattered, vacuous, slippery, stringlike, flat, and so on.

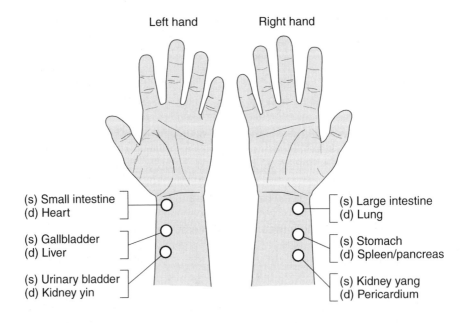

Left hand   Right hand

(s) Small intestine
(d) Heart

(s) Gallbladder
(d) Liver

(s) Urinary bladder
(d) Kidney yin

(s) Large intestine
(d) Lung

(s) Stomach
(d) Spleen/pancreas

(s) Kidney yang
(d) Pericardium

(s) = Superficial
(d) = Deep

Figure 3.4:   Location of Major Points Used in Pulse Diagnosis

All of this diagnostic information is compiled to arrive at a "pattern of disharmony," or bian zheng. A single biomedical disease can be associated with a large number of Chinese diagnostic patterns. A lower urinary tract infection, for example, might be related to one of four distinct diagnostic patterns. Each of these patterns would be treated in different ways, as it is said, "one disease, different treatments." Also, many different biomedical diseases may fall into one pattern, thus the saying, "different diseases, one treatment" (Ergil, 1996).

TREATMENT

Since an individual's combinations of yin and yang are unique, TCM practitioners must tailor their treatment to each client. The goal of treatment is to reestablish a balanced flow of energy in the person through diet, herbs, massage, acupuncture, and Qigong.

Diet

The simplest and most accessible treatment is diet. Dietary interventions are individualized on the basis of the individual's pattern of disharmony. Foods are used to rebalance the body's internal "climate" by bringing warmth to coldness, or cooling off too much heat. The thermal nature of food is described by the way a person feels after ingesting it. For example, after eating watermelon or asparagus, which are cooling foods, one feels physically and emotionally cooler. An internal feeling of warmth comes after eating warming foods such as salmon, lamb, or sweet potatoes. Neutral foods do not create a specific thermal quality and are thus good diet balancers. A diet to maintain health should be varied and include a minimum of seven different fruits and vegetables a day to avoid a cold or hot imbalance. If a person is ill and the symptoms indicate a hot condition, then the diet should emphasize cooling foods, and vice versa. In addition to the overall daily diet, specific foods are used as medicines to correct hot and cold imbalances (Zhang, 1998). See Box 3.1 for a list of common foods and their thermal effects on the body.

Foods are categorized according to one of six tastes, each taste having a specific function in the body. *Sweet* foods are often used to aid digestion and qi and influence the spleen and stomach. *Salty* foods affect the kidney and bladder and are often used to "soften" cysts or tumors and may be tried before surgery. *Sour* foods, such as lemons or tomatoes, are used to dry mucous membranes in the intestinal, urinary, reproductive, or respiratory surfaces. *Pungent* foods such as garlic and onion are used to aid digestion, stimulate circulation, and promote sweating. *Bitter* foods, such as greens or tonic water, also help

Box 3.1: Thermal Food Qualities

Cooling

Pork, duck, eggs, clams, crab, millet, barley, wheat, lettuce, celery, broccoli, spinach, tomato, banana, watermelon, asparagus, ice cream, soy sauce

Neutral

Beef, beef liver, rabbit, sardines, yam, rice, corn, rye, potato, beet, turnip, carrot, lemon, apple

Warming

Tuna, turkey, salmon, lamb, venison, chicken, chicken liver, shrimp, trout, oats, cabbage, squash, kale, scallion, celery, ginger, sugar, garlic, pepper

digestion and are used to regulate the bowels. *Astringent* foods, such as beans or potatoes, stop the flow of bodily secretions such as tears, saliva, and sweat (Schwartz, 1996).

Each food has both yin and yang energies but often one predominates. Cooling foods and those with bitter and salty flavors are yin. Warming foods are yang, as are foods with pungent and sweet flavors. When people have an excess of yin they may be sluggish, laid back, calm, slightly overweight, and emotionally sensitive. To balance these overly yin tendencies, yang foods are added to the diet to help activate the metabolism and provide more energy. People experiencing an excess in yang may be tense, loud, hyperactive, and aggressive. Their internal tension is cooled by adding yin foods to the diet.

TCM practitioners recommend certain foods for balancing and improving a variety of conditions. Foods can be potent healers, especially when dealing with temporary illnesses, but they are never used as a lone treatment for serious or chronic conditions.

Herbs

Herbal medicine (ahong yao) is an integral part of TCM. In terms of the complexity of diagnosis and treatment, it resembles the practice of Western internal medicine. Herbs may be taken in the form of tea or the substances may be powdered and made into pills, pastes, or tinctures for internal or external use. Just as in food, some herbs are warming (cinnamon) and some are cooling (mint).

With the exception of conditions that require surgery, herbs can be used to treat almost any condition in the practice of TCM. Herbs are often prescribed in complex mixtures and tend not to be used as isolated components, e.g., extractions from the parent plant. TCM practitioners believe that the healing benefits of herbs result from the synergistic interactions of all the components of the plant. The same herb can be used for many different disorders. Likewise, the same disorder in different people will be treated with different herbs, depending on assessment of the individual. Herbs are used in the following ways: antiviral, antibacterial, antifungal, and anticancer. Herbs are also used to treat pain, aid digestion, lower cholesterol, treat colds and flus, increase resistance to disease, enhance immune function, improve circulation, regulate menstruation, and increase energy (*Alternative Medicine,* 1992; Weil, 1995). Box 3.2 lists herbs commonly used as tonics in TCM. Chapter 6 covers the use of herbs in greater detail.

Box 3.2: Tonic Herbs Frequently Used in TCM

Herb	Use
Garlic	Lowers blood pressure, lowers cholesterol and triglycerides, antiseptic, antifungal
Ginger	Warming effect, stimulates digestion, decreases nausea, relieves aches and pains
Green tea	Lowers cholesterol, anticancer effects, antibacterial effects
Astragalus	Enhances immune function by increasing activity of WBCs and increases production of antibodies and interferon
Siberian Ginseng	Enhances immune function, increases energy
Ginseng	Increases appetite and digestion, tones skin and muscles, restores depleted sexual energy
Dong Quai (Tang Kuei)	Blood-building tonic which improves circulation, tones the uterus, balances female hormones
Ho Shou Wu	Cleans the blood, nourishes hair and teeth, increases energy, powerful sexual tonic

Massage

Traditional Chinese massage methods were described in texts as early as 200 B.C. Both energizing and sedating techniques are used to treat and relieve many medical conditions. Major techniques in use are (*Alternative Healing*, 1992):

- *ma*, rubbing with palm or finger tips
- *pai*, tapping with palm or finger tips
- *tao*, strong pinching with thumb and fingertip
- *an*, rapid and rhythmical pressing with thumb, palm, or back of the clenched hand
- *nie*, twisting, with both thumbs and tips of the index fingers grasping and twisting the area being treated
- *ning*, pinching and lifting in a stationary position
- *na*, pinching and lifting in a stationary position
- *tui*, pushing, often with slight vibratory effect

Widely varying illnesses are treated with traditional Chinese massage including the common cold, insomnia, leg cramps, painful menses, diarrhea, abdominal pains, headache, asthma, rheumatic pains, stiff neck, colic, nasal bleeding, and throat pains. Massage increases circulation of blood and lymph to the skin and underlying muscles bringing added nutrients and pain relief. Massage can help restore proper movement to injured limbs and joints and help restore a sense of balance. Massage is an effective method of reducing stress and tension that usually leads to a feeling of relaxation (*Alternative Medicine*, 1994; Schwartz, 1996). Chapter 11 covers massage in greater detail.

Acupuncture

Acupuncture involves stimulating specific anatomic points called *hsueh* where each meridian passes close to the skin surface. Puncturing the skin with very fine needles is the usual method but practitioners may also use pressure (shiatsu), friction, suction, heat, or electromagnetic energy to stimulate points. Moxibustion is an application of heat from certain burning substances at acupuncture points on the body. The primary goal of acupuncture is the manipulation of energy flow throughout the body following a thorough assessment by a TCM practitioner. Treatment is offered in the context of the total person and with the goal of correcting the flow of qi to restore health. Some Western health care practitioners who have learned the techniques of acupuncture miss the broader context and limit their focus to an injured or painful body part.

Acupuncture is effective in the treatment of acute and chronic pain and motion disabilities. In addition it is used in respiratory and cardiovascular conditions (asthma, COPD, palpitations, hypertension), eye, ear, nose, and throat disorders (conjunctivitis, tinnitus, Meniere's disease, rhinitis, sore throat), gastrointestinal problems (gastritis, ulcers, colitis, constipation, irritable bowel syndrome), urogenital conditions (premenstrual syndrome, endometriosis, menopausal symptoms, prostatitis, incontinence, erectile problems), skin disorders (eczema, shingles, urticaria), psychiatric problems (anxiety, depression, schizophrenia), and in addictive disorders and withdrawal syndromes. Ear acupuncture is a complete system within itself and is quite powerful for balancing the hormones and overall energy of the body. Contraindications to acupuncture are pregnancy, hemophilia, and acute cardiovascular disorders (*Alternative Healing,* 1994; Johnstone et al., 1994; Weil, 1995). Chapter 12 covers acupuncture in more detail.

Qigong

Qigong, pronounced chee-gong, is the art and science of using breath, movement, self-massage, and meditation to cleanse, strengthen, and circulate vital life energy and blood. In India the comparable practice is called yoga. Both of these traditions of self-healing have been called "moving meditation" or "meditation in motion." T'ai Chi, which is familiar to many Americans, is a more physical form of qigong. In China, millions of people from children, to workers, to elders, to patients in the hospital practice qigong daily. The techniques are easy to learn and simple to apply for people who are well or sick. Qigong decreases fatigue and forgetfulness and generates energy by enhancing bodily functions.

It is inevitable that taking a deep breath triggers a sense of relaxation. By adding the intention to relax with the breath, the effect is even greater. Adding gentle movements or self-massage to the deep breathing and relaxation generates increased self-healing abilities. The focus on deep and intentional relaxation allows for release of emotional stress, for a sense of tranquility, and for one's natural spirituality to arise (Jahnke, 1997).

RESEARCH

Although extensive research has been done in China through the institutions of TCM, much of this clinical research has been reports of observed results of various treatments. Many of these reports have been difficult to translate into Western languages and into the causal and analytic type of research modalities typical of the biomedical model. Research standards throughout the world are subject to cultural influences. Not all cultures require their medical practitioners to conduct randomized, double-blind clinical trials. Consequently, the research data is influenced by the location of the study. Research that is meaningful to the scientific communities of China and Japan may not have the same impact on European and North American biomedical communities.

Extensive research has been published on the pharmacology and toxicity of many traditional herbs. Researchers in China and Japan have been studying the therapeutic value of herbs in the following areas: chronic hepatitis, rheumatoid arthritis, hypertension, atopic eczema, various immunologic disorders including AIDS, and certain cancers. It would be useful to repeat these studies using biomedical research criteria. Research on the medical effects of qigong has been continuing since the mid-1980s and is now focusing on qigong as a biophysical rather than a mystical force. Acupuncture is one of the most thoroughly researched and documented TCM practices. Research studies are covered in more detail in the chapters devoted to these specific practices. Research opportunities in the future might include studies regarding manual healing therapies, bioelectricity, magnetic physical interventions, and the use of body-mind interactions for health purposes (*Alternative Medicine,* 1994). For the most up-to-date list of research studies available in the United States, contact the Office of Alternative Medicine (OAM) at the National Institutes of Health. Refer to Box 3.3 for a list of currently funded studies supported by the OAM.

Box 3.3: Funded Studies by Office of Alternative Medicine

Medical Condition	Modality
Unipolar depression	Acupuncture
Osteoarthritis	Acupuncture
Premenstrual syndrome	Traditional Chinese Medicine
Common warts	Chinese herbal therapy
Balance disorders	T'ai Chi
Menopausal hot flashes	Chinese herbal therapy
Postoperative oral surgery pain	Acupuncture
Breech version	Acupuncture
Chronic sinusitis in HIV infection	Tradition Chinese Medicine
Hyperactivity	Acupuncture
Intractable reflex sympathetic dystrophy	Qigong

RELATED SYSTEMS

Tibet

In Tibetan Buddhism, religion and medicine are never separated from one another. The spiritual goal of Buddhism is to understand the nature of oneself and suffering, and to develop compassion and compassionate action in one's life. Tibetan medicine, a sophisticated system, is based on general medical and philosophical assumptions as well as each individual's emotions, attitudes, lifestyle, and spiritual beliefs. It is believed that one's positive actions produce happiness and one's negative actions produce suffering. This belief in cause and effect is referred to as *karma*. In Tibetan medicine, disease results from two causes. The first cause is spiritual, something brought from past life karma. Spiritual diseases are mediated by a qualified teacher who uses meditation and yoga to balance body, mind, and spirit. The process of learning how to control one's mind to function in a balanced mode with one's body is called *dharma* (Begley, 1994).

The second cause of disease involves factors from this life including seasonal changes, personal habits and behaviors, poisons, and negative spirits. Illness is considered to be a lack of internal harmony or balance or a lack of harmony with the larger external environment. The process of diagnosis is similar to Traditional Chinese Medicine. Essential components in helping people mobilize their resources for self-healing are caring and compassion (Begley, 1994).

Other treatments include dietary changes, massage, exercise, yoga, meditation, breath work, and acupuncture. Surgery is only used when absolutely necessary. Herbal medicines are made from a variety of herbs, minerals, fruits, twigs, roots, and animals. As in the Native American tradition, the state of the practitioner's mind and the method of gathering are important to the medication's therapeutic outcome. All preparation of medicines begins with prayer (Begley, 1994).

Korea

Chinese medicine arrived in Korea in approximately 200 B.C. The close relationship between China and Korea facilitated the exchange of ideas for hundreds of years. In the tenth century A.D., Korea established its political independence from China but cultural and medical exchange continued. A contemporary innovative system developed in Korea in 1971 involves hand and finger acupuncture. Energy channels of the entire body are mapped onto the hands, where they are stimulated using short, fine needles and magnets. This system is rapidly gaining in popularity throughout the world (Ergil, 1996).

Japan

The history of medical information exchange dates back to the first century A.D. By the eighth century many Chinese medical texts were translated for use in Japan. Several factors contributed to the unique adaptation of Chinese medicine. The scarcity of herbs led to an emphasis on lower prescription doses in Japan. Palpation, as a part of the diagnostic process, includes palpation of the abdominal energy pathways. A division of specialization in Japanese medicine relegates acupuncture, massage, and herbs to separately licensed practitioners. In Japanese medicine, acupuncture involves the use of somewhat finer gauge needles and more shallow insertion (Ergil, 1996).

Europe

The history of Chinese medicine in Europe dates back to the middle of the sixteenth century A.D. when texts on acupuncture were written by European physicians who traveled and studied in China and Japan. In the 1950s and 1960s notable English acupuncturists, Dr. Felix Mann and Dr. Sidney Rose-Neil, influenced the development of acupuncture in English-speaking countries (Ergil, 1996).

United States

In 1826 Dr. Bache became one of the first American physicians to use acupuncture in his practice. When large numbers of Chinese laborers arrived in the United States, they were accompanied by TCM physicians and herbal merchants. Ah Fong Chuck became the first licensed practitioner of TCM in the United States in 1901 when he was awarded a medical license in Idaho. With the advent of World War II and the interruption of the herb supply from China, these practices disappeared or retreated into Chinatowns nationwide. In the 1970s President Nixon reopened communication with China and the practice of TCM began to gain visibility once again throughout the United States. Now, a clear interest in acupuncture, herbs, and qigong can be found among many North American people (Ergil, 1996).

INTEGRATED NURSING PRACTICE

Although as nurses we are not educated as TCM practitioners, some principles are common to both nursing and TCM. Fifteen principles of nurse healers' practice are listed in chapter 1, and it is easy to see how closely they correlate with the principles of TCM. Nursing and TCM practitioners believe that people are at once mind, body, emotions, and spirit; energy fields become unbalanced as a response to stress; energy fields are constantly interacting; people heal themselves; and the client-practitioner relationship is one of partnership.

Caring and compassion are considered to be essential components in helping people mobilize their resources for self-healing in both the practice of nursing and TCM. A critical attitude on the part of the compassionate nurse, is one of *intent* to help and comfort. Even though outcomes of illness are not primarily in the hands of health care practitioners, as nurses, we must still be willing to do our best. In addition to our valuable technical skills, we must be present in the moment for each of our clients. It means grounding and centering one's self before we enter into a healing relationship with another person. It means keeping our focus on the other person rather than being distracted by our personal internal dialogue. All levels of nursing practice incorporate principles of caring as a guiding focus for nursing intervention. Some nurses will want to continue their education through in-depth study of principles and practices of Traditional Chinese Medicine. Requirements and programs of study can be obtained from the Council of Colleges of Acupuncture and Oriental Medicine, the addresses of which are found in the Resources section.

Before we can care for our clients, we must first learn to value and care for ourselves. Drawing from TCM, self-care means seeking ways to establish and maintain balance and harmony in our lives. Exercise programs might include vigorous exercise such as aerobics, running, or swimming; moderate exercise such as dancing or walking; or gentle movement exercise such as qigong, T'ai Chi, or yoga. Touching and being touched are important to our sense of well-being. Self-massage, partner massage, and professional therapeutic massage contribute to a sense of balance and connection with others. Meditation, prayer, and worship are spiritual aspects of self-care. Breath work is both a physical way to increase relaxation and decrease stress and a spiritual way to connect with the universe.

Diet is another area where TCM can provide us with some practical guidelines. North Americans seem to have diets of extremes with fluctuation between overindulgence in food and starvation diets. It is often an all-or-none attitude that has neglected the principle of balance. Limiting the diet to a few fruits and vegetables may be as harmful as a steady diet of hamburgers. In TCM it is believed that illness can be avoided by eating a varied diet as much as possible. For example, avoiding a cold or hot imbalance is accomplished by eating a minimum of seven different fruits and vegetables each day.

For mild, temporary illnesses one might use a number of diet remedies. The cold type of the common cold and flu previously described as characterized by low-grade fever, no sweating, headache, muscle aches, stuffy nose, and a cough with clear white phlegm is treated with warming foods such as garlic, ginger, chives, pepper, pumpkin, apple, onion, and lamb. The hot type of the common cold and flu with its symptoms of high fever, sweating, headache, dry or sore throat, thirst, nasal congestion, and sticky or yellow mucus responds to cooling foods such as watermelon, eggplant, banana, plums, tomato, and tofu. The cold type of low back pain characterized by coldness and severe pain in the lower back that gradually worsens over time, is not relieved by lying down, and is aggravated by rainy days is treated with hot foods including garlic, chicken, apple, yam, celery, onion, peach, and mustard greens. The hot type of back pain that includes symptoms such as soreness of the lower back that is relieved by lying down, weakness of the legs, and frequent relapses is treated with cooling foods such as peanuts, sesame, soybeans, beef, pineapple, and grapes.

Like many other forms of alternative therapies, TCM regards breath as an important function of life. Restrictions in breathing lead to dysfunction and disease. Forming healthy breathing habits can counter stress and help balance body, mind, emotions, and spirit. See the box: Try This: Relaxation for some suggestions you can easily incorporate into your daily life.

TRY THIS: *Relaxation*

Throughout the day one may find hundreds of opportunities to integrate some deep breathing, relaxation, self-massage, and gentle movement techniques into usual activities. Try this:

- You are sitting at a stoplight. Take a deep breath.
- You are just about to fall asleep or have just awakened. Breathe deeply and allow your whole body to become completely relaxed.
- You are in the shower washing your hair. As you apply shampoo, massage your scalp vigorously; rub your ears, relax, take several deep breaths.
- As you apply lotion or oil to your body following your bath, do so with the intent of relaxing each muscle group as you gently massage your entire body.
- You are watching television. During each commercial break, massage your hands, feet, and ears. Breathe deeply and relax.
- You are vacuuming the house. Relax your shoulders, breathe deeply, and coordinate your movements with your breathing.
- You are about to enter a patient's room. Stop, breathe deeply, relax, and enter with an intent to help and heal.

Source: Jahnke, *The Healer Within* (San Francisco: HarperSanFrancisco, 1997).

REFERENCES

AAOM, Philosophy Statement. 1991. Catasauqua, PA: American Association of Oriental Medicine.

Alternative Medicine: Expanding Medical Horizons. 1994. A report to the National Institutes of Health on Alternative Medical Systems and Practices in the United States. U.S. Government Printing Office. Washington, DC.

BEGLEY, S. S. (1994). Tibetan Buddist medicine: A transcultural nursing experience. *J Holistic Nurs.* 12(3): 323–342.

ERGIL, K. V. 1996. China's traditional medicine. In M. S. MICOZZI, ed. *Fundamentals of Complementary and Alternative Medicine.* New York: Churchill Livingstone, 185–223.

JAHNKE, R. 1997. *The Healer Within.* San Francisco: HarperSanFrancisco.

JOHNSTONE, H., J. MARCINAK, M. LUCKETT, and J. SCOTT. 1994. An evaluation of the treatment effectiveness of the Chicago Health Outreach Acupuncture Clinic. *J Holistic Nurs.* 12(2): 171–183.

LAGATREE, K. M. 1996. *Feng Shui.* New York: Villard.

LONGO, A. and S. NEWHOUSE. 1984. Chinese medicine and women's health. In: K. WEISS, ed. *Women's Health Care: A Guide to Alternatives.* Reston, VA: Reston Publishing, 162–181.

MONTE, T. 1997. *The Complete Guide to Natural Healing.* New York: Perigee.

PORKERT, M. 1979. Chinese medicine: A traditional healing science. In: D. S. SOBEL, ed. *Ways of Health: Holistic Approaches to Ancient and Contemporary Medicine.* New York: Harcourt Brace Jovanovich, 147–172.

SCHWARTZ, C. 1996. *Four Paws, Five Directions.* Berkeley, CA: Celestial Arts.

WEIL, A. 1995. *Spontaneous Healing.* New York: Alfred A. Knopf.

WENSEL, L. 1984. Acupuncture for women's health. In K. WEISS, ed. *Women's Health Care: A Guide to Alternatives.* Reston, VA: Reston Publishing, 182–194.

ZHANG, Z. January–February, 1998. Do-it-yourself Chinese medicine. *Natural Health.* 90–93, 164–166.

RESOURCES

Council of Colleges of Acupuncture and Oriental Medicine
1010 Wayne Avenue
Ste. 1270
Silver Spring, MD 20910
301-608-9175

Guidebook provides a detailed description of all candidate and accredited schools in the United States.

Academy of Chinese Culture and Health Science
1601 Clay Street
Oakland, CA 94612
510-763-7787
www.acchs.edu
e-mail: acchs@best.com

American Academy of Medical Acupuncture
800-521-2262

American Association of Oriental Medicine
433 Front Street
Catasauqua, PA 18032
610-266-1433

American Foundation of Traditional Chinese Medicine
505 Beach Street
San Franciso, CA 94133
415-776-0502

Chinese Journal of Integrated Traditional and Western Medicine
English edition subscription: Relaxing Natural Health Inc.
19 Warwick Road
Watertown, MA 02172
www.nihao.com/cjim

Herbs
www.cathayherbal.com/library

4 Ayurvedic Medicine

The relationship between the body and the mind is so intimate that, if either of them get out of order, the whole system would suffer.

Ghandi

The doctor of the future will give no medicine but will interest his patients in the care of the human frame, in proper diet, and in the cause and prevention of disease.

Thomas A. Edison

BACKGROUND

Ayurveda, one of the oldest medical systems in the world, has been practiced for 4,000 years in India. It is a holistic and sophisticated system encompassing balance of body, mind, and spirit as well as balance between people, their environments, and the larger cosmos. *Ayurveda* is a Sanskrit word derived from two roots—*ayur*, which means life, and *veda,* or knowledge—and translates literally to the science of life. Ayurveda has been adapted by Hindu, Buddhist, and other religious groups and is undergoing a renaissance both in India and throughout the West.

Ayurveda is an intricate system with a tradition of integrating that which is useful from other systems. This ancient system has adapted to modern science and technology, including biomedical science and quantum physics. This blending of Ayurveda and conventional medicine has proved completely compatible (Chopra, 1991; Zysk, 1996).

CONCEPTS

Ayurveda asserts a fundamental connection between the microcosm and macrocosm. People are a creation of the cosmos and as such are minute representations of the universe, containing within them everything that makes up the surrounding world. One must understand the world in order to understand people and, conversely, understand people in order to understand the world. Ayurveda emphasizes the interdependence of the health of the individual and the quality of societal life. Therefore, measures to ensure the collective health of society, such as pollution control and appropriate living conditions, are supported (*Alternative Medicine,* 1994; Zysk, 1996).

Five Elements

Ayurveda views nature and people as made up of five elements or qualities. These elements are earth, water, fire, air, and space and contain both matter and energy. As they interact, they give rise to all that exists.The earth element is dense, heavy, and hard. In the human body, all solid structures and compact tissues are derived from the earth element. The water element is liquid and soft and exists in many forms in the body such as plasma, cytoplasm, saliva, nasal secretion, eye secretion, and cerebrospinal fluid. The fire element is hot and light and is believed to regulate body temperature as well as being responsible for digestion, absorption, and assimilation. The solar plexus is the seat of fire in the body. Fire manifests in the brain as the gray matter which allows one to recognize, appreciate, and comprehend the world. The air element is cold, mobile, and rough and in the cosmos is the magnetic field responsible for the movement of the earth, wind, and water. In the body, the air element governs cellular function, the movement of breath, and movements of the intestines. Thought, desire, and will are also governed by the air principle. The space element is clear and subtle and makes up most of our bodies. Space plays a unique role because it allows the existence of sound, which needs space in order to travel. Sound includes not only audible sound like music but subtler vibrations that resonate in our bodies (Chopra, 1991; Vanloon, 1997).

People are a composite of these five elements, which combine in various ways to govern mind, body, and spirit. Ayurveda sees the body as doshas (vital energies), dhatus (tissues), and malas (waste products). It is the dosha's job to assist with the creation of all the various tissues of the body and to remove any unnecessary waste products from the body.

Doshas

Doshas are both structures and energy and are the mediators between body tissues, wastes, and the environment and are responsible for all physiological and psychological processes. The Sanskrit names for the three doshas are Vata, Pitta, and Kapha. As the driver or mover of the entire body, the *Vata* dosha is the most important. It is composed of the elements of air and space and is involved with all elimination, physical and mental movement, and nervous function. If Vata becomes imbalanced, it can cause the other two doshas to become imbalanced. The *Pitta* dosha is composed of the elements fire and water, governs enzymes and hormones, and is responsible for digestion, body temperature, hunger, thirst, sight, complexion, courage, and mental activity. The *Kapha* dosha, composed of the elements of earth and water, is the heaviest of the three doshas. It provides the structure, strength, and stability that the body needs. It is also responsible for lubrication, sexual power, and fertility. Figure 4.1 illustrates the connections between the elements and the doshas.

Body Types

Vata, Pitta, and Kapha are present in every cell, tissue, and organ, but each person is made up of unique ratios of the three doshas. This individual constitution is determined by genetics, diet, lifestyle, and emotions. According to Ayurveda, the ten body types are:

- Single-dosha types: One dosha is predominant
  Vata
  Pitta
  Kapha
- Two-dosha types: One dosha is predominant with a strong secondary dosha
  Vata-Pitta, Pitta-Vata
  Pitta-Kapha, Kapha-Pitta
  Kapha-Vata, Vata-Kapha
- Three-dosha type: All three doshas are in equal proportions
  Vata-Pitta-Kapha

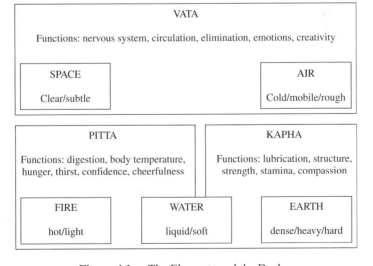

Figure 4.1: The Elements and the Doshas

Knowing one's body type is the key to balancing one's life in the way that nature intended. This balance goes beyond physical and mental health and includes personal relationships, work satisfaction, spiritual growth, and social harmony. As a general rule, the strongest dosha in one's constitution has the greatest tendency to increase, making people most susceptible to illnesses associated with an increase of that dosha (Morrison, 1995).

The basic pattern of the Vata type is "changeable." Vata people are unpredictable and often start things without finishing them. Stress usually leads to anxiety or fear. They are responsive to sound and touch and dislike loud noise. Balanced Vata people are happy, enthusiastic, and energetic. When out of balance they have a tendency to be impulsive. The characteristics of the Vata body type include:

- light, thin build
- thin, dry skin
- dark, coarse, curly hair
- irregular hunger and digestion
- difficulty putting on weight
- light, interrupted sleep
- tendency toward constipation
- aversion to cold weather, craves warmth
- bursts of mental and physical energy
- performs activity quickly
- quick to grasp new information, also quick to forget
- tendency for worry, anxiety, fearfulness
- excitability, changing moods
- enthusiasm, vivaciousness
- fast talking
- illnesses: degenerative, related to being underweight, or those interfering with movement

The basic pattern of the Pitta type is "intense." Pitta people are ambitious, outspoken, bold, orderly, and efficient. They tend to respond to the world visually and enjoy being surrounded by fine objects. Balanced Pitta people are sweet, joyous, and confident. Other characteristics of the Pitta type include:

- medium build
- fair, soft, warm skin
- fine, soft, blond, light brown or red hair

- sharp hunger and thirst, strong digestion
- cannot skip meals
- no problem gaining or losing weight
- aversion to hot weather, craves coolness
- moderate strength and endurance
- sleep is sound but short
- speech is sharp, clear, precise
- sharp intellect, good, quick memory
- enterprising character, likes challenges
- busy lifestyle, achiever
- tendency toward anger, irritability under stress, judgmental
- illnesses: inflammation, bleeding

The basic pattern of the Kapha type is "relaxed." Kapha people are stable, steady people who have a happy, tranquil view of the world. They are graceful people who wake up slowly, eat slowly, and speak slowly. They respond to the world through taste and smell and tend to place a great deal of importance on food. Other characteristics of the Kapha type include:

- solid, powerful build
- thick, pale, cold skin
- thick, wavy, lusterous hair
- tendency to obesity, hard to lose weight
- slow digestion, mild hunger
- sleep is heavy and for long period of time
- oily, smooth skin
- aversion to cold, damp weather
- steady energy, great strength and endurance
- graceful in action
- slow to grasp new information, good retentive memory
- good organizer
- affectionate, tolerant, forgiving
- tendency to be greedy and possessive
- tendency to be complacent
- speech is slow, may be labored
- illnesses: swellings, tumors, those related to overweight

Few people are single-dosha types. Most are two-dosha types, with one dosha predominant but not extreme. The dominant dosha gives people their primary reactions to the world, which are then moderated by the second dosha. Those with the two doshas of Vata-Pitta type are quick-moving, friendly, and talkative with a sharp intellect. They are not as unpredictable or irregular as the single Vata type. They enjoy challenges but stress makes them tense and hard-driven. People who have a combination of Pitta and Kapha types are stable personalities but have a tendency toward anger and criticism. They have steady energy and good stamina but are less motivated to be active. Those whose doshas are the Kapha and Vata type may have a hard time identifying themselves since the Vata and Kapha tend to be opposites. Usually they have a thin body type but with a relaxed, easygoing manner. They tend to procrastinate but can be quick and efficient when necessary. The three-dosha type tends to have good immunity, lifelong good health, and longevity (Chopra, 1991; Zysk, 1996).

Tissues/Dhatus

The seven dhatus or tissues are the structures of the body, are responsible for nourishment, and must be retained for health. They are *rasa* (plasma), *rakta* (blood cells), *mamsa* (muscle), *meda* (adipose), *asthi* (bone), *majja* (bone marrow), and *shukra* (reproductive tissue). In general, Ayurveda practitioners work to keep these tissues intact and healthy (Morningstar, 1997).

Waste Products/Malas

The malas, or wastes, are the nonretainable substances within the body. Urine, feces, and sweat, for example, need to be released and eliminated as the body rids itself of toxins. Excreting the malas cleanses, thus people are cautioned against inhibiting the body's natural functions, including sneezing, yawning, burping, urinating, defecating, and passing gases. Vata is the dosha that causes these urges, and suppression of them disturbs Vata. Ayurveda encourages expression of these urges in a way that is not offensive to other people (Morningstar, 1997).

Energy/Prana

Prana, which the Chinese call qi, in Sanskrit means "primary energy," sometimes translated as "breath" or "vital force." Prana is not only the basic life force, it is the original creative power. Prana has many levels of meaning, from the physical breath to the energy of consciousness. The five pranas are categorized according to movement, direction, and body region. The navel is considered the pranic center of the physical body. *Prana vayu,* forward-moving air, moves inward and regulates the intake of substances into the body. This prana moves energy from the head down to the navel. It is the basic energy that drives us in life. *Apana vayu,* air that moves away, moves downward and directs all forms of elimination and reproduction. It controls the movement of energy from the navel down to the root chakra at the base of the spine. *Udana vayu,* upward moving air, brings about the transformations of life energy. It governs the growth of the body and the release of positive energy. This prana moves energy from the navel up to the head. *Samana vayu,* balancing air, moves from the periphery to the center and moves energy from the entire body back to the navel. It aids in all types of digestion—food, oxygen, and emotional and mental experiences. *Vyana vayu,* outward moving air, moves from the center to the periphery and regulates energy out from the navel through the entire body. It directs the circulation of nutrients throughout the body (Frawley, 1997).

VIEW OF HEALTH AND ILLNESS

When the doshas are balanced, individuals experience health on all levels: mental, emotional, physical, and spiritual. It is much more than the mere absence of disease. Mentally healthy people have good memory, comprehension, intelligence, and reasoning ability. Emotionally healthy people experience evenly balanced emotional states and a sense of well-being or happiness. Physically healthy people have abundant energy with proper functioning of the senses, digestion, and elimination. From a spiritual perspective, healthy people have a sense of aliveness and richness in life, are developing in the direction of their full potential, and are in good relationship with themselves, other people, and the larger cosmos.

Balancing one's doshas does not mean trying to achieve an equal portion of Vata, Pitta, and Kapha. One cannot change the ratio of doshas that are present from conception. Health is the balance of each dosha that is right for that particular individual. Doshas, however, are responsive to people's habits, such as diet, exercise, and daily routines, which can either deplete or increase the doshas. While both states of imbalance lead to ill-health or disease, increased doshas are more problematic than decreased doshas.

Imbalance in the doshas is the first sign that mind, body, and spirit are not perfectly coordinated. One type, called natural imbalance, is due to time and age. Natural imbalances are typically mild and normally do not cause problems. Each dosha becomes more predominant during certain times of day, as energy moves through six cycles in each 24-hour period: Veta predominates from 2 to 6, day and night; Kapha during the hours of 6 to 10; and Pitta from 10 until 2. Each dosha also predominates during particular seasons and stages of life. Kapha is predominate during childhood and during the spring season, Pitta during summer and middle age, and Vata during fall and the latter part of one's life.

Unnatural balances of the doshas can be caused by a variety of factors, each of which falls into one of three broad categories of disease. Adhyatmika diseases originate within the body and include hereditary and congenital diseases. Adhibhautika diseases originate outside the body and include trauma, bacteria, and viruses. Adhidaivika diseases originate from supernatural sources, including those diseases that are otherwise unexplainable, such as illnesses originating from seasonal changes, divine sources, planetary influences, and curses (Zysk, 1996). While some of these causes are beyond individual control, lifestyle and diet are within one's control. Preventing disease and improving overall health depends on the recognition of dosha imbalance and an understanding of the factors that increase and decrease each of the doshas.

Imbalanced Vata shows up as rough skin, weight loss, anxiety, restlessness, insomnia, decreased strength, constipation, arthritis, hypertension, rheumatic disorder, and cardiac arrhythmia. Pitta imbalance includes a yellowish complexion, excessive body heat, insufficient sleep, weak digestion, inflammation, inflammatory bowel disease, skin disease, heartburn, and peptic ulcer. Kapha imbalance presents as a pale complexion, coldness, lethargy, excessive sleep, depression, sinusitis, respiratory disease, asthma, and excessive weight gain (Zysk, 1996).

A number of factors aggravate or increase each of the doshas. Factors increasing Vata are excessive exercise, wakefulness, falling, cold, late autumn and winter, fear or grief, agitation or anger, fasting, and pungent, astringent, bitter foods. Factors increasing Pitta are anger, fasting, strong sunshine, midsummer and early autumn, and pungent, sour, or salty food. Kapha is increased by factors such as sleeping during the daytime, spring and early summer, heavy food, mild products, sugar, and sweet, sour, or salty foods (Zysk, 1996).

DIAGNOSTIC METHODS

The first question asked is not "What disease does this person have?" but "Who is this person?" The complete process of diagnosis takes into account physical, mental, and spiritual components integrated with the social and environmental worlds in which the person lives. In addition to using x-rays or other biomedical diagnostic tools, Ayurvedic practitioners diagnose by observing people, touching them, taking pulses, and interviewing them.

Pulse Diagnosis

Pulse diagnosis is a highly specialized skill that requires great sensitivity. The process involves placing the index, middle, and ring fingers of the right hand on the radial arteries of the right hand of men and the left hand of women. The general feel of the pulse is related to body type. A Vata pulse, felt by the index finger, is irregular or wavering, resembling the movment of a snake. A Pitta pulse, felt at the middle finger, feels forceful and throbbing, resembling the movement of a frog. A Kapha pulse, felt at the ring finger, is said to be gliding, resembling the movement of a swan. A three-dosha pulse resembles the movement of a woodpecker. This basic form of pulse reading gives the practitioner a vital clue to the person's body type. Pulse diagnosis is remarkably comprehensive. Experienced physicians cannot only diagnose present diseases but can also tell what diseases the person has experienced in the past and which are likely to develop in the future (Chopra, 1991; Zysk, 1996).

Tongue Diagnosis

Tongue diagnosis can also reveal the functional status of internal organs. A healthy tongue should be pink, clear, and shiny. A discoloration and/or sensitivity of a particular area of the tongue indicates dosha dysfunction. Kapha imbalance is evidenced by a whitish tongue, Pitta imbalance a yellow-green tongue, and Vata imbalance a brown to black tongue (Lad, 1998).

Urine Diagnosis

Ayurvedic practitioners do urine examinations as another way to understand dosha imbalances. A midstream specimen is collected first thing in the morning. Healthy urine should be clear without much foam. Kapha imbalance gives the urine a cloudy appearance, Pitta imbalance imparts a dark yellow color, and pale yellow and oily urine indicates a Vata imbalance. The practitioner also puts a few drops of sesame oil in the urine and examines it in the sunlight. The shape of the drops signifies which dosha is imbalanced: a snake-like shape with wave movement indicates Vata, an umbrella shape with multiple colors, Pitta, and a pearl shape, Kapha. The movement of the oil in the urine indicates the prognosis of the disease. If the drop spreads immediately, the illness is probably easy to cure. If the oil drops to the middle of the urine sample, the illness is more difficult to cure. If the oil sinks to the bottom, the illness may be impossible to cure (Lad, 1998; Zysk, 1996).

Body Observation

The practitioner carefully examines the skin, nails, and lips. Cool, hot, rough or dry skin indicate imbalance. Imbalance can be visualized in the nails by longitudinal striations, bumps, or a parrot beak at the end of the nail. Dry, rough lips or inflammatory patches on the lips are another sign of imbalance

Coldness, dryness, roughness, and cracking indicate Vata imbalance. Hotness and redness indicate Pitta imbalance. Kapha imbalance is indicated by wetness, whiteness, and coldness (Zysk, 1996).

TREATMENT

Specific lifestyle interventions are a major preventive and therapeutic approach in Ayurveda. Each person is prescribed an individualized diet and exercise program depending on dosha type and the nature of the underlying dosha imbalance. Herbal preparations are added to the diet for preventive or regenerative purposes as well as for the treatment of specific disorders. Yoga, breathing exercises, and meditative techniques are also prescribed by the practitioner (*Alternative Medicine,* 1994).

Nutrition

In Ayurveda, a balanced diet is different from the Western perspective of a balanced diet derived from the basic food groups of meat, dairy, fruit, grains, and vegetables. Ayurveda recognizes six tastes: sweet, sour, salty, pungent, bitter, and astringent. A balanced Ayurveda diet must contain all six tastes at every meal but in different proportions depending on dosha type. The word "taste" includes not only the perceptions on the tongue but also the immediate effect of the substances within the body. Each of the six tastes is derived from two of the five elements as illustrated in Figure 4.2. Sour, salty, and pungent have the fire element and so increase body temperature, dilate body channels, and allow energy and toxins to flow out from the body. Sweet, bitter, and astringent have no fire and thus are cooling, promoting relaxation. Sweet, sour, and salty have the water element and soften tissues, lubricate mucus membranes, and increase water retention (Vanloon, 1997).

Ayurveda describes the actions of each of the six tastes. *Sweet* promotes the vitality of body tissues, soothes the five senses, and adds bulk and firmness. Used to excess, sweet creates obesity, weak digestion, and a tendency to excessive sleep and heaviness. *Sour* improves the taste of food, increases digestion, and awakens the mind. In excess, sour wastes muscles and causes a buildup of toxins in the blood. *Salty* promotes digestion, moisturizes the body, softens all organs and acts as a laxative and sedative. In excess, salty causes stagnation of blood, wasting of the muscles, wrinkling of the skin, and digestive hyperacidity. *Pungent* cleanses the mouth, opens the vessels, improves blood flow, and cures disorders of excess fluid in the body. In excess, pungent causes fatigue, emaciation, dizziness, and thirst. *Bitter,* though it does not taste good in itself, restores the sense of taste, detoxifies, relieves thirst, and is anti-

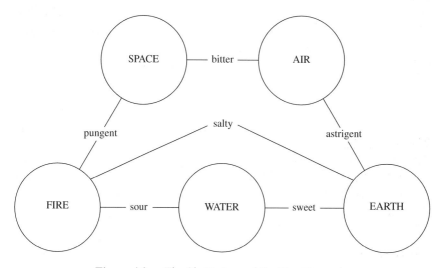

Figure 4.2:   The Six Tastes and the Five Elements

bacterial, germicidal, and antipyretic. In excess, bitter causes wasting away of the tissues, weakness, and dryness. *Astringent* is drying, firming, and sedating. It stops bleeding and aids in healing of wounds. In excess, astrigent causes premature aging, constipation, retention of wastes, spasms, convulsions, and weakens vitality (Vanloon, 1997).

Three pairs of gunas or qualities are inherent in food: heavy or light, oily or dry, and heating or cooling. Examples are (Chopra, 1991):

- Heavy: wheat, beef, cheese
- Light: barley, chicken, skim milk
- Oily: milk, soybeans, coconut
- Dry: honey, lentils, cabbage
- Heating: pepper, honey, eggs
- Cooling: mint, sugar, milk

It is not necessary to memorize which foods reduce which doshas as there are any number of books offering long lists of foods matched to the dosha, taste, and guna. Many people seem to know naturally what their bodies need for balance. See Box 4.1 for the relationship between the doshas, tastes, and gunas. To counter an excess of Vata, diet recommendations consist of warm food with moderately heavy textures, salt, sour, and sweet tastes, and added oil. Examples of foods to include are asparagus, carrots, green beans, avocados, bananas, melons, rice, wheat, chicken, seafood, chickpeas, and tofu.

Box 4.1: Foods in Relation to Doshas

Vata

Balances		Aggravates	
Salt	Hot	Pungent	Light
Sour	Oily	Bitter	Dry
Sweet	Heavy	Astringent	Cold

Pitta

Balances		Aggravates	
Bitter	Heavy	Pungent	Hot
Sweet	Cold	Sour	Light
Astringent	Dry	Salty	Oily

Kapha

Balances		Aggravates	
Pungent	Light	Sweet	Heavy
Bitter	Dry	Sour	Oily
Astringent	Hot	Salty	Cold

Sources: Ayurvedic Foundations, 1996; Chopra, 1991; Zysk, 1996

To counter an excess of Pitta, diet recommendations are for cool or warm (but not hot) foods with moderately heavy textures and bitter, sweet, and astringent tastes. Examples of foods to include are broccoli, cabbage, lettuce, apples, grapes, raisins, barley, oats, ice cream, chicken, shrimp, chickpeas, and tofu. Coconut, olive, and soy oil are acceptable. For an excess of Kapha, diet recommendations include warm, light food, cooked without much water, pungent, bitter, and astringent tastes, and a minimun of butter and oil. Examples of foods to include are cauliflower, celery, leafy green vegetables, apricots, pears, dried fruits in general, barley, corn, rye, skim milk, chicken, shrimp, sunflower seeds, and raw honey (Chopra, 1991).

Every food can be characterized by taste and guna. In addition to a balanced diet in terms of fats, carbohydrates, and proteins, people need variety in salty, sour, sweet, pungent, bitter, and astringent foods. The goal of diet management is to avoid aggravating any of the doshas and keep them calm and balanced.

Herbs

In Ayuveda, natural medicines are primarily herbal but may include animal and mineral ingredients, and even powdered gemstones. Many thousands of herbs are prescribed by practitioners. Like food, herbs are classified according to the six tastes. Herbs, however, are more potent and specific in their action than is food. Some herbs, used for preventive and regenerative purposes, are readily available. The use of herbs for treating disease must be medically supervised. As in Traditional Chinese Medicine, the entire plant is used. It is believed that the plant contains other chemicals that buffer the active ingredient thus reducing possible side effects (Chopra, 1991).

Like foods, herbs balance doshas. Vata balancing herbs include ginseng, licorice, Indian Penny wort, Bala, and Sitopladi. Aloe vera, comfrey root, Indian Gooseberry, and saffron are used to balance Pitta, while elecampane, honey, and sitopladi balance Kapha. Herbs usually take longer to work than Western medications prescribed by practitioners. Historically, Ayurvedic herbs have had little exposure outside India but are now becoming more familiar with the rapid explosion of herbal medicine in North America. Following are a few of the more common herbs found in health food stores. Sitopladi is a very good herbal formula for colds and flu. Indian Penny wort (brahmi) enhances a person's ability to focus mentally and learn new material. Guggulu is a powerful purifying agent, well known for lowering of blood cholesterol levels. Shilajit, with its antispasmodic qualities, is effective in acute and chronic respiratory illnesses. Bala, or Indian Country Mallow, is helpful in all types of nervous system disorders and certain types of heart disease. These few examples of herbs give one an idea of how they are used as natural body medicines. Chapter 6 presents herbs in more detail. Numerous books on the market and various web sites describe the use of herbs in alternative medicine.

Exercise

According to Ayurveda, exercise should conform to one's dosha type. Kapha people can perform moderately heavy exercise such as aerobics, running, dancing, and weight training. Because of their physical strength, Kaphas excel at endurance sports. Pitta people, who have more drive than endurance and an intense competitive spirit, should have a moderate amount of exercise. Brisk walking or jogging, hiking, swimming, and skiing are appropriate. People with a Vata dosha might enjoy jogging, but exercises like stretching, yoga, and T'ai Chi are better choices. They have bursts of energy but tire quickly and may push themselves past their limits. Walking is probably the best exercise for all people as it calms all dosha types. Ayurveda recommends a brisk half-hour walk every day (Chopra, 1991; Lad, 1998).

For people over the age of 80 or under 10 as well as those people who have serious Vata and Pitta imbalance, exercise should be very gentle. Exercise should always leave a person ready for work as opposed to exercise being work itself. Several other exercise precautions must be noted. One should not engage in exercise sooner than half an hour before and one to two hours after a meal. Exercising in the evening is discouraged because it is better for the body to slow down and prepare for sleep. Exercise is discouraged in the wind or cold since heavy breathing of cold, damp air is unhealthy for the respiratory tract. Also discouraged is exercise during the intense heat of the day, since environmental heat causes an even greater rise in body temperature.

The key to exercise is moderation and regularity. Ayurveda suggests that all exercise should be done at one-half of one's capacity. That means working out just until sweat appears on the forehead, under the arms, and along the spinal column. This amount of exercise improves digestion, prevents constipation, improves circulation, stimulates metabolism, regulates body temperature, and maintains body weight. Exercise keeps one's senses and mind alert and attentive as well as being effective in inducing relaxation and sleep. Overexercise, as indicated by panting and heavy sweating, may cause dehydration, muscle aches, breathlessness, and even chest pain. It is believed that overexercise eventually contributes to arthritis, sciatica, or heart conditions (Lad, 1998).

Yoga, developed in the Ayurvedic tradition, is one of the most effective forms of exercise for the body as well as nourishment for the mind and spirit. Hatha yoga, the most familar form of yoga in North America, is a combination of body positions, breathing exercises, and mental focus on the here-and-now. Stretching helps relax and tone the muscles, improves circulation, improves concentration, and helps one regain energy. Yoga is increasingly recognized for maintaining general health as well as helping people to manage chronic disorders such as headaches, insomnia, hypertension, and depression. Further information about yoga is found in chapter 15.

Breathing

Practicing controlled breathing is a valuable technique that leads to a healthier lifestyle. Several techniques can be utilized to relax the mind and body. Simple breathing helps people become aware of their breath and often relieves tension. Simple breathing involves closing the eyes and observing the breath, becoming more aware of its pattern and changes. Slow, easy breathing is continued for several minutes until a sense of relaxation is achieved. Alternate nostril breathing, Pranayama, is another technique which can ease difficulty in breathing by making the respiratory rhythm more regular, which in turn soothes the entire nervous system. Pranayama is helpful prior to meditation because it focuses attention inward. Pranayama is performed while seated with the eyes closed. Figure 4.3 illustrates the position. The index and middle fingers of the right hand are placed in between the eyebrows.The thumb closes the right nostril while the person breathes in through the left nostril. The left nostril is then closed with the ring finger and the right nostril is opened for the out breath and the next in breath. The right nostril is then closed and the out breath occurs through the left nostril. After doing a couple of rounds, breathing naturally gets deeper and smoother.

Meditation

An important part of daily life in Ayurveda, meditation is considered a powerful tool to help maintain health. Meditation is a moment-to-moment awareness that is cleansing to the body, mind, and spirit. It is finding the quiet in the mind. As the mind is brought into a silent and receptive state, new energy comes into being, which is conducive to a state of health and peace. Further information about meditation is found in chapter 16.

Massage

Marma therapy is a massage technique focusing on 107 sensitive points, called marmas, located on the skin. These points are similar to the acupuncture points called hsueh in Traditional Chinese Medicine. Marma therapy predates the Chinese approach and is likely the parent to acupuncture and acupressure. Marmas are activated through various methods. One is through yoga movements which gently stretch specific marma points. Warm oil dripped on the center of the forehead on a major marma point can be profoundly soothing. A daily self-massage with oil can reach all the marmas on the skin. Once taught, these techniques can be practiced at home.

Aromatherapy

Aromatherapy is based on olfactory stimuli used to help balance the doshas as each responds to specific signals. Specialized olfactory cells provide instant connnection of odors with the brain. The hypothalamus responds through regulation of bodily functions, the limbic system responds with emotions, and the hippocampus responds with memories, which explains how smells can elicit memories so vividly. In general, Vata is balanced with warm, sweet, and sour aromas such as basil, orange, rose geranium, clove, and other spices. Pitta is balanced by sweet, cool aromas like rose, mint, cinnamon, sandalwood, and jasmine. Kapha is balanced by warm aromas with spicy overtones such as juniper, eucalyptus, camphor, and clove. People whose doshas are out of balance are given specific oils to restore dosha balance. Aromatherapy may be used at

Figure 4.3:   Pranayama/Controlled Breathing

any time but is often prescribed at night as it helps induce sleep (Chopra, 1991). Aromatherapy is discussed further in chapter 9.

Music

India has a long tradition of merging music and medicine. Unlike most Western music in which the notes are distinct, the tones tend to blend together, creating a soothing, unifying sound. As with taste and smell, doshas can be balanced with certain tones and rhythms. The three doshas peak at different times of the day and traditional Indian music smooths the process of these transitions. An example of a rough transition is the inability to fall asleep because one's mind is racing with many thoughts. Ten minutes of music can be used as a gentle wakeup in the morning, after a meal to settle digestion, just before bedtime to aid sleep, and during the recovery period from an illness (Campbell, 1997).

Purification

Panchakarma, or purification therapy, involves five procedures, any or all of which can be chosen based on the person's general condition, the season, and the nature of the disease. The five therapies of Panchakarma are experienced over a period of a week and involve purifying the body through the use of sweating, emetics, purgatives, enemas, and nasal inhalations. Commonly administered by an Ayurvedic physician with the help of a number of assistants, the benefits of Panchakarma are relief from long-standing symptoms, renewed health, and extended longevity (Morningstar, 1997; Zysk, 1996).

RESEARCH

Many Western researchers seem to believe that they look at reality in an objective way. In contrast, Ayurvedic researchers believe that nothing happens in a vacuum. Everything that happens, happens in relationship to what is occuring around it. The principle of research is that knowledge cannot be separated from its context.

In extensive studies of Ayurveda in both Indian and Western medical literature, researchers have demonstrated that:

- students in hatha yoga classes showed improvement in flexibility, strength, equilibrium, and stamina (Jharote, 1973).
- changes in metabolic rate, oxygen exchange, lung capacity, and red and white blood cell counts are associated with general yogic training (Gopal et al., 1974).

- a three-month study in the Netherlands found that 79 percent of people who used Ayurvedic therapies demonstrated improvements with a number of disease conditions including rheumatoid arthritis, asthma, chronic bronchitis, eczema, psoriasis, hypertension, constipation, headaches, chronic sinusitis, and non-insulin-dependent diabetes (Janssen, 1989).
- study participants have demonstrated reductions in blood pressure, cholesterol, and reactions to stress when using Ayurvedic measures (Murphy, 1992; Schneider et al., 1992).
- studies on Ayurvedic herbs have shown them to have a wide range of potentially beneficial effects for the prevention and treatment of certain cancers (Sharma et al., 1990), the treatment of psychiatric disorders (Alexander et al., 1989), and in the treatment of aging (Glaser et al., 1992).
- mechanisms underlying these effects are believed to include free-radical scavenging effects (Fields et al., 1990), immune system modulation, brain neurotransmitter modulation, and hormonal effects (Glaser et al., 1992).

INTEGRATED NURSING PRACTICE

Although most of us have not been educated in Ayurvedic medicine, as nurses we can integrate a number of principles into our professional practice. Ayurveda teaches self-discovery and self-understanding; it encourages people to learn how they maintain their health and how and when they become sick; and it advocates lifestyle changes to maximize one's well-being (Morrison, 1995).

The first step to encourage self-understanding is helping people learn their dosha or body type. See Box 4.2 for the check list and follow these steps to determine dosha type:

- Make a check mark next to the description that best describes how you have been most of your life. If you fall between two descriptions, check both of them.
- Consider the qualities carefully. There are no right or wrong answers. Be honest and check how you are, not how you would like to be.
- Look for lasting trends. For example, if your sleep has been heavy and for long periods of time most of your life but you are now sleeping light and fitfully, the change is likely to be due to imbalance rather than dosha type. Check your usual pattern.

- Notice whether each dosha has some checks because everyone has Vata, Pitta, and Kapha as part of their body type.
- Total the number of checks for each dosha. The dosha with the greatest number should be your body type. If the highest two doshas are close, you are probably a two-dosha type. If all three dosha scores are close, you have a three dosha type.

Determining dosha type allows people to begin to understand how their health is affected by internal and external influences as they consider their unique blend of doshas. As people become more familiar with their bodies, they can observe and experience the effect of what they eat and do each day, how they think and feel, the state of their metabolism, digestion, and elimination, the relationships they engage in, their jobs, and the environment in which they find themselves. Because all of these factors are interdependent, problems in one area can cause problems in other areas.

People's dosha balance can be disrupted in a number of ways. An inappropriate diet and lifestyle for your dosha type will cause a slowly developing

---

Box 4.2: Learn Your Dosha

Vata Type
- light, thin build
- thin, dry skin
- dark, coarse, curly hair
- irregular hunger and digestion
- difficulty putting on weight
- light, interrupted sleep
- tendency toward constipation
- aversion to cold weather, craves warmth
- bursts of mental and physical energy
- performs activity quickly
- quick to grasp new information, also quick to forget
- tendency for worry, anxiety, fearfulness
- excitability, changing moods
- enthusiasm, vivaciousness
- fast talking

Box 4.2: Learn Your Dosha (*continued*)

Pitta Type

- medium build
- fair, soft, warm skin
- fine, soft, blond, light brown or red hair
- sharp hunger and thirst, strong digestion
- cannot skip meals
- no problem gaining or losing weight
- aversion to hot weather, craves coolness
- moderate strength and endurance
- sleep is sound but short
- speech is sharp, clear, precise
- sharp intellect, good, quick memory
- enterprising character, likes challenges
- busy lifestyle, achiever
- tendency toward anger, irritability under stress, judgmental

Kapha Type

- solid, powerful build
- thick, pale, cold skin
- thick, wavy, lusterous hair
- tendency to obesity, hard to lose weight
- slow digestion, mild hunger
- sleep is heavy and for long period of time
- oily, smooth skin
- aversion to cold, damp weather
- steady energy, great strength and endurance
- graceful in action
- slow to grasp new information, good retentive memory
- good organizer
- affectionate, tolerant, forgiving
- tendency to be greedy and possessive
- tendency to be complacent
- speech is slow, may be labored

excess or deficiency in doshas. If you suffer significant trauma, however, the dosha levels can change immediately and dramatically. Dosha imbalance can also occur from an accumulation of toxins or when too many experiences of a particular dosha take place without enough experiences from the other doshas. Once people understand their baseline dosha type, they can assess imbalances which may contribute to disease. Remind people that the strongest dosha in their constitution has the greatest tendency to increase. For example, if you have a Kapha dosha type, you have a natural tendency to those things which have Kapha qualities, thus increasing your Kapha energy. If you have a lifestyle that includes overeating, not exercising, and sleeping excessively, and you have a desk job, your Kapha dosha can become excessive. You may need to consciously add opposite qualities to pacify or balance your Kapha energy such as decrease your food intake, eat more pungent and bitter vegetables and astringent fruits, and increase your exercise (Morrison, 1995).

Achieving balance of the doshas does not happen quickly—people need to work at it consciously. In some cases, lifestyle changes may be difficult, such as the nature of your job, while others may be easier, such as a change in leisure activities. Typically, people find that diet, exercise, and leisure activities are the most amenable to change. For example, television and computers increase Vata through stimulation of the eyes and ears and increase Kapha by the passive nature of these activities. If the television program makes you angry or your computer program will not do what you wish, your Pitta may be stimulated. Limiting the time spent watching television and being selective with programs may help you balance your doshas and move toward a healthier state. Likewise, if you spend a lot of time at your computer, you need to take frequent breaks, move and stretch your body, and rest your eyes (Morrison, 1995).

If your strongest dosha is Vata, you need to develop more regularity in your daily routines such as eating regular meals, having an established bedtime, and slowing down and taking time to think. Because you have a tendency to dry skin, oil your skin regularly. People with Vata doshas are drawn to sensory experiences involving movement, speed, and action, and you may enjoy loud music and computer games. To maintain a healthy balance, make an effort to balance those activities with quiet, creative pursuits such as writing, photography, or painting. Similarly, because you are attracted to vigorous exercise, try to engage in gentle exercise every day. Ayurveda suggests that all exercise be done at one-half of one's capacity. If you know that you are exhausted after a 40-minute aerobic class, then you should do only 20 minutes of the class. People with Vata doshas enjoy spending their vacations sightseeing, touring, and filling their days and nights with many activities and returning home exhausted. A more beneficial vacation would be in a beautiful, sunny, and warm environment where you rest and limit your activities. If you are a Vata type, your clothes are mostly dark shades that may reflect a tendency to become depressed. Bright yellow colors and pastel shades may brighten your mood (Morrison, 1995).

If you are a Pitta type, you need to loosen up on setting and achieving goals and learn to enjoy here-and-now moments. You can learn to achieve your ambitions without pressuring yourself. Your need to organize yourself, and everyone else, must be kept under control lest you become easily frustrated when things do not go as planned. You are stimulated by competitive, mentally challenging situations that may increase your aggression or your determination to win. Learn to use constructive criticism rather than confrontation. Engaging in noncompetitive leisure activities such as gardening may help prevent an excess of Pitta. Vacations in cooler climates and water and winter sports will cool your tendency to be warm. Avoid organizing your vacations in the greatest of detail and try to enjoy whatever happens. Red clothing overstimulates Pitta and may contribute to a more aggressive approach to others. Cool, soft, pale colors are more balancing to the Pitta dosha (Morrison, 1995).

If you are a Kapha type, you need to vary your daily experiences to avoid becoming stuck in a rut. Try to make small changes in routine every day. Get up early and go to bed late to limit your tendency to sleep many hours. Since you may prefer to sit and do nothing, find activities that are mentally and physically stimulating. Kapha is balanced by vigorous exercise but you will most likely have to force yourself. Because you have good stamina, you can exercise for a longer time than people who are Vata or Pitta. You would prefer a vacation lying on a beach doing nothing but soaking up the sun. You will find, however, that sightseeing and touring will be more stimulating and balancing for you. All colors, except greens and dark blues, balance Kapha. You will find that bright, strong colors are exciting and balancing.

Helping people understand their doshas is an ongoing process. As people observe their mind, body, spirit, and relationships, they learn how they respond to different qualities in everyday activities. After determining dosha type, have people review their lifestyle in terms of diet, work, leisure activities, exercise, daily routines, quiet times, sleep, and relationships. Applying the principles of Ayurveda, people can begin making choices about the qualities they wish to incorporate into their lives. Rather than focusing on negatives, what they want to stop doing, have them focus on positives, what they want to start doing. Suggest that they limit their exposure to those qualities they do not want, and enjoy those that will aid their well-being. Change begins with small steps and is a gradual process. Some people will want to seek the advice of an Ayurvedic practitioner to individualize a lifestyle change program. Remind people that their mind and body always strive toward health and that every individual needs time, nurturing, routine, and gentle discipline to achieve a more complete level of well-being (Morrison, 1995).

TRY THIS: *Massage*

Sesame Oil Massage

Use the refined sesame oil sold in health food stores, not the heavy Chinese sesame oil. If you wish, you may use olive oil instead. Warm a quarter cup of oil in the microwave for 10–15 seconds being careful not to overheat it.

Mini-Massage (1–2 minutes)

Use one tablespoon of warm oil and rub it into your scalp. Use small, circular motions with the flat of your hand. Using your palm, massage the forehead from side to side and gently massage your temples using circular motions. Gently rub the outside of the ears. Massage both the front and the back of the neck.

Use a second tablespoon of warm oil and massage both feet using the flat of the hand. Massage each toe with your fingertips. Vigorously massage the soles of your feet. Sit quietly for a few seconds to relax and then shower or bathe as usual.

Full Body Massage (5–10 minutes)

Massage the scalp, ears, and neck with one tablespoon of warm oil as described above.

Using more oil, vigorously massage your arms using long strokes on the long parts and circular motions at the joints.

Adding oil as necessary, massage the chest, stomach, and lower abdomen using gentle circular strokes in a clockwise direction. Massage as much of your back and spine as you can reach.

Massage the legs as you did the arms using vigorous movements

With the remaining bit of oil, massage the feet as described above. Bathe with warm water and mild soap.

Source: Chopra, *Perfect Health* (New York: Harmony Books, 1991).

REFERENCES

ALEXANDER, C. N. et al. 1989. Transcendental meditation, mindfulness, and longevity: An experimental study with the elderly. *J Pers Soc Psychol.* 57: 950–964.

Alternative Medicine: Expanding Medical Horizons. 1994. A report to the National Institutes of Health on Alternative Medical Systems and Practices in the United States. U.S. Government Printing Office. Washington, DC.

Ayurvedic Foundations. 1996. Vata, Pitta, Kapha Pacifying Programs. http://www.ayur.com/dosha/tridosha.html

CAMPBELL, D. 1997. *The Mozart Effect.* New York: Avon Books.

CHOPRA, D. 1991. *Perfect Health.* New York: Harmony Books.

FIELDS, J. Z. et al. 1990. Oxygen free-radical scavenging effects of an anticarcinogenic natural product, Maharishi Amrit Kalash. *The Pharmacologist.* 32: 155.

FRAWLEY, D. October–November, 1997. The secrets of prana. *Yoga International.* 38: 25–29.

GLASER, J. L. et al. 1992. Elevated serum DHEAS levels in practitioners of the transcendental meditation (TM) and TM-Sidhi programs. *J Behav Med.* 15(4): 327–341.

GOPAL, K. S. et al. 1974. Biochemical studies in foreign volunteers practicing hatha yoga. *J Research Indian Med.* 9(3): 1–8.

JANSSEN, GWHM. 1989. The application of Maharishi Ayur-Veda in the treatment of ten chronic diseases: A pilot study. *Nederlands Tijdschrift Voor Integrale Geneeskunde.* 5: 586–594.

JHAROTE, M. L. 1973. Effect of yoga training on physical fitness. *Yoga-Mimamsa.* 15(40): 31–35.

LAD, V. 1998. An Introduction to Ayurveda. http://ayurveda.com/info/factors.html

MORNINGSTAR, A. December–January, 1997. Journey to health. *Yoga International.* 33: 38–43.

MORRISON, J. H. 1995. *The Book of Ayurveda.* New York: Simon & Schuster.

MURPHY, M. 1992. Appendix C, scientific meditation studies. In *The Future of the Body.* Los Angeles: Jeremy Tarcher, 603–611.

SCHNEIDER, R. H. et al. 1992. In search of an optimal behavioral treatment for hypertension. In E. H. JOHNSON, W. D. GENTRY, S. JULIUS (eds.) *Personality, Elevated Blood Pressure, and Hypertension.* Washington DC: Hemisphere Pub. Corp.

SHARMA, H. M. et al. 1990. Antineoplastic properties of Maharishi 4, against DMBA-induced mammary tumors in rats. *J Pharmacology, Biochemistry, and Behavior.* 35: 767–773.

VANLOON, G. October–November, 1997. The six tastes. *Yoga International.* 38: 48–50.

ZYSK, K. 1996. Traditional ayurveda. In M. S. MICOZZI, ed. *Fundamentals of Complementary and Alternative Medicine.* New York: Churchill Livingstone, 233–260.

RESOURCES

Center for Mind Body Medicine (Ayurveda)
1110 Camino del Mar, Suite G
Del Mar, CA 92014
619-794-2425

Maharishi Ayurveda Health Center for Stress Management and Behavioral Medicine
P.O. Box 344
Lancaster, MA 01523
508-365-4549

Shivani Ayurvedic Personal Care Products
P.O. Box 377
Lancaster, MA 01523
800-237-8221

Auromere Ayurvedic Imports
1291 Weber St.
Pomona, CA 91768
909-629-0108

Websites
www.ayurvedic.com
www.yogaclass.com

5 Native American Healing and Curanderismo

Morning Prayer
I thank You for another day. I ask that You give me the strength to walk worthily this day so that when I lie down at night I will not be ashamed.

Evening Prayer
At the end of each day, face west and say: Thank you for all the things that happened today, the good as well as the bad.

For emotional, physical, and mental health
Lie down with your navel toward the Earth and your head to the north, saying: Grandmother Earth, please send your healing energy through this body and bring it back into balance.

To find an answer to a problem
Face east and think about your problem saying: Grandfather Sun, you come each day to dispel the darkness. In that same way I ask you to shed your light so that I may see where to take the next step.

Prayers by Bear Heart,
Native American Shaman

Although each Native American Indian–based healing system is unique, they share a number of characteristics. This chapter presents the commonalities found among tribes. The population of today's Native American tribes is only a fraction of what it was before Europeans invaded this continent. Forty-five percent of all Indians living on reservations live below the poverty level. Native Americans have the highest infant mortality rate of any group in the United States, and life expectancy among Indians on reservations is under fifty years of age. Alcoholism is a significant problem for a variety of reasons both social and genetic. Many customs have been lost forever. Despite these impediments, many of the traditions and ceremonies practiced by Native Americans for centuries are still in evidence today (Bear Heart, 1996).

BACKGROUND

Non-Indian people can learn a great deal from the Native American approach to life and traditional healing. To learn, people must be open to the ancient wisdom and understand it in the context of the entire Indian experience. It is not something to be trivialized by simply purchasing medicine objects and trying them out at home. As one Sioux leader said, "First they took our land, now they want our pipes . . . all the wannabees, these New Agers, come with their crystals and want to buy a medicine bag to carry them around in. If you want to learn our ways, come walk the red road with us, but be silent and listen" (Johnson, 1994, p. 6).

In their earliest encounters, white physicians devalued the skills of Native healers. This association has, in a way, come full circle. Western medicine is now advancing toward a holistic point of view that Native Americans have been practicing for thousands of years. Today, medicine women and men continue with a system that is parallel to conventional medicine. Some people are traditional, meaning that they adhere strictly to the old ways of life and reject any form of biomedicine. Others have acculturated, or adapted to the mainstream culture, and use both Indian medicine and conventional medicine. A third group of Native Americans are assimilated and have virtually abandoned all traditional ways in favor of the dominant culture and utilize only biomedicine (Levin, 1997).

Most tribal people have one or more types of health care specialists that frequently overlap. Some Native healers use herbs, some heal with songs, and some with spiritual rituals. A midwife or a medicine woman or man might focus on natural medicines such as herbs and hands-on techniques but also use prayer and ceremony. Shamans or holy people emphasize spiritual healing but are often also knowledgeable about natural medicines. Kahunas are people, usually of Hawaiian ancestry, who have developed a level of spirituality that joins them with many of the spirit powers allowing direct communication about the healing process (*Alternative Medicine,* 1994; Sun Bear et al., 1989).

Shamans and medicine people are seen as channels the Creator has provided and trained. Some are born into families with medical or ritual skills, while others discover this path through a dream or vision. Selection is based on signs of devotion, wisdom, humility, and honesty. Once called, the individual seeks training, usually by apprenticing to a medicine person for a number of years. All knowledge comes from the Creator, and the elders are charged with the responsibility of keeping knowledge about healing foods, herbs, and medicine and passing it on. Trusted with all secrets, rituals, and legends of their people, Native healers are considered to be inspired individuals with great importance to the tribe. Training is complete when the teacher says it is complete and when the candidate has practiced the skills publicly and with success (*Alternative Medicine,* 1994; Johnson, 1994).

CONCEPTS

Spirituality

Spirituality and medicine are inseparable in Native American tradition. Essentially no distinction is made between religious and medical practices. "Making medicine" is an important part of traditional life. It is how people give thanks to the Spirit who helps, guides, nourishes, and clothes them. Medicine is the constant pipeline to the Creator. In Indian tradition, making medicine is a process for achieving a variety of positive outcomes: a good hunt, plentiful crops, connecting with someone, healing someone, a successful birthing, and so on. Medicine is the way people keep their balance; it provides them with the opportunity to grow in new and more healthy ways (Sun Bear et al., 1989).

Native Americans believe in a singular living God, but also believe that same God may be contacted through many ways, from many cultures. In Native languages, God is given such names as Great Spirit, Creator, Great Being, Great Mystery, Above Being, The One Who Oversees All Things, and He Who Gives Life. The missionaries mistakenly thought that Indian people worshiped trees, eagles, the Pipe, and many other things. What was misinterpreted was the use of these objects as gifts from the Creator, put here to help. Using these gifts is one way to create an atmosphere conducive to addressing the Creator (Bear Heart, 1996).

Gratitude is a central aspect of Native American culture. Every day is a spiritual, sacred day. One morning prayer is, "I thank You for another day. I ask that You give me the strength to walk worthily this day so that when I lie down at night I will not be ashamed" (Bear Heart, 1996, p. 164). Thanks are given to the Great Power who makes all things possible. People give thanks, not only for the good events but also for the bad things that happen throughout the day, because they believe that the more they show their appreciation, the more blessings they will receive.

Native peoples do not own or possess land but rather see themselves as caretakers of the earth for the Great Spirit. The land is considered the Mother since all things come from her body. Animals, birds, trees, and grass all come from Mother Earth and are powerful living beings, just like human beings. When Native people take something from the earth, such as herbs or even a stone, they always give an offering, usually tobacco, in return and say a prayer that the item taken will be used in a good manner (Bear Heart, 1996).

Healing

Medicine women and men see themselves as channels through which the Great Power helps others achieve well-being in mind, body, and spirit. The only healer is the One who created all things. Medicine people consider that they have certain knowledge to put things together to help the sick person heal and that knowledge has to be dispensed in a certain way, often through ritual or ceremony. Healers receive their knowledge through fasting and asking for guidance from Above. During the period of fasting, the Great Being might reveal a chant or the location of a particular herb and give instructions on how to use it for different illnesses (Bear Heart, 1996).

Time is often considered an ally in recovery. With the passage of time, fears and problems sometimes fade. Love is a key element in the healing process. The healer enters into the healing relationship with love and compassion. The two individuals experience a joining or merging as this process unfolds. This merger symbolizes the cementing together of people and the Divine Spirit (Mails, 1988).

Circle

The circle represents the cycles of life which have no beginning, no end, and no time element. The Great Spirit causes everything to be round. The sun, earth, and moon are round. The sky is deep like a bowl. Things that grow from the ground like the stem of a plant or plant roots are round. The circle, symbol of infinity and interconnectedness, is seen in the sweat lodge, the bowl of the Sacred Pipe, the Sacred Hoop, and the Medicine Wheel. In addition, the camp is circular, tepees are circular, and people sit in a circle in all ceremonies. When people come together in a circle, a spirit of oneness and a sense of sacredness comes upon them.

The Medicine Wheel is both an important conceptual scheme and a major ceremonial observance. The Sacred Hoop makes up the circumference with the interior of the circle being divided into four quadrants. Each quadrant represents a direction, a totem, an element, a color, a kingdom, a quality, a season, and a gateway to the individual. The four colors—white, black, yellow, and red—represent the races of all humanity. See Figure 5.1 for an illustration of the Medicine Wheel.

Number Four

The number four is significant to Native American people and is incorporated into their daily lives through prayers, ceremonies, and activities. It is believed to be the number of completeness. Everything that grows from the earth consists

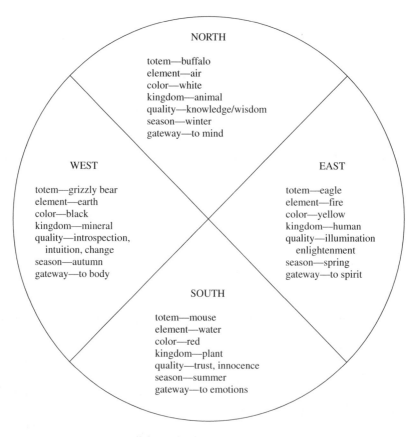

Figure 5.1:   The Medicine Wheel. Source: Meadows, 1991; Milne, 1995.

of four parts: roots, stems, leaves, and fruit. Earth, air, fire, and water are the four elements. Four types of things take breath: those that crawl, those that fly, those that walk on four legs, and those that walk on two legs. There are four directions, four seasons, and four races of people—white, black, yellow, and red.

VIEW OF HEALTH AND ILLNESS

Health is viewed as a balance or harmony of mind and body. The goal is to be in harmony with all things, which means first being in harmony with oneself. Harmony is thought to neutralize problems and help one's life to become beautiful. Good health makes it easier for all people to do their part in the universe, to serve others, and to fulfill their personal life visions.

Life is considered in all of its dualities: winter/summer, cold/hot, day/night, mind/body, spiritual/physical, work/play, etc. Native people believe that the two sides of everything deserve equal attention and that both should be nourished with love. A healthy person who is walking in balance is energized and alert, and in the presence of disease will still feel alive and fulfilled (Mails, 1988).

Traditionally, Native American people lived long, happy, healthy, and balanced lives. They did everything to respect and honor Mother Earth and the Great Spirit. They ate wholesome food and considered all food to be blessed as a gift of life from the Creator. They got up with the sun and went to bed with the moon. Exercise was a natural part of their lives, integrated into daily activities. These good health habits, a sense of joy, and a purpose in life are key factors for living into old age (Sun Bear et al., 1989).

Illness occurs when balance is disrupted. It is believed that most illness begins in the head and people must get rid of ideas which predispose illness. If the mind is negative, the body will be drained, making it more vulnerable. When people open up to the universe, learn what is good for them, and find ways to be happier, they can begin to work toward a longer and healthier life. Many ancient people had ways to get rid of this negativity. The Mayan people of Mexico would stand in a stream of flowing water and talk out all their angers, fears, sorrows, or troubles over the water. The moving water would take all the emotions they poured out of themselves into the current and away from them. The Bear Dance was a way the Indian people of northern California rid themselves of negativity. A man in a bear costume would dance around a circle of people who would use switches to hit him as they spoke about the things in their lives that were bothering them. When the bear had everyone's negativities, he went down into the stream, washing them away. Some Native people of the southwest had dancers armed with swords who went through the village singing, chanting, and rattling, driving out the negative forces as they went. Behind them people came with brooms to sweep away anything that was left over. Most Indian tribes had some way of letting people get rid of negativity so that they could go on and build new positive patterns (Sun Bear et al., 1989).

Dreaming is a powerful way for people to learn what is good for them. Dreams are a personal connection to the upper, spiritual realms. Divine guidance is thought to come through dreams and visions. In a period of illness, people may actually dream the healing. Dreaming is important in the healing practices of medicine women and men since treatment information is often provided through dreams. Dream weavers, dream catchers, or dream nets are special medicine objects that catch the dream and hold it for the person.

DIAGNOSTIC METHODS

Healers must diagnose the source of the problem because they want to treat the cause, not just the effect. They always look at the total person whether they are treating someone for physical illness or emotional problems. They look at the overall picture, determine what is out of balance within the whole, and then pinpoint the trouble spots. Some healers diagnose by going into trance. While in trance, "hand tremblers" pass their shaking hands over the body of the person; when the hands stop trembling, the locale of the illness is found and the cause is usually identified. "Star gazers" also enter trance states to read cause in the stars. "Listeners" do not go into trance but listen to the person's story and on that basis identify the cause of the illness (*Alternative Medicine,* 1994).

TREATMENT

When people fall ill, they often experience anxiety and fear that may incapacitate them. The healer is not so burdened and is able to supply coherence, calmness, and hope. Power flows through the healer to the patient. Healers use medicine objects to assist them, and treatments consist of ceremony, touch, herbs, and sometimes peyote.

Items used to help make medicine are called *medicine objects.* Medicine objects can be anything that relates to the Great Spirit in a sacred way. The medicine bag contains healing objects, which vary in size and number but typically are such things as feathers, claws, bird or animal bones, an assortment of herbs or roots, smudges, or paints. The medicine bag may also contain personal items that represent oneself and personal experiences and are sacred to the individual. Native Americans are protective of their medicine bags. The bags carry a part of themselves and are among their most prized companions. The Medicine Wheel is a sacred circle usually built from stones. It is entered for the purpose of healing, giving thanks, praying, or meditating. The Pipe is one of the most sacred medicine objects and is an instrument of prayer.

The Indian art of healing is ceremonial in nature. Different ceremonies are conducted according to the type of illness or the severity of the person's condition. Healing ceremonies are led by medicine people or holy people. The primary purpose is to allow connection with the Great Healer, since physical health often fails without the aid of spiritual means. A secondary benefit is a cleansing of the body, mind, and spirit. A healing session is never a casual encounter. It is arranged through a formalized procedure after discussion by the patient, family, advisors, and healer. Acceptance by the healer is followed by instructions on preliminary actions which may include fasting, abstinences, prayers, or the preparation of offerings or feasts.

Smudging

Smudging is a cleansing and purifying process using smoke from burning herbs, usually sweet grass, sage, or cedar. People and all sacred objects are smudged so all can be centered and focused on the healing process. The smoke clears negativity, purifies the energy field of people and places, and is a prayer to the Creator. In addition to use in healing ceremonies, smudging is used in the morning or evening as part of daily devotion. Smudging is a practice known to many religions; examples include the use of frankincense in Catholic churches and sticks of incense in Buddhist temples (Sun Bear et al., 1989).

Sweatlodge

The sweatlodge is a ceremony to cleanse body, mind, heart, and spirit. It may be held as its own ceremony or in preparation to another ceremony, such as a vision quest. Typically the sweatlodge is held in a round structure covered with overlapped pieces of tarpaulin or blankets with a small door flap. When the flap is down, the place is nearly dark and almost sealed off from the outer air. Near the lodge is a fire pit, where rocks are heated and then passed into the lodge. Water from a bucket is splashed on the stones, creating a dense steam referred to as the Breath of Spirit. Depending on the illness, a variety of herbs are burned on the sweat rocks. Sacred songs and prayers go on for several hours. Everyone in the sweatlodge prays hard for the one needing healing, but it is the responsibility of the one being healed to pray that healing energies come to her/him and ask the Spirit to give guidance to the medicine person (Bear Heart, 1996; Sun Bear et al., 1989).

The sweatlodge is also a powerful ceremony to keep people healthy, and many view it as the first line of defense in preventing illness. It is a bringing together of the four elements: earth, air, fire, and water. Through sweating and praying, the body is cleansed of toxins, the mind of negativities, the heart of hatred, and the spirit of doubt. The sweatlodge is a sacred place as if it were a church or temple (Bear Heart, 1996).

Drumming and Chanting

Drumming and chanting are powerful ways to bring oneself in balance with self, others, and the world. Drumming harmonizes people with the heartbeat of Mother Earth. It is a pulse rather than a tempo. As people dance to the pulse of the drum, they dance in harmony with the Creator and with one another. Symbolically, the drum represents all life. The wood was once a tree, and the skin covering the drum was once life. They are related to life that has gone on, yet they are helping the lives that are still here. Chanting is a form of prayer through music. Holyway chants are used to attract good, to cure, and to repair. Ghostway chants are used to remove evil, and lifeway chants are used to treat injuries and accidents (*Alternative Medicine,* 1994; Bear Heart, 1996).

Sing

A sing is a healing ceremony that lasts from two to nine days and nights. It is guided by a highly skilled specialist called a singer. Used in healing, sings are attended by as many people in the community as are able because just being present is considered healing. Some songs are only for children and call on spirits who take care of little children. Some spiritual songs take care of adults only. Other songs focus on specific problems, such as the song for small burns that will cool them and keep them from blistering. To learn a single chant can take up to several years. It takes some people 40 years of singing before they master the chants and the accompanying herbal preparations. (*Alternative Medicine,* 1994; Johnson, 1994).

Pipe Ceremony

The Pipe ceremony takes many different forms depending on how this sacred knowledge was given to the various tribes. The Pipe is one of the most sacred medicine objects and represents the universe to Native American people. The bowl represents the Earth Mother and the female powers of the universe. The stem represents the plant kingdom and the male powers of the universe. When the bowl and stem are joined together, the Pipe is sacred. The tobacco smoked in the Pipe is an instrument of prayer and has come to signify the sacredness of the ritual. As the smoke of the Pipe rises, it creates an atmosphere of prayer by symbolizing prayers going up to the Creator (Sun Bear et al., 1989).

Pipes are used for private and group prayers. Prayers are transmitted in the smoke of the burning tobacco. Participants in the Pipe ceremony are as centered and focused as possible, since everything they think and feel is part of the prayers being offered. As in many other ceremonies, the number four has special significance. The Pipe is offered to the four directions and is often passed in four ritual repetitions (Lewis, 1990).

Vision Quest

An extremely powerful ceremony is the Vision Quest. Traditionally, it is a time of fasting, praying, isolation, and exposure to the elements, all of which contribute to a mystic experience with the goal of understanding self and communicating with the Great Spirit. Questions are asked, such as How can I best serve the people? How can I best serve Mother Earth? How can I best serve future generations? The Vision Quest tells people who they are, what they are really supposed to do, what their life goal should be, and the purpose and meaning of their lives. The Vision Quest begins with a sweatlodge for purification, after which the person is taken to an isolated place in nature and begins the period of silence and fasting. During the Vision Quest, the individual focuses only on prayer and vision and in this way is pushed into the spirit world. After the Vision Quest, the person returns to the Sweatlodge and a Pipe Ceremony (Johnson, 1994; Lewis, 1990).

Healing Touch/Acupressure

Native Americans have always considered touch to be therapeutic. The Creator touches patients and transfers power to them through medicine people or shamans who are healing instruments. Touching, an expression of loving care, is essential for the healing process. It cleanses the affected area and relieves pain. The willingness to touch on the part of the healer demonstrates no fear of contamination. Healing touch is a powerful way to remove barriers and create or restore relationships (Bear Heart, 1996; Mails, 1988).

Some tribes have used a form of acupressure since ancient times. Compared with traditional Chinese practitioners, Native Americans used fewer pressure points but the process is similar. Prior to using acupressure, medicine people warm their hands over a fire so that the Great Being can send healing warmth through them to the patient. It is believed that no harm will be done to a person as long as the pressure is applied slowly and in a relaxed way. Medicine people are taught that acupressure should only be done with the utmost gentleness and love (Mails, 1988).

Herbs

Native Americans have long used herbs in maintaining health and treating disease. Botanical remedies are supplemented with ceremony and prayer during the healing process. The beneficial properties of herbs as medicines often depend on the greenness or ripeness of the plant and the part of the plant to be used such as roots, barks, twigs, bulbs, rhizomes, fruit seed, tubers, leaves, and flowers. Knowing the best time for cutting and digging each type of plant, for peak effectiveness, is part of the knowledge of the Native healer. Whether it be in summer, winter, spring, or autumn, the timing must be appropriate for each plant. An herb gathered with prayers, at the correct time and prepared properly will restore a person from illness to health (Hutchens, 1991).

Ancient Native people considered nature to be their pharmacy. They did not have aspirin but they did have willow bark, which contains salicylic acid. The active ingredient in squaw tea is ephedrine, the main ingredient in many cold cures now on the conventional market. The active ingredient in foxglove is digitalis, which was used to brew tea to help people with heart problems. Particular molds, similar to those forming the basis for penicillin, were used to treat infections. Purple coneflower (echinacea) is an immune system booster and antibiotic that is held in high esteem by many people today. Goldenseal, which is a good disinfectant that promotes scab formation, is one of the most important Native American medicinal plants. Currently, it is also used as a gargle for sore throat or as a mouth rinse for canker sores, tonsillitis, and infected gums (Lewis, 1990; Weil, 1995).

Peyote

An hallucinogenic herb, peyote, has been used by the Indians of North America for a long time. Native people do not use peyote to "get high" but rather to see teaching visions. Peyote makes people highly sensitive to sight and sound and more aware of what is around and inside of them. It is used to heal all kinds of sickness, for clairvoyance, and in the worship of the Great Being. It is believed that the Creator put peyote on earth as a medicine to help people. It is viewed somewhat like an aspirin, a cure for all kinds of physical as well as mental and emotional problems (Bear Heart, 1996).

Role of Medicine Women and Men

Although they are the primary care providers in many places, the responsibilities of medicine women and men go beyond healing illness. They also evaluate advice and treatment given by other health care practitioners. They often have a strong influence on the acceptance or rejection of the treatment plans from conventional health care providers. They may also function as tribal social mediators, dispensing traditional wisdom and suggesting action. Medicine people reaffirm and strengthen tribal identity through the recounting of myth and song. They have an extensive knowledge of their communities and of family relationships and interaction.They are the formulators and teachers of the old religion and creators of the new. Medicine people are figures of authority and awe as instruments of the Creator (Lewis, 1990).

RESEARCH

Formal research into healing ceremonies is almost nonexistent. Anecdotally, many ailments and diseases have reportedly been cured by medicine people and shamans. These disorders range from skin rashes and asthma through heart disease, diabetes, and cancer. More current research regarding scientific data on the use of herbs is available. This information is presented in chapter 6.

CURANDERISMO

Curanderismo, from the Spanish verb *curar,* to heal, is a cultural healing tradition found in Latin America and among many Hispanic Americans in the United States. In Mexico, many beliefs are shared with Native American cultural traditions. Curanderismo, as described here, is most characteristic of Mexican Americans. Although it is a traditional healing system, it utilizes Western biomedical beliefs, treatments, and practices. It is also believed, however, that in certain types of illness and healing, Native healers are more accomplished than practitioners of conventional medicine (*Alternative Medicine,* 1994; Trotter, 1996).

Natural/Supernatural Illnesses

Illnesses are classified into two types: natural and supernatural. The natural source of illness includes genetic disorders, dysfunction of the body, improper self-care, infection, and psychological conditions. Supernaturally induced illnesses are said to be caused by either evil spirits or by a person practicing magic and placing a hex on the victim. Supernatural illnesses, which may look like natural illness, occur when these negative forces damage a person's health. It is believed that conventional medical practitioners are unable to intervene with supernatural illnesses (Trotter, 1996).

Curanderos (men) and curanderas (women) believe that they work by virtue of *el don,* a gift of healing, often believed to be a gift from God. In some areas, becoming a healer is a matter of inheritance while in others areas it is a matter of being called. Healers routinely deal with physical ailments as well as with problems of a social, psychological, or spiritual nature (Trotter, 1996).

Three Levels of Healing

Three levels of care are practiced among curanderos and curanderas. These three levels are the material level, the spiritual level, and the mental level. Healers have the gift for working at only one of these levels since each requires distinct areas of knowledge, methods of diagnosis, and types of healing. The majority of the healers work at the material level, and most combine shamanic healing, herbal medicine, and first aid techniques (*Alternative Medicine,* 1994; Trotter, 1996).

The material level involves the use of physical or supernatural objects to heal or to change the person's environment. Physical healers include midwives, bone setters, herbalists, and people who treat sprains and tense muscles. Objects and rituals are used for their curative powers. Objects include herbs, religious symbols (crucifix, pictures of saints, incense, holy water), and secular items (cards and ribbons). Several types of rituals are used for supernatural cures. One of the most frequently used is a cleansing ritual that includes prayers and invocations designed to remove the negative forces that are causing the illness and a purification of the environment with incense. At the same time, the patient is given the spiritual strength necessary to achieve recovery (Trotter, 1996).

The spiritual level of healing is similar to shamanic healing rituals. It is believed that spiritual beings who exist in another dimension are interested in making contact with the physical world. These spirit entities come from once-living humans. Spiritual-level healers become a direct link or medium with these spirits. They enter a trance state and make contact with the spirit world. Some spirits have left tasks undone in their physical lives; some wish to help or harm others; and some wish to communicate with their friends and relatives. Healers believe that spirits can manipulate a person's health by directing positive or negative forces at them from the spiritual realm (Trotter, 1996).

The mental level is the least encountered level of practice. Healers have the ability to transmit, channel, and focus mental vibrations in a way that directly affects a person's mental or physical condition. If healers are working with physical illness, such as cancer, they channel vibrations to the afflicted area to retard the growth of abnormal cells and accelerate the growth of healthy cells. If healers are working with mental conditions, they send vibrations into the person's mind to manipulate energies and modify behavior. Mental healing can be accomplished in person or over long distances (Trotter, 1996).

Most research done on curanderismo is traditional anthropological research such as participant observation and interviewing. Many of the home remedies have been tested for biochemical and therapeutic activities and have demonstrated therapeutic actions that match the healers' uses. Research regarding herbs is presented in chapter 6.

INTEGRATED NURSING PRACTICE

Just as Native American healers see themselves as channels through which the Great Power helps others achieve a sense of wellness, some nurses see God or the Divine Being at work in their professional practice. Although clients may be unaware of this spiritual impetus, these nurses believe that the spiritual dimension provides the energy and momentum for their practice. Other nurses believe that their desire to care for others is what provides direction for their practice. The art of nursing, for many, is in being there, with another person or persons, in a context of caring. As we return to our nursing roots in using our hands, heart, and head in creating healing environments, we approach the Native American ideal of healing practices.

Like Native Americans, nurses have traditionally looked at the total person in their care. The context of people's lives is critically important to the nurse-healing model. In addition, nurses also believe that feelings or energy or caring flows from nurses to clients. People in distress or who are ill are anxious and fearful. When we are centered and balanced as nurses, we can share our sense of calmness in the face of crisis. Before entering a client's home or room, take a moment to center with a couple of deep, cleansing breaths and focus on what you are about to do with this person who is your client. When you are with the client, touch may be an appropriate intervention. For some people who are suffering or in crisis, a touch on the arm or holding their hand may be the most effective nursing intervention you will provide. It is important to remember that touch must always be appropriate and acceptable to the client.

Just as Native American tribes have rituals for cleansing the mind of negative thoughts and feelings which predispose to disease, we can help clients modify unhealthy thinking patterns. Negative thinking not only occurs in our brains, but occurs in our bodies; negative thoughts cause instantaneous chemical changes in every cell. Continuous cellular disruption may contribute to the onset of illness and disease. To counteract negative thinking, some people find it helpful to look at themselves in the mirror and say aloud, three good things about themselves. People might say "I'm a good friend," "I'm an honest person," "I'm a caring person," "My hair looks beautiful today," "I am becoming healthier every day," and so on. The goal is to say different positive qualities about themselves each day. Keeping a journal about feelings immediately after the exercise and feelings throughout the day is helpful in evaluating the impact of positive statements on negative thinking.

Positive affirmations are another way to counteract negative thinking. In this nursing intervention you encourage people to make a list of positive things that are occuring in their lives or things that they would like to have occur. Affirmations are always stated as if they were a fact, even when they are still a dream. For example, if you have financial problems, instead of thinking "I'm never going to get ahead. My debts are just too big," you might make affirmations such as "I am financially secure," "I pay my bills easily," "Money comes in when I need it," "I am at ease about the subject of money." Affirmations can be made about work, school, relationships, feelings, commitments, future goals, and even pleasurable activities. Encourage clients to write a list of affirmations over a period of several days. People often tape record their affirmations and listen to the tape every day. Some people find that it makes a commute to work more pleasant. Other people find a time and place to say them aloud every day. Since people tend to live their lives according to their expectations, changing expectations from negative to positive can improve the level of wellness.

Although it might not be reasonable to find a stream of flowing water to take away angers, fears, sorrows, or troubles, you can teach people to visualize that process. Direct clients through the relaxation process and have them mentally walk into a stream or actually stand in a shower that is comfortable in terms of temperature and force of the flow. As they stand in the stream, have them visualize the water washing out all their physical, mental, emotional, or relational problems. Similar to the Indian art of healing, this nursing intervention may be beneficial for clients who feel weighted down with their problems or sorrows.

Gratitude is important in Native American culture. As a nurse, you can help others become more grateful for their life experiences. Many people find it extremely beneficial to keep a gratitude journal. At the close of every day, they write at least three things that happened during the day for which they are thankful. They may be thankful for a beautiful sunrise, a smile from a stranger, a hug from a child, an A on an exam, a wonderful dinner, an intimate moment with their partner, and so on. Focusing on gratitude is another way to become more in harmony with oneself and is thought to neutralize problems and negative thinking.

Most people have objects that are significant to them. Although these objects are not medicine objects in the Native American tradition, they may bring with them a sense of comfort and perhaps protection. Encourage and support clients to have religious symbols or holy books around them if those items are important. Secular items can also be of great comfort, such as pictures of family and friends, get well cards, poems, beloved books, and so on. Most of us may not have sweatlodges or sings as part of our healing practices, but many clients have a community of family or friends who may be sending their love and concern or praying for their healing. Actively support those activities that provide love and hope to counteract the fears and doubts that accompany illness.

Like Native Americans, nurse psychotherapists find the circle to be a beneficial design. Group therapy typically occurs with all the participants sitting in a circle, which contributes to the group's sense of oneness and connectedness. Circle arrangements foster cooperation rather than competition. It is often helpful to use a circle arrangement for nursing team conferences or interdisciplinary clinical conferences.

Integrated nursing practices related to herbs are covered in chapter 6, those related to acupressure in chapter 12, and those related to dreams in chapter 18.

TRY THIS: *Positive Thoughts*

Often we endure such runs of negative thoughts that we are unaware of the process until we have been "beating ourselves up" for 10–15 minutes. To become more aware of this habitual process, tap your left finger on a firm surface for every negative thought. When your finger becomes quite sore, you will have another level of awareness of your negativity. Negative thoughts can be countered with positive ones. When you catch yourself thinking and feeling a negative thought, such as how fat your body is or how dumb you are, **STOP.** Now look for and substitute a positive thought or feeling in the place of the one you removed, such as how lovely your hair looks or how well you have succeeded at something. Now listen to yourself saying the positive phrase out loud. Continue in this way, adding other phrases and wishes for yourself.

REFERENCES

Alternative Medicine: Expanding Medical Horizons. 1994. A report to the National Institutes of Health on Alternative Medical Systems and Practices in the United States. U.S. Government Printing Office. Washington, DC.

BEAR HEART. 1996. *The Wind Is My Mother.* New York: Berkely Books.

HUTCHENS, A. R. 1991. *Indian Herbalogy of North America.* Boston: Shambhala.

JOHNSON, S. 1994. *The Book of Elders.* San Francisco: HarperSanFrancisco.

LEVIN, C. L. 1997. Tribal values and western medicine. *Native Peoples.* 10(4): 56–58.

LEWIS, T. H. 1990. *The Medicine Men.* Lincoln, NE: University of Nebraska Press.

MAILS, T. E. 1988. *Secret Native American Pathways.* Tulsa, OK: Council Oak Books.

MEADOWS, K. 1991. *The Medicine Way.* Rockport, MA: Element Books.

MILNE, C. 1995. *Sacred Places in North America.* New York: Stewart, Tabori, and Chang.

SUN BEAR, C. MULLIGAN, P. NUFFER, and WABUN. 1989. *Walk in Balance.* New York: Simon & Schuster.

TROTTER, R. T. 1996. Curanderismo. In M. S. MICOZZI, ed. *Fundamentals of Complementary and Alternative Medicine.* New York: Churchill Livingstone, 259–277.

WEIL, A. 1995. *Natural Health, Natural Medicine.* Boston: Houghton Mifflin.

RESOURCES

The Bear Tribe
P.O. Box 9167
Spokane, WA 99209-9167
509-326-6561
(workshops, apprentice programs, vision quests)

Dance of the Deer Foundation, Center for Shamanic Studies
P.O. Box 699
Soquel, CA 95073
408-475-9560
www.shamanism.com
email: shaman@shamanism.com
(dance, shamanic healing, prayer circles, dream work)

Feathered Pipe Ranch Foundation
Box 1682
Helena, MT 59624
406-442-8196
(variety of programs to help people learn their wholeness and interconnectedness)

Willow Rain Herb Farm
P.O. Box 15
Grubville, MO 63041
(herbs grown and prepared in a sacred manner)

The School of Lost Borders
P.O. Box 55
Big Pine, CA 93513
(vision quests)

UNIT III
BOTANICAL HEALING

The Lord hath created medicines out of the
earth: and he that is wise will not abhor them.

Ecclesiasticus 38:4

6 Herbs and Nutritional Supplements

Let thy food be thy medicine and thy medicine be thy food.

Hippocrates

The Great Spirit is our father, but the earth is our mother. She nourishes us; that which we put into the ground, she returns to us, and healing plants she gives us likewise.

Big Thunder

Also known as botanical medicine or phytotherapy (*phyto* means plant), herbal medicine is used by 80 percent of the world's population. According to a national survey by *Prevention* magazine, adults in the United States spend an average of $54 a year on herbs resulting in a $3.24 billion-a-year business (Zurlinden, 1998). In some cases, herbal alternatives are giving prescription drugs a run for their money. In the early 1990s, Prozac was the superstar of antidepressant prescription drugs. In recent years, the focus shifted to St. John's wort, one of the best-selling over-the-counter (OTC) herbal medicines in the United States. Herbal remedies are also beginning to compete with prescription drugs that lower cholesterol. For many conditions, herbs are the treatment of choice because they are milder and have fewer side effects than prescription drugs. In the past, herbal medicines were available only in health food stores, but they now can be found in mainstream supermarkets and pharmacies.

BACKGROUND

Throughout history, almost all societies have used plants for therapeutic purposes. For example, the oldest surviving garlic prescription, carved into a clay tablet, dates from 3000 B.C. Over thousands of years, a medical pharmacopoeia developed in every culture, from Asia to the Americas, to Europe and Africa. Over an extensive period of time, Chinese herbalists documented the healing properties of more than 7,000 herbs and thousands of herbal combinations. St. John's wort has a 2,500-year history of safe and effective use and was prescribed as medicine by Hippocrates (460–377 B.C.) himself. Galen (A.D. 130–200) described 130 herbal antidotes and medicines, and Dioscorides (first century A.D.) wrote about the medicinal properties of 500 plants and described how to prepare 1,000 simple remedies. The ancient Egyptians used peppermint and spearmint to relax the digestive tract, while Chinese and Ayurvedic doctors used mint to treat colds, coughs, and fevers (Castleman, 1996).

When Europeans came to the Americas, they found that Native Americans had a vast pharmacopoeia of medicinal plants such as birch, blackberry, coneflower, ginseng, goldenseal, and ginger, handed down from generation to generation. Early Jesuit missionaries in Canada discovered American ginseng in the early 1700s and exported it to Asia where it became a highly revered tonic. The Shakers (Church of the United Society of Believers), who were great friends of Native Americans, were the first to cultivate medicinal plants in mass quantities and became the first reputable pharmaceutical manufacturers in the United States. Until the Civil War disrupted their efforts, they sold 354 varieties of therapeutic herbs. During the early twentieth century, tincture of echinacea was highly valued for its antibiotic properties until synthetic antibiotics became available. Kava, used to calm the nervous system and decrease anxiety, was even sold during the 1920s in the Sears, Roebuck and Co. catalog. Many herbs used in ancient times are still in use today throughout the world. Herbal medicine has generally been more widely accepted outside the United States, where health care providers often combine it with conventional therapy (Castleman, 1996; Kaye and Billington, 1997).

Researchers are intensifying their efforts to collect and screen more natural products for their medicinal properties. Gordon Cragg, chief of the National Cancer Institute's natural-products branch (Hallowell, 1997) states, "Nature produces chemicals that no chemist would ever dream of at the laboratory bench." The most concentrated and diverse number of healing herbs are found in a wide band around the equator. Unfortunately, destruction of these natural plant habitats, especially tropical rain forests, are driving many species to extinction before they can be found and studied.

In the 1960s, the Food and Drug Administration (FDA) developed the current U.S. regulations regarding medications. At that time, herbal medicine had little popularity and thus was virtually ignored by the FDA. Herbs are viewed as dietary supplements and are controlled by the 1994 Dietary Supplement Health and Education Act. Under this act, dietary supplements cannot make specific medical claims as can prescription and OTC drugs. General statements such as "improves memory" or "promotes regularity" can be used as long as a disclaimer notes that the herb is not approved by the FDA and that the product is not intended to diagnose, treat, cure, or prevent any disease.

It is unlikely that most herbal medicines will ever win FDA approval since the process costs approximately $100 million per drug. Large pharmaceutical companies are willing to invest this fortune in new drugs that can be patented and sold at high profits. In contrast, granting exclusive rights or patents to most herbs, such as garlic or ginseng, is nearly impossible, which takes away the financial incentive to get them approved for medicinal use. The lack of profit, rather than the lack of efficacy of herbs, keeps drug companies from advocating change toward FDA approval of herbs.

Much of what is known about herbs comes from Germany, where an expert panel called Commission E, set up in 1978, has reviewed all available literature on 300 medicinal herbs, issuing recommendations for their use. Several smaller pharmaceutical companies in the United States, such as Shaman Pharmaceuticals, are working closely with native herbalists in a number of countries. In addition, the National Cancer Institute (NCI) is screening plants for compounds active against the AIDS virus and nine major types of cancer. Since 1986, the NCI has received samplings of thousands of plants from ethnobotanists throughout the world. Indigenous people have been testing and using healing plants for thousands of years but only recently has their knowledge been sought by Western researchers.

CONCEPTS

Synergism

The active chemicals in herbs work synergistically; that is, the action of two or more substances achieves an effect of which each is individually incapable. Most herbal medicines rely on the complex interplay of many chemicals for the therapeutic action and many lose their activity when purified and isolated. For example, a number of antimicrobial compounds are found in tea tree oil, but studies indicate that no single compound in the oil accomplishes its remarkable germ-fighting ability; rather, the interaction of at least eight distinct chemicals in the oil seems to produce the effects. This complexity makes it nearly impossible for an infectious microbe to build up resistance to tea tree oil. One of the primary problems with conventional antibiotics is the ability of many microbes to develop resistance, thus rendering the drug useless. Antioxidant defenses also operate synergistically. For example, a number of carotenoids working together have higher anticancer properties than a single carotenoid. Thus beta-carotene supplements may not provide the same protection as eating fruits and vegetables rich in beta-carotene. Other substances in the plant may help the body to assimilate its benefits as well as buffer any side effects. Including the whole plant in the final product often ensures that some measure of the natural "checks and balances" will be retained (Britton and Kircher, 1998).

Various herbs and other substances may also work synergistically with one another. A rather dramatic example of this effect occurred during the testing of plant samples from the rain forest of Ecuador for chemicals that could be used to treat diabetes. The leaves from the plant were immersed in an alcohol extract and then a water extract. The debate among the researchers concerned whether to throw a live crab into the extract, just as native healers did. Some believed it might make a difference while others believed the crab was simply ritualistic. Amazingly, the only extract that showed therapeutic effect was the one with the crab in it. It turns out that a component in a crab's shell is needed to extract the active chemical compound from the plant (Cray, 1997).

Phytonutrients

Phytonutrients are chemicals present in plants that make the plants biologically active and are responsible for giving plants their color, flavor, and natural disease resistance. Phytonutrients are products of photosynthesis or are substances that serve as defense mechanisms against attacks by insects and other predators. These active components of plants usually occur in groups that complement the protective and healing effects of each other. Descriptions of the most important phytonutrients and their uses are found in Table 6.1.

Antioxidants

Antioxidants are a group of vitamins, minerals, enzymes, and herbs that help protect the body from naturally occurring free radicals. As the body goes through its normal processes, and oxygen is used to provide cellular fuel, some of the oxygen molecules lose one of their pair of electrons. When they do, the formerly stable oxygen molecules become dangerous free radicals that try to stabilize themselves by stealing another electron from stable molecules, thus damaging them and creating more free radicals. Because free radicals react so easily with other compounds, they can effect significant changes in the body. Many different factors can lead to the production of free radicals. Internal sources, in addition to oxygen consumption, include emotional stress and strenuous exercise. External sources include air pollution, cigarette smoke, factory and car exhaust, smog, pesticides, herbicides, food contaminants,

Table 6.1: Phytonutrients

Name	Properties	Use/Effects
Carbohydrates	Main energy source and structural support of plants	In some herbs, such as coltsfood and marshmallow, the cellulose combines with other chemicals to form mucilage, a gummy substance, which, when ingested by humans, soothes and protects irritated or inflamed internal tissue.
Fatty oils	Mixture of triglycerides, glycerol, and fatty acids	Cathartic effect of castor oil useful for constipation and colic in young children.
Essential oils	Vaporize when heated; combinations give plants their particular smell	Garlic is an antiseptic, thyme is an expectorant, chamomile relieves gaseous distention and painful intestinal spasms.
Tannins	Chemical substances with astringent and antiseptic properties	Form a protective layer on the skin and mucous membranes and are useful in treatment of burns and local inflammation; used for eye and mouth infections.
Bitter principles	Group of chemicals that have an extremely bitter taste	Through a reflex action via tastebuds, stimulate appetite and flow of digestive juices, stimulate liver activity and flow of bile, some act as diuretics. Viewed as overall tonics.
Alkaloids	Group of nitrogen-containing compounds with most therapeutic plant substances: analgesic, local anesthetic, sedating, antispasmodic, heart constricting, and/or hallucinatory; poisonous to varying degrees	Affect both the nervous and circulatory systems. Most familiar are atropine, caffeine, cocaine, morphine, nicotine, and quinine.
Isoflavones	Compounds similar to human estrogen and found primarily in soy products	May prevent prostate, breast, and other hormone-related cancers; lower cholesterol, relieve menopausal symptoms, prevent osteoporosis by increasing bone density.

continued

Table 6.1: *(continued)*

Name	Properties	Use/Effects
Carotenoids	Yellow, orange, or red pigments in photosynthetic plants, converted into vitamin A in the liver	Three most important to humans: • Beta-carotene may aid in cancer prevention by neutralizing free radicals. Used in conjunction with topical sunscreens, better prevention of sunburn and skin damage. • Lycopene may prevent prostate cancer and decrease risk of heart attacks. • Lutein may be useful in prevention of macular degeneration, a leading cause of blindness in the elderly.
Glycosides	Complex organic substances; some of most potent herbal remedies and among most toxic substances known	Cardiac glycosides include foxglove and lily of the valley, which affect cardiac contractions and used to correct arrhythmias. Mustard glycosides are used externally and have antiseptic and analgesic effects. Cyanogenic glycosides release hydrogen cyanide when chewed or digested resulting in antispasmodic, purgative, and sedative effects. Found in some nuts, vegetables, and the seeds of some fruits. Hydrogen cyanide, sometimes called prussic acid, is highly poisonous. Phenolic glycosides include salicylic derivatives found in willow and other plants and is main ingredient in aspirin—antiseptic, analgesic, and antiinflammatory effects. Coumarine glycosides strengthen capillary walls and act as anticoagulant. Anthraquinones glycosides are used as laxatives. Flavonoid glycosides, known as bioflavonoids or flavonoids, improve circulation, stimulate bile production, lower cholesterol levels, and strengthen the liver.

Sources: Balch and Balch, *Prescription for Nutritional Healing*, 2d ed. (Garden City Park, NY: Avery Publishing, 1997); Lindsay and Claywell, "Considering soy: Its estrogenic effects may protect women," *Lifetimes*, 2(1): 41–44.

chemotherapy, and radiation. All cause the overproduction of free radicals. Oxidative damage can be visualized when one bites into an apple, leaves it for a few minutes, and then notices that the exposed part becomes brown or oxidized. Humans, however, cannot "see" the damage being done by free radicals in the body. An excess of free radicals is, in part, responsible for the effects of aging and is implicated in cancer and a variety of chronic and degenerative conditions, including arthritis and heart disease (Balch and Balch, 1997).

Free radicals are normally kept under control through the production of enzymes that act as free radical scavengers to search out and neutralize dangerous free radicals. As people age, they produce fewer of these enzymes, and may benefit from dietary antioxidants such as vitamin C, vitamin E, carotenoids, the mineral selenium, and the hormone melatonin. Herbs with antioxidant properties include bilberry, ginkgo, grape seed extract, green tea, and flavonoids. Fruits and vegetables are the primary sources for antioxidants, though they are also available in the form of supplements.

Plant-Derived Products

Before pharmaceutical companies was herbal medicine. In many parts of the world, treating illness with herbs is still the only medicine available. Even though only a tiny fraction of plants have been studied for medicinal benefits, plant-derived products are used regularly by conventional physicians. Twenty-five percent of all prescription drugs sold in the United States are derived from plants. Examples of herbal remedies that have been synthesized into modern drugs are reserpine from Indian snakeroot, digoxin from foxglove, quinine from Peruvian bark, aspirin from willow tree bark, morphine from opium poppy, cocaine from coca leaves, and atropine from deadly nightshade. Recently, researchers discovered taxol, found in Pacific yew bark, which is currently being used in the treatment of early and advanced breast cancer and ovarian tumors. Taxol has also been found to decrease the chances of developing breast cancer in women who are at high risk. Unfortunately, taxol has also been associated with an increased risk for pulmonary embolism and endometrial cancer. Another recent advance is the drug vincristine, which has been isolated from the Madagascar periwinkle. Vincristine has been found to arrest cell division so dramatically that it is being used to treat acute leukemia and Hodgkin's disease (Hallowell, 1997; Weiner and Weiner, 1994).

Safety

Not all plant life is beneficial. Most plant-related poisonings are due to accidental consumption of toxic ornamental plants such as jade, holly, poinsettia, schefflera, philodendron, and dieffenbachia rather than from herbs. Data compiled by the American Association of Poison Control Centers indicates that in any two-year period of time, plants cause two or three deaths and approximately 50 major poisonings. In contrast, prescription medications cause close to a thousand deaths from poisoning and almost 7,000 major nonfatal poisonings per year (Castleman, 1996). Unrelated to direct poisoning are adverse drug reactions (ADRs), defined as any unintended and undesired effect of a drug with usual therapeutic doses. After excluding errors in drug administration, noncompliance, overdose, and drug abuse, a significant study found that ADRs may be the fourth to sixth leading cause of death in the United States. This incidence has remained stable over the last 30 years, a fact not widely recognized by the general population (Lazarou et al., 1998).

The vast majority of herbal medicines present no danger. Some can, however, cause serious side effects if taken in excess or, for some, if taken over a prolonged period of time. For example, comfrey, a digestive remedy, and coltsfoot, used to treat cough, can cause liver damage if taken in large doses. Herbs can also interact with drugs, and caution should be used when combining herbs with prescription and OTC medications. Pregnant women should be cautioned not to take herbs internally except for mild herb teas (Fugh-Berman, 1997; Kaye and Billington, 1997).

TREATMENT

Medicinal herbs are available at health food stores, herb shops, supermarkets, and pharmacies. They can be used as a preventative, a tonic, or a treatment. Herbs can be prepared and used in a number of ways. *Extracts* or *tinctures* are made by pressing herbs with a heavy press and soaking them in alcohol or water, which after evaporation yields a concentrated extract. Extracts are generally measured in drops and diluted in a small amount of water for ingestion. A preparation of the delicate parts of plants, that is, leaves, flowers, and seeds, is called an *infusion,* a process similar to making tea. Hot water is poured over the herb, steeped for 3–5 minutes, and strained before drinking. Honey or lemon may be added to taste. *Decoction* is the preparation of the more resilient parts of plants, such as the bark, roots, and berries. These parts of the herb are usually boiled for 10–20 minutes and strained before drinking. A *compress* is a cloth soaked in a warm or cool herbal solution and applied directly to an injured area. An herbal *poultice* is made by mixing powered herbs with enough hot water to make a thick paste that is then applied directly to the skin. Poultices are used to reduce swelling, relieve pain, decrease muscle spasms, draw out toxins from the body, increase circulation, and speed healing (Balch and Balch, 1997). Table 6.2 lists some of the more common herbs as well as their action, dosage, and side effects.

Table 6.2: Common Herbs

Name	Properties/Use	Form/Dose	Contraindications/Side Effects
Capsaicin	For tenderness and pain of osteoarthritis, fibromyalgia, diabetic neuropathy, shingles	Cream topically applied	May be a brief burning or stinging sensation with first use Wash hands after applying; avoid touching eyes
Chamomile	For anxiety, stomach distress, stomach ulcers, infant colic, drug withdrawal	Infusion; Tincture: 1 teaspoon TID	NOT for those allergic to ragweed
Chondroitin	Helps slow cartilage degradation in osteoarthritis	400 mg TID	
Echinacea	Antiviral, antibiotic for colds, flu, and other infections	400 mg for 5–14 days, peaks at 5 days	NOT for people with autoimmune disease, NOT for pregnant and lactating women Bitter taste
Evening Primrose oil	For PMS, mastalgia, hypertension, multiple sclerosis, alcholism	250–500 mg/day	
Feverfew	For prevention of migraines	0.2% parthenolide 100–300 mg/day	NOT for use with prescription headache drugs NOT for use by pregnant and lactating women Chewing leaves can cause mouth sores and loss of taste; capsule preferred
Garlic	Antibiotic, antiviral, antifungal, anticoagulant; for any infection, hypertension, high blood lipid levels	Varying recommendations	NOT for people with clotting disorders May cause stomach upset
Ginger	For nausea and vomiting of various causes, hypertension, high cholesterol; enhances insulin	500–1000 mg q 4 hrs Motion sickness: 1500 mg 30 prior	People taking anticoagulant should check with MD prior to use

continued

121

Table 6.2: *(continued)*

Name	Properties/Use	Form/Dose	Contraindications/Side Effects
Ginkgo	For attention and memory problems, headaches, timitus, intermittent claudication, erectile problems	24% flavonoids & 6% terpenes. 60–80 mg TID or QID	May cause mild GI upset
Ginseng	For mood swings, improved physical performance, reduction of fasting blood glucose, stimulation of immune system, ease cocaine withdrawal	200 mg BID. Minimum 4–6 weeks	NOT for use when acutely ill with cold or flu NOT to be used with hypoglycemia Nervousness, insomnia, euphoria, hypertension
Glucosamine	Improves pain and movement in osteoarthritis	500 mg TID	People taking diuretics may need higher doses of herb
Goldenseal	Antibiotic, antiseptic, antiinflammatory for wound healing, colds and flu, hypertension, uterine bleeding, enhances insulin	2 capsules TID for maximum 3 weeks	NOT for use during pregnancy—may cause premature uterine contractions Only for short-term use; long-term use may irritate or inflame mucosa
Green tea	Antioxidant, protects against cancer, lowers cholesterol, helps regulate blood sugar and insulin levels	3–4 cups/day	NOT to be used in large quantities during pregnancy People with anxiety disorder or irregular heartbeat should limit use to no more than 2 cups daily
Kava	For anxiety, insomnia, low energy, muscle tension	100 mg TID	In large amounts—intoxicating and potential for abuse
Milk Thistle	Antioxidant for all liver disorders; psoriasis	Varying recommendations	No known side effects

St. John's Wort	For mild to moderate depression, viral infections including HIV and herpes	900 mg/day Minimum 4–8 weeks	NOT for pregnant and lactating women, not for children NOT for use with other antidepressants May cause photosensitivity; avoid foods with tyramine and OTC cold and flu remedies, amino acid supplements
Saw Palmetto	Urinary antiseptic, for benign prostatic hyperplasia	160 mg BID	Use only after proper diagnosis from primary practitioner May cause dizziness, dry mouth, tachycardia, angina, testicular pain
Selenium	Antioxidant especially when combined with vitamin E, may prevent some types of tumors, aids in production of antibodies, protects liver	200 mcg	Metallic taste in mouth, garlicky breath odor Excessively high levels may lead to liver and kidney impairment
Tea Tree Oil	Antifungal, antiseptic, for acne, minor burns and cuts, athlete's foot, nail infections, herpes, douche for yeast infections	Full strength or dilute in water or oil	Do NOT ingest
Valerian	For insomnia, muscle pain, menstrual and intestinal cramps, benzodiazepine withdrawal	400 mg before bed 0.5% essential oil	NOT to be used with alcohol Nonaddictive; bitter taste
Yohimbe	For decreased sex drive, erectile problems	Varying recommendations	NOT for people with hypertension, kidney disease NOT to be used with tyramines, OTC cold remedies, caffeine, amphetamines May cause hypertension, anxiety, panic attacks, hallucinations

RESEARCH

Most herbal medicines have not been tested as thoroughly as prescription drugs in the United States. In contrast, many scientific studies have been conducted outside the United States on a variety of herbal remedies. Commission E, in Germany, has reviewed all available literature on 300 medicinal herbs and issued recommendations for their use. Good data can be found on the efficacy of about two dozen herbs, data which is backed up by well-designed clinical trials. Research studies demonstrate the effectiveness of herbs in the following conditions:

- Ginkgo, which some say is the most important of all herbs, has been the subject of at least 400 scientific papers. Ginkgo has been found to improve memory, concentration, absent-mindedness, and confusion and is a promising herb for the treatment of dementia (LeBars et al., 1997).
- Ginkgo may be helpful for sexual problems such as erectile dysfunction, delayed ejaculation, anorgasmia, and decreased sex drive (Cohen and Bartlik, 1997; Sikora, 1989).
- St. John's wort is an effective treatment for mild to moderate depression. A meta-analysis of 23 controlled trials with 1,757 outpatients found that St. John's wort was almost three times more effective than placebo and comparable to standard antidepressants (Linde et al., 1996).
- Garlic lowers cholesterol levels by 18–21 percent compared to a 3–5 percent reduction in control groups (Bordia et. al., 1981; Isaacsohn et al., 1998; Vorberg and Schneider, 1990).
- Studies on the effect of garlic on mild hypertension have been mixed as to reduction of diastolic blood pressure (Auer et al., 1990; Silagy and Neil, 1994).
- Several trials indicate that feverfew may be effective in the prevention of migraines (Johnson et. al., 1985; Murphy et al., 1988).
- Of 45 people treated with topical capsaicin for fibromyalgia, those receiving capsaicin reported less tenderness at their trigger points and a significant increase in grip strength (McCarty et al., 1994). Sixty-nine percent of people with diabetic neuropathy reported pain improvement with capsaicin cream (Capsaicin Study Group, 1991).
- Saw Palmetto improves urinary flow rate in men with mild to moderate symptoms of benign prostatic hyperplasia in 50–88 percent of the cases (Braeckman, 1994; Champault et al., 1984; Wilt et al., 1998).
- A review of 26 controlled clinical trials of echinacea found positive results for 30 of the 34 treated groups in terms of preventing or curing upper respiratory infections, enhancing the immune system, and reducing the side effects of cancer therapies (Melchart, 1994).

• Milk thistle is thought to speed the production of new liver cells and bind to the outside of liver cells, slowing the entry of liver-damaging toxins. It appears to be effective in people with hepatitis and cirrhosis (Ferenci et al., 1989; Mascarella et al., 1993; Salmi and Sarna, 1982).

• Rosemary extract prevents DNA damage in cell cultures induced by aflatoxin, a potent agent known to cause liver cancer (Offord et al., 1997).

• Ginger is helpful in postoperative nausea and vomiting, morning sickness, and motion sickness (Bone et al., 1990; Fisher-Rasmussen et al., 1990; Mowrey, 1982).

• Valerian, when compared to placebo, has a significant positive effect on sleep latency and subjective quality of sleep (Lindahl and Lindwall, 1989).

• In a double-blind trial, people with irritable bowel syndrome had significant improvement in bowel symptom scores using both individualized and standard Chinese herbal formulas when compared to the control group (Bensoussan et al., 1998).

• Bee venom appears to slow down the body's inflammatory response by inhibiting the amount of free radicals or by stimulating the adrenal glands to release cortisol. The National Multiple Sclerosis Society is sponsoring a study of bee venom to determine whether it is effective in reducing fatigue and muscle spasms (Cerrato, 1998).

• Traditional Chinese Medicine uses moxibustion (burning herbs to stimulate acupuncture points) of the herb mugroot near the woman's fifth toe to promote version of fetuses in breech presentation. The effect may be through increasing fetal activity (Cardini and Weixin, 1998).

• Laboratory research on the anticancer activity of perillyl alcohol, distilled from lavender has recently begun human clinical trials at the University of Wisconsin at Madison.

• Kudzu Kuzu is in clinical trials for decreasing the craving for alcohol.

• Heantos, a mixture of 13 herbs, is in clinical testing at Johns Hopkins University and the National Institute of Drug Abuse for the treatment of heroin, opium, and cocaine addiction.

INTEGRATED NURSING PRACTICE

Because herbs are marketed as "natural" or promoted as foods, consumers may assume incorrectly that herbs are safe and without side effects. It is important that you remember that natural remedies be approached with respect. They work because they have strong pharmacological activity. It is important that you teach people that though herbs are generally much safer than prescription drugs, if abused or overused they can cause harm.

Although herbs can be quite effective, it is important to caution people about becoming fanatical. If they have a life-threatening illness such as asthma or if they experience chest pain or if they notice more benign symptoms that persist for longer than a few days, they should seek medical attention. While it may be healthy to take echinacea if they feel a cold coming on, any serious ailment should be diagnosed by a health care practitioner before undertaking a herbal cure. Self-diagnosis and self-care are by nature subject to limits. Conventional medicine is best used in crisis situations, and herbs are best used in noncrisis situations. Professionals can save consumers from treating something that does not exist or failing to treat something that does. Further, health practitioners can help individuals evaluate the extent of their progress on the herbal regimen. Consultation is especially important if people are taking other medications; while some herbs can work with prescription drugs, others may not. Some herbs potentiate the effects of drugs, so people may need a lower dose of their regular medication. Suddenly stopping a prescription medication and/or a drug interaction with herbs can be hazardous to one's health. Pregnant and lactating women should always consult their primary care practitioner before taking any herbal medicines.

As a nurse, you need to educate consumers about potential actions and interactions of herbal remedies. People cannot expect to take an herb for a few days to undo ten years of poor health habits nor replace a healthy diet with herbal supplements. If people eat a healthy, varied diet that is high in fresh foods, especially fruits, vegetables, and whole grains, they do not need to take other supplements unless they have special needs (Weil, 1998).

Sometimes walking into a health food store or pharmacy is highly confusing. Many people are overwhelmed by the wide assortment of products and brands. As a nurse, you can teach consumers the following basic guidelines in selecting herbal medicines.

- Store clerks are not experts. They do not have an adequate scientific background to counsel people.
- Go with a name brand. Since the industry is unregulated, it is best to choose products made by large, reputable companies that have been in business for a long time. Many excellent products are produced in Germany and France, where they must meet strict production standards.
- Check the label. Look for the word "standardized," which tells you that the product consistently contains a certain percentage of a specific chemical.
- Check to see if the claims are reasonable. Be wary of promises of instant cures for complicated disorders. If something sounds too good to be true, it probably is.
- Consider the product's form. A liquid, powder, or solid extract is generally best. Bulk herbs can lose their potency quickly. Many herbal tinc-

tures are 50 percent grain alcohol, which may be a problem for people with a history of alcohol abuse or for those who take drugs that can interact with alcohol.

- Be wary of ultra-combination products. If the product has more than six ingredients, it probably contains a small amount of each. The fact that herbs are combined does not make the product necessarily better. If you need ginkgo to boost your memory, it is better to get it full strength than to get a product diluted with ginseng, garlic, and other herbs.

- Take the right dose. Do not take higher doses than the label recommends. Exceeding the recommended dose can lead to toxicity. Most herbal remedies are not to be given to children under the age of one unless directed by an experienced practitioner. Children ages 1 to 6 are typically given one-third the adult dose while children ages 6 to 12 receive one-half the adult dose. People over 65 years may need to reduce the dosage also.

- Watch for side effects. If you have any unusual symptoms, such as allergies, rashes, heart palpitations, or headaches, stop taking the herb immediately and see a health care practitioner.

- Give it time to work. Evaluate how the product makes you feel. After 30 days, ask yourself whether the product has made a difference in your health. If you are not sure, stop taking the herb to gauge the difference.

- Inform your primary health care practitioner about the herbal remedies you are taking.

- If you plan on regularly using herbal remedies, invest in a good herbal reference guide to insure proper information. One suggestion is James A. Duke's book, *The Green Pharmacy* (Rodale Press, 1997), or Daniel Mowrey's book, *Scientific Validation of Herbal Medicine* (Keats Pub, 1990), or consult with the one of the organizations in the resource list. The U.S. Department of Agriculture provides free access to 80,000 records on herb taxonomy and use of herbs worldwide, developed by Dr. James A. Duke.

Traditional Chinese remedies are taken as an herbal drink. Many Americans, however, complain about the bitter taste and inconvenience of steeping the herbs for hours at a time. Dr. James H. Zhou, formerly a professor at Yale University School of Medicine and founder of HerbaSway, has developed a line of Chinese herbal teas and elixirs in pleasant-tasting liquid concentrates which are becoming more popular among Western consumers.

As a nurse, it is also important that you warn consumers about remedies that can be risky. Chaparral, sold as teas and pills to fight cancer and "purify blood," has been linked to serious liver damage. Dieter's teas, containing such ingredients as senna, aloe, rhubarb root, buckthorn, cascara, and castor oil, act as laxatives that, when consumed in excessive amounts, can disrupt potassium levels and contribute to cardiac arrhythmias. Ephedra, also called ma huang, is an herb used most often for asthma. It is a cardiac and nervous system stimulant containing ephedrine, which can cause anxiety, psychotic episodes, hypertension, stroke, tachycardia, arrhythmias, and cardiac arrest. Mixing ephedra with caffeine or other substances, as the OTC energy-boosting products do, can increase its dangers. Ephedra should not be combined with theophylline, thyroid hormone, tricyclic antidepressants, methylphenidate, or any other drugs that can cause tachycardia or hypertension. Several states have banned supplements containing ephedrine because of the dangers (Fugh-Berman, 1997).

The American public is demanding more information about herbal remedies. In the best of all worlds, consumers would have an educated professional—a nurse, a pharmacist, or a doctor—to help guide them through the process of using herbal remedies. That is the situation in Germany, where health care practitioners and pharmacists must be knowledgeable about natural remedies, their approved uses, their potential side effects, and how they should be prescribed. It has not been true in the United States but is sure to change in the near future. Schools of nursing and schools of medicine are including courses on alternative medicine in their curriculum. The College of Pharmacy at the University of Illinois at Chicago has become a collaborating center with the World Health Organization's traditional medicine program and offers a required course in herbal therapy.

As nurse-author Carolyn Kresse Murray, (1996, p. 59) has said, "Part of patient advocacy is making sure you help your patient with all his [her] therapies. Equipping yourself with knowledge about herbal therapies is another way to keep him [her] from harm."

TRY THIS: *Herbal Remedies*

Borage Tea

Used for reducing fever and also for increasing milk in nursing mothers.

How to: Combine a small handful of fresh leaves with 2 1/2 cups boiling water. Steep 10 minutes, strain, and drink warm.

Chamomile

An excellent home remedy for indigestion, heartburn, and infant colic. It also soothes skin and has mild relaxant and sedative properties.

TRY THIS: *Herbal Remedies (continued)*

How to: For an infusion, use 2–3 heaping teaspoons of dried or 1/3 cup of fresh flowers per cup of boiling water. Steep 10–20 minutes. Strain and drink up to 3 cups a day. Diluted infusions may be given to infants for colic.

For a relaxing herbal bath, fill a cloth bag with a few handfuls of dried or fresh flowers and let the water run over it.

For allergic skin rashes, tightly pack a jar of flowerheads, cover with olive oil, cover and set in a sunny place for 3 weeks. Strain and apply to rashes.

Comfrey

External use only. Promotes the growth of new cells and has a mild anti-inflamatory action. Used in wound and burn treatment.

How to: Mix powdered root with water to make a paste. Apply to injured area and cover with clean bandage. Change daily.

Ginger

Decreases nausea, boosts the immune system, lowers blood pressure.

How to: Use 2 teaspoons of powdered or grated root per cup of boiling water. Steep 20 minutes, strain, add juice from half a lemon and honey to taste. Drink hot up to 3 cups a day. Dilute ginger infusion to treat infant colic. If you buy whole root, refrigerate it.

Mint

Relaxes the digestive tract; used to treat colds, coughs, and fevers.

How to: For an infusion, use 1 teaspoon of fresh herb or 2 teaspoons of dried leaves per cup of boiling water. Steep 10 minutes, strain, and drink up to 3 cups a day. Peppermint has a sharper taste than spearmint and feels cooler in the mouth.

For a relaxing herbal bath, fill a cloth bag with a few handfuls of dried or fresh leaves and let the water run over it.

Rosemary

Stimulates circulation and relaxes tired and sore muscles.

How to: For tired, sore feet, make a footbath by adding 10 drops of essential oil to a basin of hot water large enough to hold both feet. Stir the oil into the water with your hand.

REFERENCES

AUER, W. et al. 1990. Hypertension and hyperlipidaemia: Garlic helps in mild cases. *Br J Clin Pract.* 69: 3–6.

BALCH, J. F. and P. H. BALCH. 1997. *Prescription for Nutritional Healing,* 2d ed. Garden City Park, NY: Avery Pub.

BENSOUSSAN, A. et al. 1998. Treatment of irritable bowel syndrome with Chinese herbal medicine. *JAMA.* 280(18): 1585–1589.

BONE, M. E. et al. 1990. Ginger root: A new antiemetic. The effect of ginger root on postoperative nausea and vomiting after major gynecological surgery. *Anaesthesia.* 45: 669–671.

BORDIA, A. et al. 1981. Effect of garlic on blood lipids in patients with coronary heart disease. *Am J Clin Nutr.* 34: 2100–2103.

BRAECKMAN, J. 1994. The extract of Serenoa repens in the treatment of benign prostatic hyperplasia: A multicenter open study. *CurrTher Res.* 55(7): 776–785.

BRITTON, J. and T. KIRCHER. 1998. *The Complete Book of Home Herbal Remedies.* Buffalo, NY: Firefly Books.

Capsaicin Study Group. 1991. Treatment of painful diabetic neuropathy with topical capsaicin. *Arch Intern Med.* 151: 2225–2229.

CARDINI, F. and H. WEIXIN. 1998. Moxibustion for correction of breech presentation. *JAMA.* 280(18): 1580–1584.

CASTLEMAN, M. 1996. *Nature's Cures.* Emmaus, PA: Rodale Press.

CERRATO, P. L. 1998. A therapeutic bee sting? *RN.* 57–58.

CHAMPAULT, G., J.C. PATEL, and A. M. BONNARD. 1984. A double-blind trial of an extract of the plant Serenoa repens in benign prostatic hyperplasia. *Br J Clin Pharmacol.* 18: 461–462.

COHEN, A. J. and B. D. BARTLIK. 1997. Ginkgo biloba for drug-induced sexual dysfunction. Presented at the American Psychiatric Association Annual Meeting. San Diego.

CRAY, D. 1997. Money that grows on trees. *Time.* Fall Special Issue. 150(19): 21.

FERENCI, P. et al. 1989. Randomized controlled trial of silymarin treatment in patients with cirrhosis of the liver. *J Hepatol.* 9: 105–113.

FISHER-RASMUSSEN, W. et al. 1990. Ginger treatment of hyperemesis gravidarum. *Eur J Ob Synecol Repro Biol.* 38: 19–24.

FUGH-BERMAN, A. 1997. Clinical trials of herbs. *Complementary and Alternative Therapies in Primary Care. Primary Care.* 24(4): 889–903.

HALLOWELL, C. 1997. The plant hunter. *Time.* Fall Special Issue. 150(19): 17–22.

ISAACSOHN, J. L. et al. 1998. Garlic powder and plasma lipids and lipoproteins. *Arch Intern Med.* 158: 1189–1194.

JOHNSON, E. S. et al. 1985. Efficacy of feverfew as prophylactic treatment of migraine. *Br. Med J.* 291: 569–573.

KAYE, C. and N. BILLINGTON. 1997. *Medicinal Plants of the Heartland.* Vienna, IL: Cache River Press.

LAZAROU, J., B. H. POMERANZ, and P. N. COREY. 1998. Incidence of adverse drug reactions in hospitalized patients. *JAMA.* 279(15): 1200–1205.

LEBARS, P. L. et al. 1997. A placebo-controlled, double-blind, randomized trial of an extract of ginkgo biloba for dementia. *JAMA.* 278: 1327–1332.

LINDAHL, O. and L. LINDWALL. 1989. Double-blind study of a valerian preparation. *Pharmacol Biochem Behav.* 32: 1065–1066.

LINDE, K. et al. 1996. St. John's wort for depression—an overview and meta-analysis of randomized clinical trials. *Br Med J.* 313: 253–258.

LINDSAY, S. H. and L. G. CLAYWELL. 1998. Considering soy: Its estrogenic effects may protect women. *Lifelines.* 2(1): 41–44.

MASCARELLA, S. et al. 1993. Therapeutic and antilipoperoxidant effects of silybin-phosphtidyl-choline complex in chronic liver disease: Preliminary results. *Curr Ther Res.* 53(1): 98–102.

MCCARTY, D. J. et al. 1994. Treatment of pain due to fibromyalgia with topical capsaicin: A pilot study. *Semin Arthritis Rheum* 23(6): 41–47.

MELCHART, D. et al. 1994. Immunomodulation with Echinacea—A systematic review of controlled clinical trials. *Phytomedicine.* 1: 245–254.

MOWREY, D. B. 1982. Motion sickness, ginger, and psychophysics. *Lancet.* 655–657.

MURPHY, J. J., S. HEPTINSALL, and J. R. A. MITCHELL. 1988. Randomized double-blind placebo-controlled trial of feverfew in migraine prevention. *Lancet.* ii: 189–192.

OFFORD, E. A. et al. (1997). Mechanisms involved in the chemoprotective effects of rosemary extract studied in human liver and bronchial cells. *Cancer Letters.* 114: 275–281.

SALMI, H. A. and S. SARNA. 1982. Effect of silymarin on chemical, functional, and morphological alterations of the liver. *Scand J Gastroenterol.* 17: 517–520.

SIKORA, R. et al. 1989. Ginkgo biloba extract in the therapy of erectile dysfunction. *J Urol.* 141: 188A.

SILAGY, C. A. and H. A. W. NEIL. 1994. A meta-analysis of the effect of garlic on blood pressure. *J Hypertens.* 12: 463–468.

VORBERG, G. and B. SCHNEIDER. 1990. Therapy with garlic: Results of a placebo-controlled, double-blind study. *Br J Clin Pract.* 69:7–11.

WEIL, A. January–February 1998. Ask the experts. *Natural Health.* 24–28.

WEINER, M. A. and J. A. WEINER. 1994. *Herbs That Heal.* Mill Valley, CA: Quantum Books.

WILT, T. J. et al. 1998. Saw palmetto extracts for treatment of benign prostatic hyperplasia. *JAMA.* 280 (18): 1604–1609.

ZURLINDEN, J. March 9, 1998. Herbal treatments. *Nursing Spectrum.* 11(5): 17.

RESOURCES

American Botanical Council
P.O. Box 201660
Austin, TX 78720
512-331-8868
www.herbalgram.org

American Herbalists Guild
P.O. Box 70
Roosevelt, UT 84066
435-722-8434
www.healthy.net/herbalists
email: ahgoffice@earthlink.net

East/West School of Herbalism
P.O. Box 712
Santa Cruz, CA 95061
800-717-5010
408-336-5010

FDA Consumer Information Line
800-FDA-4010
www.fda.gov

HerbaSway
800-672-7322
203-269-9703 fax
www.arxc.com/herbaswy/herbaswy.html
email: herbs@herbasway.com

Herb Research Foundation
1007 Pearl St., Suite 200
Boulder, CO 80302
800-748-2617
303-449-2265
www.herbs.org
email: info@herbs.org

Journal of Ethnopharmacy
Elsevier Science Ireland, Ltd.
Madison Square Station, Box 882
New York, NY 10159
212-989-5800

Journal of Natural Products
American Society of Pharmacognosy
555 31st St.
Downers Grove, IL 60515
708-971-6417

National Institute of Medical Herbalists
56 Longbrook St.
Exeter, Devon, United Kingdom
EX4 6AH
011-44-39-242-6022

Ontario Herbalists Association
11 Winthrop Place
Stoney Creek, Ontario, Canada L8G 3M3
905-536-1509

U.S. Department of Agriculture
http://probe.na/usda.gov

U.S. Pharmacopeia
Office of External Affairs
12601 Twinbrook Parkway
Rockville, MD 20852
301-881-0666

7 Naturopathy

All things are connected
Whatever befalls the earth
befalls the sons of the earth.
Man did not weave the
web of life.
He is merely a strand in it.
Whatever he does to the web
He does to himself.

Chief Seattle, upon
surrendering his
tribal lands in 1856

It is more important to know what sort of
person has a disease than to know what
sort of disease a person has.

Hippocrates

Naturopathic medicine is not only a system of medicine but also a way of life
with emphasis on client responsibility, client education, health maintenance,
and disease prevention. It may be the model health system of the future with the
movement toward healthy lifestyles, healthy diets, and preventive health care.

BACKGROUND

The basic precepts of naturopathy are similar to those in ancient medical systems throughout the world. Naturopathy can trace its philosophical roots to the
Hippocratic school of medicine around 400 B.C. Hippocrates had a holistic approach to clients and instructed his students only to prescribe wholesome treatments and avoid causing harm or hurt. Furthermore, Hippocrates thought that
the entire universe followed natural laws and the role of the physician was to
understand and support nature's own cures (Pizzorno, 1996).

Naturopathic medicine grew out of the nineteenth-century medical systems of America and Europe. The term itself was coined by Dr. John Scheel of New York City in 1895, although it was Benedict Lust who formalized naturopathy in 1902 as both a system of medicine and a way of life. By the early 1900s, more than 20 naturopathic schools of medicine were operating in the United States. In the 1920s and 1930s, naturopathic journals encouraged a diet high in fiber and low in red meat, the same type of diet promoted by the National Institutes of Health and the National Cancer Institute in the 1990s. With the development of antibiotics and vaccines in the 1940s and 1950s, the popularity of naturopathy began to decline as people began to rely on these medical breakthroughs. The 1970s saw a renewal in the importance of nutrition, healthy lifestyles, and environmental cleanup programs. This interest continued to grow into what is now the American interest in alternative medicine (Cassileth, 1998; Pizzorno, 1996).

PREPARATION

In order for naturopathic medicine to establish itself as a legitimate health care system, it needed to establish accredited schools and conduct credible research. Currently five schools exist in the United States and Canada: Bastyr University in Seattle, Washington, National College of Naturopathic Medicine in Portland, Oregon, the Southwest College of Naturopathic Medicine and Health Science in Scottsdale, Arizona, University of Bridgeport in Connecticut, and the Canadian College of Naturopathic Medicine in Toronto, Ontario. The Council on Naturopathic Medical Education is the accrediting agency for programs in the United States and Canada (Milbank Memorial Fund, 1998).

The scope of naturopathic practice is determined by state law. Currently, eleven states and five Canadian provinces issue licenses for naturopathic physicians (NDs). The laws typically allow standard diagnostic procedures, a range of therapies, vaccinations, and limited prescriptive rights. Some states allow the practice of natural childbirth. In states that do not license NDs, anyone can call herself/himself a naturopathic doctor after completing some correspondence courses. These individuals may give seminars and advise people on healthy lifestyles, but they are not permitted to diagnose illness or to prescribe treatment. When seeking an ND as a primary care physician, people must ask for verification of graduation from an accredited naturopathic medical school (Milbank Memorial Fund, 1998).

The education of naturopathic physicians is extensive and similar to conventional medical education. Four years of medical school follow a college degree in a biological science. The first two years of medical school include courses in anatomy, cell biology, nutrition, physiology, pathology, neurosciences, histology, pharmacology, biostatistics, epidemiology, and public health as well as alternative therapies. Some differences are significant. For example, conventional medical students may have only four course hours of nutritional education, while naturopathic medical students have 138 course hours in nutrition. The third and fourth years of medical school are oriented toward clinical experience in diagnosis and treatment. Today's naturopathic doctor is an extensively educated, primary care physician able to utilize a broad range of conventional and alternative therapies (*Alternative Medicine,* 1994; Pizzorno, 1996).

CONCEPTS

Naturopathic medicine holds the same view of human physiology, bodily functions, and disease process as conventional medicine. While many alternative health care professions are defined by the therapies used, naturopathy is defined more by basic concepts.

Healing Power of Nature

It is believed that the body innately knows how to maintain health and heal itself. Natural laws of life operate inside and outside the body and the physician's job is to support and restore them by using techniques and medicines that are in harmony with the natural processes. These natural methods are geared to strengthen the body's own healing ability. Faith, hope, and beliefs may be the most significant aspects of any treatment. Many studies have documented the ability of the mind to affect the process of disease, either positively or negatively. Physicians consider issues such as "What does it mean, for this person, to be in balance?" and "What are the healing powers available for this person?"

First Do No Harm

Iatrogenic illness, the creation of additional problems from medical treatment, is a major health problem in the United States. Steel and colleagues (1981) found that at least one-third of all inpatients suffered some ill effect from the medical treatment plan. Nine percent of the patients' lives were threatened or they suffered a major disability and two percent of patients died from the iatrogenic disorder. More recently Lazarou, Pomeranz, and Corey (1998) found that adverse drug reactions appear to be between the fourth and sixth leading cause of death in the United States. Furthermore, drug-related injuries occur in almost seven percent of hospitalized patients.

As Hippocrates said, "Above all else, do no harm." Naturopathic physicians prefer noninvasive treatments that minimize the risk of harmful side effects. Issues considered are "Will a delay in treatment be of benefit?" and "What is the potential for harm with this particular treatment plan?"

Find the Cause

Naturopathic physicians look for the underlying causes of disease and try to help patients eliminate them. These causes are often found in people's lifestyles, habits, and/or diets. Physical, mental, emotional, and spiritual factors are important in determining cause. Issues considered are "What are the causative factors contributing to 'dis-ease' in this person? Of these causative factors, which are avoidable or preventable? What are the limiting factors in this person's life?"

Physician as Teacher

The word *doctor* comes from the Latin *docere,* meaning to teach. Unlike many conventional medical physicians who have little time to teach, the primary focus of naturopathic physicians is teaching people how to achieve health and avoid disease. The emphasis is on people learning to assume responsibility for themselves and their well-being. A growing awareness among consumers views good health as dependent to a great extent on treating the body properly. Consumers are looking for health care practitioners who can teach them how to treat all aspects in a healthy manner, and naturopathic physicians are an appropriate choice for many. Issues to be considered include "What type of patient education is the physician providing? In what ways does the physician encourage and support patient responsibility?"

VIEW OF HEALTH AND ILLNESS

Naturopathy views health as more than the absence of disease. Health is a dynamic process that allows people to thrive despite various internal and external stresses. Health arises from a complex interaction of physical, mental, emotional, spiritual, dietary, genetic, environmental, lifestyle, and other components. Health is characterized by positive emotions, thoughts, and actions. Healthy people are energetic and creative as they live goal-directed lives. Health does not come from doctors, pills, or surgery, but rather from people's own efforts to take appropriate care of themselves (Pizzorno, 1996).

Naturopathic physicians recognize the role of bacteria and viruses in illness but view these as secondary factors. They believe that most disease is the direct result of ignoring natural laws. These violations include eating processed foods, having little exercise and rest, living a fast-paced lifestyle, focusing on negative thoughts and emotions, and being exposed to environmental toxins. Disease-promoting habits lead people away from optimal function toward progressively greater dysfunction in body, mind, and spirit. Naturopathy recognizes death is inevitable, but believes progressive disability is often avoidable (Pizzorno, 1996).

DIAGNOSTIC METHODS

Naturopathic physicians practice as primary care providers. They see people of all ages suffering from all types of disorders and diseases. They make conventional medical diagnoses using standard diagnostic procedures such as physical examinations, laboratory tests, and radiology. They also perform a detailed assessment of lifestyle, looking for physical, emotional, dietary, genetic, environmental, and family dynamics contributing to a disorder. Since health or disease is a complex interaction of factors, naturopathic physicians treat the whole person, taking all these elements into account. Careful attention to each person's individuality and susceptibility to disease is critical to accurate diagnosis. When necessary, naturopathic physicians, like family practice physicians, refer patients to other health care professionals for hospitalization, surgery, or other specialized care (Pizzorno, 1996).

TREATMENT

Naturopathic physicians do not provide emergency care nor do they do major surgery. They rarely prescribe drugs and they treat clients in private practice and outpatient clinics, not in hospitals. Some physicians practice natural childbirth at home or in a clinic.

The therapeutic approach of the naturopathic doctor is to help people heal themselves and to use opportunities to guide and educate people in developing healthier lifestyles. The goal of treatment is the restoration of health and normal body function, rather than the application of a particular therapy. Virtually every natural medical therapy is utilized, most of which are described in this text. Physicians mix and match different approaches, customizing treatment for each person. The least invasive intervention to support the body's natural healing processes is a primary consideration. These interventions include dietetics, therapeutic nutrition, herbs (European, Native American, and

Chinese), physical therapy, spinal manipulation, acupuncture, lifestyle counseling, stress management, exercise therapy, homeopathy, and hydrotherapy. Counseling is an important intervention because mental, emotional, and spiritual factors are part of the holistic approach. Lifestyle modification is crucial to the success of naturopathy. While it is relatively easy to tell a person to stop smoking, get more exercise, and reduce stress, such lifestyle changes are often difficult for people to make. The naturopathic physician is educated to assist people in making the needed changes. This process involves helping people acknowledge the need to change habits; identifying reinforcers for unhealthy habits; setting realistic and progressive goals; establishing a support group of family, friends, and others with similar difficulties; and giving people positive recognition for their gains (Pizzorno, 1996).

RESEARCH

The American Association of Naturopathic Physicians publishes the *Journal of Naturopathic Medicine,* which includes articles on original research, research reviews, and news and review articles relating to naturopathic medicine. Naturopathic schools of medicine have active research departments investigating a number of healing therapies. Because treatment programs are individually designed, it is nearly impossible to compare naturopathic medicine with conventional medicine, since simply too many variables are involved. Scientific research in particular therapies has been conducted in China, India, Germany, France, and England. In the United States, substantial scientific information is readily available on the effectiveness of diet and lifestyle in modifying the risk of severe illness such as heart disease and cancer. Hundreds of scientific papers address diet, nutritional supplements, herbs, exercise, and acupuncture. Some of the other natural healing therapies have not been fully investigated from the Western scientific perspective. It may be many years before science is sophisticated enough to understand some of these therapies (*Alternative Medicine,* 1994; Loecher and O'Donnell, 1997; Murray, 1994).

INTEGRATED NURSING PRACTICE

Interestingly, the bond between nursing and naturopathy is demonstrated by the enrollment in U.S. Naturopathic Colleges of Medicine; one-third of the students are nurses who have chosen this path to continue their post-baccalaureate education. The profession of nursing, like naturopathy, has traditionally embraced the concept of the healing power of nature and the belief that the locus of restoring health is within each person and cannot be "given" to a client by health care practitioners. Drugs, herbs, procedures, surgeries, or mind-body techniques may be helpful or necessary, but by themselves do not cure disease. People must, and do, rebalance and repair themselves. The profession of nursing was founded on this philosophy and view of life as noted by Florence Nightingale's basic premise that healing is a function of nature that comes from within the individual. She saw the role of the nurse as putting the "patient in the best condition for nature to act on him" (1969).

Nursing has always focused on education of those who have been entrusted to our care. We believe that through education we empower others by providing the knowledge, skills, and support to tap into their inner wisdom and make healthy decisions for themselves. This concept is basic to the practice of nursing and is evidenced in the American Nurses Association's Standard of Nursing Practice where health teaching is one of the standards. The goal of nursing, as in naturopathy, is one of healing and, if possible, the restoration of health. Because nurses spend so much more time with clients than do physicians, we are often in a position to prevent or respond quickly to iatrogenic illnesses. To this end, it is critically important that we monitor closely the impact of medications on the recipients. We must know the physiological action, expected effects, side effects, and adverse effects of every medication we administer. We must assess and reassess clients who are receiving medications. Likewise, we must understand procedures and their potential problems for all clients in our care. It is up to each one of us to maintain clinical skills through self-study and continuing education.

TRY THIS: *Visualization*

Visualization is one of many interventions used by nurses. This visualization is called "Winched up the Hill." Next time you are faced with a hill to ascend, imagine a winch at the top and a chord from it to your solar plexus. Invite the winch to draw you upward, easily and effortlessly. At first it may make little difference, but persevere with the visualization at every opportunity until you train yourself to tune into this extra source of energy. Respect the power of intent and subtle energies.

Source: Rutherford, *Principles of Shamanism* (San Francisco: Thorsons, 1996).

REFERENCES

Alternative Medicine: Expanding Medical Horizons. 1994. A report to the National Institutes of Health on Alternative Medical Systems and Practices in the United States. U.S. Government Printing Office. Washington, DC.

CASSILETH, B. R. 1998. *The Alternative Medicine Handbook.* New York: W. W. Norton.

LAZAROU, J., B. H. POMERANZ, and P. N. COREY. 1998. Incidence of adverse drug reactions in hospitalized patients. *JAMA.* 279: 1200–1205.

LOECHER, B. and A. O'DONNELL. 1997. *New Choices in Natural Healing for Women.* Emmaus, PA: Rodale Press.

Milbank Memorial Fund. 1998. *Enhancing the Accountability of Alternative Medicine.* New York: Milbank Memorial Fund.

MURRAY, M. T. 1994. *Natural Alternatives to Over-the-Counter and Prescription Drugs.* New York: William Morrow & Co.

NIGHTINGALE, F. 1969. *Notes on Nursing.* New York: Dover Press.

PIZZORNO, J. E. 1996. Naturopathic medicine. In M. S. MICOZZI, ed. *Fundamentals of Complementary and Alternative Medicine.* New York: Churchill Livingstone, 163–181.

RUTHERFORD, L. 1996. *Principles of Shamanism.* San Francisco: Thorsons.

STEEL, K., P. M. GERTMAN, C. CRESCENZI, and J. ANDERSON. 1981. Iatrogenic illness on general medical service at a university hospital. *N Eng J Med.* 304: 638–642.

RESOURCES

American Association of Naturopathic Physicians
601 Valley Street, Suite 105
Seattle, WA 98109
206-328-8510
www.infinite.org/naturopathic.physician

British Naturopathic and Osteopathic Association
Frazer House
6 Netherall Gardens
London NW3 5RR
01458-840 072

Naturopathic Medicine Network
www.pandamedicine.com

8　Homeopathy

The art of healing comes from Nature,
not the physician . . . every illness has its
own remedy within itself. . . . A man could
not be born alive and healthy were there
not already a Physician hidden in him.

Paracelsus, 1493–1541,
Swiss alchemist and physician

Miracles do not happen in contradiction
of nature, but in contradiction to what
we know about nature.

Saint Augustine

Homeopathy is derived from the Greek words *omoios,* meaning "similar"
and *pathos* meaning "feeling." It is a self-healing system, assisted by
small doses of remedies or medicines, that is useful in a variety of acute
and chronic disorders. The practice of homeopathy in the United States
has increased tremendously since the 1980s, corresponding to the increase
in other forms of alternative medicine. An estimated 3,000 health care
practitioners currently use homeopathy, and a survey in 1993 (Eisenberg)
showed that 1 percent of the general population, or 2.5 million Americans,
sought help from a homeopathic practitioner. Homeopathic medicine is
practiced worldwide, especially in Europe, Latin America, and Asia. In
Great Britain, visits to homeopaths are increasing at a rate of 29 percent a
year. Forty-two percent of British physicians refer people to homeopaths.
Forty percent of Dutch physicians, 25 percent of German physicians, and
32 percent of French physicians use homeopathy. India has more than 100
homeopathic medical colleges and more than 100,000 homeopathic practitioners (Jacobs and Moskowitz, 1996; Lerner, 1996)

In the United States, the homeopathic drug market has grown into a
multimillion-dollar industry. The National Center for Homeopathy estimates
that Americans spend $165 million a year for homeopathic preparations and
that sales are rising by 20–25 percent a year. Most of these remedies are not

regulated by the FDA and are available as over-the-counter medications (*Alternative Medicine,* 1994; Milbank, 1998).

BACKGROUND

Homeopathy, as a therapeutic system, is approximately 200 years old. It was developed by Samuel Hahnemann (1755–1843), a German physician and chemist. Homeopathy came to most of Europe, the United States, Russia, and Latin America in the 1830s. During epidemics of cholera, typhus, and scarlet fever, homeopathy was significantly more effective than the conventional medical approaches of the times. In 1869, the American Institute of Homeopathy opened free dispensaries for the poor and voted to admit female physicians, unheard of in conventional medicine. By the 1890s, 15 percent of American physicians used some homeopathic remedies in their practice, learned in the 22 homeopathic medical schools and practiced in more than 100 homeopathic hospitals (Castleman, 1996; Lerner, 1996).

During and after the Civil War, the practice of medicine began to change with technical achievements such as anesthesia, antisepsis, surgery, microbiology, vaccines, and antibiotics. State legislatures began to license physicians and accredit medical schools. The American Medical Association (AMA) invited homeopaths to become members in exchange for licensing, seeking to create a monopoly against lay healers, midwives, and herbalists. When the homeopaths chose not to join forces, the AMA began to persecute homeopathy, and in 1914, proposed uniform standards of medical education and assumed the power of accreditation, using it to phase out homeopathic colleges. Between the 1920s and 1970s, homeopathic education in the United States was almost nonexistent (Jacobs and Moskowitz, 1996).

PREPARATION

About half of the homeopaths in the United States are physicians. The others are licensed health care practitioners such as nurse practitioners, dentists, naturopathic physicians, chiropractors, acupuncturists, and veterinarians. Training in homeopathy is offered through professional courses at the National Center for Homeopathy in Alexandria, Virginia. The certification process involves a specified number of hours of training, three years of clinical practice, and written and oral examinations. Certification earns the right to place the designation "DHt" after one's name. Licensure to practice homeopathy varies among the states. At the present time, five states—Arizona, Connecticut,

Delaware, Nevada, and New Hampshire—have medical boards regulating homeopaths. Other states regulate practitioners through the "scope of practice" guidelines issued by medical boards (Frye, 1997; Milbank, 1998).

CONCEPTS

Law of Similars

Hahnemann proposed the use of the Law of Similars, which claims that a natural substance that produces a given symptom in a healthy person, cures it in a sick person. The substance whose symptom-picture most closely resembles the illness being treated is the one most likely to initiate a curative response for that person. Hence the name homeopathy—"similar feeling."

If taken in large amounts, these natural compounds will produce symptoms of disease. In the doses used by homeopaths, however, these remedies stimulate a person's self-healing capacity. As Andrew Weil states, "The difference between a poison and a medicine is the dose" (Frye, 1997). An example is seen in the use of Ipecac which in large doses causes severe nausea and vomiting. Women who are experiencing the nausea and vomiting of pregnancy, however, can use small doses of Ipecac to cure those same symptoms (Jacobs, 1984; Skinner, 1996).

Law of Infinitesimals

Natural healing compounds are specially prepared for homeopathic use through a process of serial dilution. The compound is first dissolved in a water-alcohol mixture called the "mother tincture." One drop of the tincture is then mixed with 10 drops of water-alcohol, and this process is repeated hundreds or thousands of times depending on the potency being prepared. At each step of the dilution, the vial is vigorously shaken, called *succussion,* which seems to be an essential step. The homeopathic belief is that the more the substance is diluted, the more potent it becomes as a remedy.

The remedies are diluted beyond the point at which any molecules of the substance can theoretically still be found in the solution. This paradox, that the remedy becomes more potent through dilution, is the reason many biomedical scientists reject homeopathic medicine. Just as biomedical pharmacologists do not understand the mechanisms of many conventional drugs, it is not presently understood how homeopathic remedies work. A number of theories are proposed. A remedy may be like a hologram. No matter how many times a substance is diluted, a smaller but complete essence of the substance remains.

Modern chaos theory supports the observation that major changes occur in living organisms when bodily substances are activated only slightly. The basic assumption of chaos theory is that minute changes can have huge effects. Advances in quantum physics have led some scientists to suggest that electromagnetic energy in the remedies interact with the body on some level. Researchers in physical chemistry have proposed the memory of water theory in which the structure of the water-alcohol solution is altered during the process of dilution and retains its new structure even after the substance is no longer present. It seems likely that remedies work through a bioenergic or subatomic mechanism that we are not as yet capable of understanding. The situation may be likened to any number of advances in the understanding of energy such as radio, television, microwave ovens, and cordless telephones that previously were virtually unimaginable (*Alternative Medicine,* 1994; Frye, 1997; Jacobs and Moskowitz, 1996).

VIEW OF HEALTH AND ILLNESS

Homeopathy is a method for treating the sick rather than a set of hypotheses about the nature of health and illness. The assumption is, however, that a vital force—known as qi or prana in other traditions—exists. It is necessary to have adequate nutrition, exercise, rest, good hygiene, and a healthy environment to adapt and maintain homeostasis. In other words, health is the ability of people to adapt their equilibrium in response to internal and external change. Illness is primarily a disturbance of the vital force manifesting as symptoms of distress. Vital force or life energy is the ultimate origin of health and illness, alike, ending only with the death of the person (Jacobs and Moskowitz, 1996).

Symptoms of illness represent people's attempts to heal themselves. Thus, homeopathy views symptoms as an adaptive reaction that is the best possible response that can be made in the present circumstances. For example, a cough is the body's attempt to clear the bronchi; inflammation is the body's effort to wall off and burn out invading foreign bodies; and fever is the body's way to create an internal environment that is less conducive to bacterial or viral growth. Given this perspective, the therapeutic approach is to aid the body's efforts to adapt to stress or infection. Thus, for someone with a high fever, homeopaths may recommend belladonna, which increases the natural healing response of body heat. The Law of Similars is a stimulation of immune and defense responses leading to spontaneous resolution of symptoms as the illness is conquered. In like manner, two of the few conventional therapies that seek to stimulate the body's own healing reaction, immunization and allergy treatment, have the homeopathic Law of Similars as their basis. Other applications in conventional medicine include the use of radiation in the treatment of cancer and Ritalin in the treatment of hyperactive children. The majority of interventions in biomedicine, however, attempt to oppose symptoms by exerting a greater and opposite force. Medicines are designed to "cure" by suppressing symptoms such as the use of aspirin in an effort to control or limit people's fevers. The danger is that, over time, suppressive treatments may actually strengthen disease processes instead of resolving them (Weil, 1995).

DIAGNOSTIC METHODS

Homeopathic diagnosis is holistic and detailed. The initial assessment may last several hours. Practitioners assess the whole person, looking at every aspect of physical, emotional, and mental life. A multitude of factors are considered, such as nutritional status, emotional imbalance, and environmental stress. It is believed that no part can be isolated from the whole person. The homeopathic interview itself is a powerful healing experience because clients are encouraged to tell their story in its entirety. They are encouraged to speak for as long a time as possible. This process of sharing pain and suffering begins the healing process. During the interview, the practitioner observes everything about the person including posture, dress, facial expression, tone of voice, rate of speech, etc. The physical exam is a head-to-toe assessment with the inclusion of laboratory work as needed to establish a diagnosis. Answers to questions are elicited in an attempt to fully understand the significance of the symptoms:

- Subjective symptoms such as pain, vertigo, fatigue, or anger
- Localization of symptoms such as one-sided, wandering, radiating, or diffuse
- Factors that modify the symptoms, making them better or worse, such as time of day, hot or cold, weather, diet, or emotional state
- Quality of symptoms such as burning, aching, throbbing
- Rate of onset or resolution of the symptoms such as sudden or gradual
- Symptoms that appear simultaneously or in sequence

Symptoms are classified into three categories—the general physical symptoms, the local symptoms, and the mental and emotional symptoms. General physical symptoms include such things as sleep, appetite, energy, temperature, or generalized bodily pain. Local symptoms occur in particular parts of the body such as swelling in the right elbow or pain in the left leg. Included in local symptoms are those related to a specific organ function such as shortness of breath or palpitations. Mental and emotional symptoms include anxiety, irritability, anger, tearfulness, isolation, or suspiciousness. This composite picture of the person is far more important than any isolated laboratory findings or abstract disease category in formulating the diagnosis (Frye, 1997). Homeopathic practitioners do not hesitate to refer to biomedical specialists for conventional drugs or surgery.

TREATMENT

As in other complementary practices, the initial question is always "Who is the person?" rather than "What is the disease?" This focus ensures an individualized approach to treatment. Each person with the same presenting complaint may be treated with different remedies, depending on the totality of physical, mental, and emotional symptoms. A person with a sore throat may be prescribed one of six or seven common remedies for sore throats, depending on whether the pain is worse on the right or left side, what time of day it is worse, how thirst and appetite are affected, and the individual's emotional state (*Alternative Medicine,* 1994).

The science and the art of homeopathy is to find the remedy with the ability to mimic most closely the sick person's pattern of symptoms. Practitioners use only one remedy at a time, since administering different remedies for different symptoms makes it difficult to know which remedy was effective. Not only are the smallest possible doses used, typically only one dose is given, which allows time for the remedy to complete its action without further interference. If necessary, a dose may be repeated or another remedy may be tried. A temporary worsening of the symptoms may occur after receiving the remedy, which is usually mild and short-lived and may be an indication that the correct remedy was chosen (Frye, 1996).

Homeopathy is used to treat both acute and chronic health problems as well as for health promotion. It cannot cure conditions resulting from structural, long-term, organic changes such as cirrhosis, diabetes, chronic obstructive lung disease, advanced neurological diseases, or cancer. In some of these cases, homeopathy can palliate the symptoms and increase the client's comfort level.

Traumatic injuries affect nearly everyone in similar ways and thus the remedies are fairly standard. Epidemic infectious diseases also tend to affect most victims in the same way and individuals are usually treated with the same remedy. Common infectious illnesses such as urinary tract infections, respiratory infections, or ear infections demonstrate more individual symptoms and require more individualization in selecting the remedy. Chronic illness such as ulcerative colitis, rheumatoid arthritis, asthma, and skin disorders are considered to be constitutional. Thus these disorders require the most skillful assessment, individualized prescription, and follow-up (Frye, 1997).

The Homeopathic Pharmacopoeia of the United States, listing more than 2,000 remedies, is the official standard for preparation and prescription. Most remedies come from plants used in traditional herbal medicine. A few remedies come from animal sources and others from naturally occurring chemical compounds. Box 8.1 lists examples of remedies. Some, such as mercury and belladonna, would be poisonous in large doses but are safe in the superdilute homeopathic doses. These remedies rank among the safest medicines available (Castleman, 1996).

Box 8.1: Examples of Homeopathic Remedies

Plant	Mineral	Animal
Herbs: comfrey, eyebright, mullein, yellow dock	**Metals:** copper, gold, lead, tin, zinc	**Venoms:** jellyfish, insects, spiders, mollusks, crustaceans, fish, snakes, amphibians
Foods and spices: cayenne, garlic, mustard, onion	**Salts:** calcium sulfate, sodium chloride, potassium carbonate	**Secretions:** ambergris, musk, cuttlefish ink
Fragrances, resins, residues: amber, petroleum, charcoal, creosote	**Acids:** hydrochloric, nitric, phosphoric, sulfuric	**Milks**
Mushrooms, lichens, mosses	**Elemental substances:** carbon, hydrogen, iodine, phosphorus, sulfur	**Hormones**
	Constituents of earth's crust: silica, aluminum oxide, ores, rocks, lavas, mineral waters	**Glandular and tissue extracts**
		Disease products: vaccines, abscesses, tuberculosis, gonorrhea, syphilis

Source: Castleman, Nature's Cures (Emmaus, PA: Rodale Press, 1996); Jacobs and Moskowitz, in Fundamentals of Complementary and Alternative Medicine, M. S. Micozzi, ed. (New York: Churchill Livingstone, 1996), 67–78.

RESEARCH

As in other areas of medical research, the two questions are "How does it work?" and "How well does it work?" Many researchers are studying the physics of how homeopathic remedies work. At this time it seems likely that remedies work through a bioenergic or subatomic mechanism that is not yet understood or measurable. Research in the areas of quantum physics, physical chemistry, and biochemistry may someday be able to answer the question of how the remedies work.

Since the mid 1980s, more research regarding the efficacy of remedies has been conducted, especially in Scotland, Britain, France, Germany, and the Netherlands. These clinical trials have suggested a positive effect of homeopathic remedies on pollen allergy, fibromylagia, flu, varicose veins, and acute childhood diarrhea. A double-blind study with people suffering from rheumatoid arthritis showed that 82 percent of those who had been given a homeopathic remedy experienced some relief of symptoms, while only 21 percent of those who had been given a placebo experienced a similar degree of improvement (*Alternative Medicine,* 1994).

A meta-analysis of 105 clinical studies of homeopathy published in 1992 found that 81 of the studies reported a positive result for homeopathic treatments. A meta-analysis of 89 clinical trials published in 1997 also found that homeopathic remedies have a more positive clinical effect than a placebo (Milbank, 1998).

INTEGRATED NURSING PRACTICE

Nurses, like homeopathic practitioners, emphasize listening to clients' stories of their lives. It is within the context of people's lives that we identify patterns of response to illnesses and disorders and formulate nursing diagnoses. Nursing diagnoses and outcome criteria focus our attention on adaptations that may help people live healthier lifestyles. The study of mental health nursing in our basic educational program teaches us the value of listening and attending to people's pain, as an intervention to help them begin the process of healing. These principles are common to both nursing and homeopathy, illustrating, once again, the broad base of nursing practice. Some nurse practitioners, valuing the contributions of homeopathy to well-being, continue their education and achieve licensure to practice homeopathic medicine. As nurses educated in Western approaches, we are more likely to suppress symptoms in an attempt to "cure" the disease. In many situations, it may be more beneficial to follow the homeopathic approach and view symptoms as the body's attempt to heal itself. We may find clients improve more quickly when non-life-threatening symptoms are supported rather than suppressed, such as low to moderate grade fevers or productive coughs.

People who are interested in homeopathic remedies can find low potency remedies in health food stores. Higher potency remedies are obtained from homeopathic pharmaceutical companies under the direction of experienced homeopathic prescribers. Since remedies are inactivated by direct sunlight and heat, teach people to store the preparations in a dark, dry place, away from other strong-smelling substances. When taking a remedy, they should have nothing by mouth for at least 30 minutes before and after the dose. Many homeopaths discourage the use of coffee, mint, camphor, and other strongly aromatic substances while undergoing treatment, since such substances may reverse the effects of the remedy. Camphor is a component in chest rubs as well as in many cosmetics, skin creams, and lip balms. If the remedy is in the form of a pellet, it should be held under the tongue and allowed to dissolve slowly. If the remedy is a liquid, it is held in the mouth for 1 to 2 minutes before swallowing.

Prescription medications, especially those given for potentially life-threatening disorders such as asthma, should not be stopped abruptly when beginning homeopathic care. As the person improves, however, a downward titration of the biomedical prescription may be needed. Acupuncture and chiropractic medicine should not be started at the same time as homeopathic remedies, but if already instituted, may be continued (Jacobs and Moskowitz, 1996).

A number of homeopathic remedies can be used to speed recovery and prevent recurrences of acute conditions such as colds, stomachaches, coughs, and headaches. Although many remedies are used for conditions that subside on their own, they can dramatically speed recovery and often prevent recurrences. Since homeopathic medicines are considerably safer than conventional drugs, it often makes sense to use them as the first resort and to consider using conventional drugs if the homeopathic remedies work too slowly or not at all. People should read all the information on the label to select the right remedy. If it says, for example, that the remedy is best used when the symptoms appear suddenly, then that remedy is not likely to be effective for a condition that emerged almost unnoticed over several days. You can teach clients the following three guidelines for the use of homeopathic remedies (Ullman, 1997):

1. The more the better: The more the symptoms match that of the remedy, the more likely it will work.
2. The less the better: The more dilute the remedy, the more powerful it is.
3. It's working if you feel better within 24 hours. If not, you may have the wrong remedy and may need a different remedy or may need to see a health care practitioner.

Many people keep homeopathic remedies on hand and ready to use. The TRY THIS box lists the top ten remedies that help with the most common physical problems and emotional difficulties.

TRY THIS: *Top Ten Remedies*

Bryonia (wild hops): for coughs that are worsened by simple breathing; headaches that are increased by bending over, walking, or even moving the eyes; constipation with dry, hard stools.

Allium cepa (onion): for colds or respiratory allergies where symptoms resemble the reaction of a person exposed to the mist of an onion: watery eyes, clear nasal discharge, and sneezes, all of which are aggravated by exposure to heat.

Pulsatilla (windflower): need is based on the type of person, rather than a specific ailment. Helpful for people who are highly emotional, weepy, impressionable, easily influenced, fearful of abandonment, and worried about what others think of them. May also be used for digestive disorders, allergies, earaches, headaches, insomnia, and PMS.

Ignatia (St. Ignatius bean): for people who experience anxiety or grief.

Arsenicum album (arsenic): used for many conditions especially when symptoms are worse after midnight, when burning symptoms are predominant, when great thirst occurs, or when the person is high strung and restless.

Belladonna (deadly nightshade): for fevers or inflammation that begin rapidly, with a red or flushed appearance, and the person is hypersensitive to touch or light.

Gelsemium (yellow jessamine): for classic flu symptoms accompanied by lack of thirst. Helpful for headaches in the back part of the head.

Nux vomica (poison nut): useful after overdosing with food or drink, indigestion, constipation, and headaches that are worse at night and on waking.

Aconitum (monkshood): for colds, flu, coughs, and sore throats with rapid onset.

Rhus toxicodendron (poison ivy): helpful for arthritis syndromes, flu, sprains and strains, and sore throats. For people who feel pain on initial motion that eases with continued motion and symptoms worse in cold or wet weather.

Source: Ullman, Homeopathy's Top Ten, *Natural Health* (July–August, 1997), 60–64.

REFERENCES

Alternative Medicine: Expanding Medical Horizons. 1994. A report to the National Institutes of Health on Alternative Medical Systems and Practices in the United States. U.S. Government Printing Office. Washington, DC.

CASTLEMAN, M. 1996. *Nature's Cures.* Emmaus, PA: Rodale Press.

EISENBERG, D. M. et al. 1993. Unconventional medicine in the United States. *N Eng J Med.* 328: 246–252.

FRYE, J. 1997. Homeopathy in office practice. *Primary Care.* 24(4): 845–864.

JACOBS, J. 1984. Homeopathy and women's health. In K. WEISS, ed. *Women's Health Care: A Guide to Alternatives.* Reston, VA: Reston Pub, 196–207.

JACOBS, J. and R. MOSKOWITZ. 1996. In: M. S. MICOZZI, ed. *Fundamentals of Complementary and Alternative Medicine.* New York: Churchill Livingstone, 67–78.

LERNER, M. 1996. The memory of water, the promise of homeopathy. *Advances: J Mind-Body Health.* 12(1): 69–75.

Milbank Memorial Fund. 1998. *Enhancing the Accountability of Alternative Medicine.* New York: Milbank Memorial Fund.

SKINNER, S. 1996. How homeopathy works. *RN.* 59(12): 53–56.

ULLMAN, D. July–August 1997. Homeopathy's top ten. *Natural Health.* 60–64.

WEIL, A. 1995. *Spontaneous Healing.* New York: Alfred A. Knopf.

RESOURCES

American Board of Homeotherapeutics
6231 Leesburg Pike, Suite 506
Falls Church, VA 22044

American Institute of Homeopathy
7297-H Lee Highway
Falls Church, VA 22042

Homeopathic Educational Services
2124 Kittredge St.
Berkeley, CA 94704
501-649-0294
www.homeopathic.com

International Foundation for Homeopathy
2366 Eastlake Ave. East, Suite 301
Seattle, WA 98102
206-324-8230

National Center for Homeopathy
810 North Fairfax, Suite 306
Alexandria, VA 22314
703-548-7790
www.homeopathic.org

9   Aromatherapy

> The art of medicine sometimes consists
> of amusing the patient while Nature
> cures the disease.
>
> *Voltaire*

Aromatherapy is the therapeutic use of essential oils of plants in which the odor or fragrance plays an important part. It is an offshoot of herbal medicine with the basis of action the same as that of modern pharmacology. The chemicals found in the essential oils are absorbed into the body resulting in physiological or psychological benefit (Stevensen, 1996). Aromatherapy is the use of essential oils to treat symptoms and as such has no theory of health and illness nor a system of diagnosis.

Scientists have long known that certain scents have the power to evoke strong physical and emotional reactions but rarely has that knowledge been used in conventional medicine. Healthy humans can smell as many as 10,000 different odors, ranging from the deep fragrance of jasmine to the putrid stench of sewage. Most people, however, do not realize how much the sense of smell affects their daily lives.

Aromatherapy has been forgotten and ignored for many years but is now one of the fastest growing alternative therapies in Europe and the United States. The term *aromatherapy* has become more than a buzzword since the mid 1980s. In the United States, it is now a generic term in the public domain and, as such, cannot be trade-marked by an individual or business (Meadows, 1997).

Essential oils come from all over the world—lavender from France, sandalwood and jasmine from India, rose from Turkey and Bulgaria, geranium from the island of Reunion, eucalyptus and tea tree from Australia, and mint from the United States. Today, only 3 percent of essential oils are used in therapy; the remaining 97 percent are used in the perfume and cosmetic industry. With increased popularity, aromatherapy has become a $300 million-a-year market in the United States (Aromatherapy Unlimited, 1997).

BACKGROUND

Almost all ancient cultures recognized the value of aromatic plants in maintaining health. Ancient Egyptians used scented oils daily to soften and protect their skin from the harsh, dry climate. They created various fragrances for personal benefit as well as for use in rituals and ceremonies. Fragrances were considered a part of the personal purification necessary to reach a realm of higher spirituality. Oils were dispersed into the air to purify the environment and provide protection from evil spirits. Egyptians were the first to perfect embalming with the use of aromatic plants and oils (Young, 1996).

Priests and physicians used oils thousands of years before the time of Christ. The Ebers Papyrus, discovered in 1817, dates back to 1500 B.C. and mentions more than 800 different formulas of herbal prescriptions and remedies. The Romans diffused oils in their temples and political buildings and bathed in hot tubs scented with oils. Ancient Arabian people studied the chemistry of plants and developed the process of distillation for extraction of essential oils. Throughout Asia perfumes were prized for both medicinal and cosmetic properties. Hundreds of references are made to oils in the Bible such as frankincense, myrrh, and cinnamon. Many were used as protection against disease and for anointing and healing the sick. Hippocrates, the father of Western medicine, reportedly said, "The way to health is to have an aromatic bath and scented massage every day" (Castleman, 1996; Maxwell-Hudson, 1994).

In the twelfth century, trade routes from the Middle East brought spices, herbs, and exotic scents to Europe, leading to the compilation of many books on therapeutic plant remedies. In the Americas, shamans also used herbs and aromatics in the bathing of patients to transform their energy field. Smoke from plants was often blown over patients as part of the healing ceremony (Stevensen, 1996).

Although oils were used with great effectiveness in ancient times, they were largely forgotten by the Western world until resurrected in the twentieth century by a French cosmetic chemist, Maurice-Rene Cattefosse. While working in his laboratory in 1920, he had an accident that resulted in a third degree burn of his hand and forearm. He plunged his arm into a vat of lavender oil, thinking that it was water. To his surprise, the burning stopped within a few moments. With the continual application of lavender oil over the next few weeks, the burn healed completely without a trace of a scar. This incident was the beginning of Cattefosse's fascination with the therapeutic properties of essential oils. He carried out experiments using oils to cure burns, treat wounds, and prevent gangrene and in 1937 coined the term *aromatherapie* (Maxwell-Hudson, 1994).

PREPARATION

Since the 1980s, numerous schools of massage and aromatherapy have opened in Britain. Training in aromatherapy has grown, and courses in it are part of the nursing degree program in some nursing colleges and universities. Aromatherapists practice in a number of settings including private practices, general medical clinics, and hospitals. Currently, no law specifies a minimum level of training and practice in the United Kingdom (Stevensen, 1996).

Some people in the United States, after a weekend course, call themselves "aromatherapists." They may know little about plant chemistry and the specific ways in which the oils need to be formulated. Their self-proclaimed title is fine if they use oils only for fragrance and perfume. Using oil formulas for a specific therapeutic action is inappropriate, however, for individuals with this limited knowledge. The Institute of Aromatherapy in Denville, New Jersey, was approved in 1997 by the New Jersey Department of Education and the state of South Carolina, making it the first state-approved aromatherapy school in the United States. Their 200 in-class hours are designed to provide a comprehensive knowledge of aromatherapy including classes in botany, psychoneuroimmunology, and plant chemistry (Aromatherapy Unlimited, 1997).

CONCEPTS

Essential Oils

Essential oils are volatile liquids that are distilled or cold pressed from plants. Although chemically they are oils and as such do not mix with water, the term *oil* is somewhat misleading, since they feel like water rather than oil. Varying amounts of essential oil can be extracted from a particular plant, which influences the price of the oil. For example, it takes 220 pounds of rose petals to furnish less than two ounces of the essential oil. Other plants such as lavender or eucalyptus give a much greater proportion. One-half ounce of rose oil may cost $200 while the same amount of orange oil may cost only a few dollars. A little oil goes a long way, however (Stevensen, 1996). Oils may be extracted from various parts of plants such as:

Leaves: eucalyptus, peppermint
Flowers: lavender, rose
Blossoms: orange, neroli
Fruits: lemon, mandarin
Grasses: lemongrass
Wood: camphor, sandalwood
Barks: cinnamon
Gum: frankincense
Bulbs: garlic, onion
Dried flower buds: clove

Essential oils are stored in tiny pockets between plant cell walls. As the plant releases the oil, it circulates through the plant and sends messages that help it function efficiently. Oils activate and regulate such activities as cellular metabolism, photosynthesis, and cellular respiration. They may also trigger immune responses to assist in coping with stressful changes in the environment and climate. Some oils protect the plant from predators, especially microorganisms and in so doing are essentially antibacterial, antiviral, and antifungal. Some oils protect the plant by repelling harmful insects while others attract insects or animals that are useful for propagation (Castleman, 1996; Wilson, 1995).

Plant oils are highly concentrated, and it is important to respect their power. One drop of oil is the medical equivalent of one ounce of the parent plant material used in herbal medicine. Essential oils are chemically diverse and may contain a mixture of more than 100 organic compounds including esters, alcohols, aldehydes, ketones, phenols, acids, and so on. Each oil may contain more of some compounds than others, which gives the oil its particular therapeutic use. Box 9.1 lists some of the major chemical components and their therapeutic effects.

Box 9.1: Chemical Compounds of Essential Oils and Their Therapeutic Actions

Chemical Compound	Therapeutic Action
Aldehydes	Anti-infectious, boost immune system, sedative
Eugenol	Antiseptic, stimulant
Ketones	Sedative, liquefy mucous, stimulate cell regeneration
Phenols	Antiseptic
Esters	Antispasmodic, calming
Sesquiterpenes	Antihistamines, anti-inflamatory
Acids	Anti-infectious, boost immune system
Oxides	Expectorant, antiparasitic
C10 terpenes	Antiseptic

Source: Stevensen, Aromatherapy, *Fundamentals of Complementary and Alternative Medicine,* M. S. Micozzi, ed. (New York: Churchill Livingstone, 1996), 137–148; Young, *An Introduction to Young Living Essential Oils and Aromatherapy* (Salt Lake City: Essential Press Pub., 1996).

How Essential Oils Work

The sense of smell is an important part of aromatherapy. Inside the human nose is a small cavity called the *vomero nasal organ* (VMO), which is lined with a cell type that is unlike any other cell in the human body. The VMO is far less prominent in people than in animals who depend more heavily on smell for guidance. Pheromones are chemical substances produced by one animal that cause a specific reaction in another, usually of the same species, through smell. The VMO appears to specialize in detecting pheromones without people's conscious awareness. In other words, people do not "smell" pheromones in the same way they smell freshly baked apple pies or essential oils. The scent, however, is registered at some brain level and people respond to it emotionally and/or physically (Crenshaw, 1996).

In addition to the VMO, the nose contains 5 million smell-sensing cells that allow people to consciously register smells. Each cell has 6–12 hairlike receptors (cilia) that hang down into the stream of air rushing into the nose. These olfactory receptors are the only sensory pathways that open directly to the brain. The cilia detect scents and the nerve cells relay this information directly to the limbic system triggering memories and influencing behavior. The amygdala of the limbic system, which stores and releases emotional memories, is most sensitive to odor or fragrance. Thus, the sense of smell can evoke powerful memories in a split second and change people's perceptions and behaviors. Olfactory stimulation can trigger negative responses such as intense fear or panic or can trigger positive feelings with increased release of endorphins and neurotransmitters. Odors stimulate the pituitary gland and hypothalamus and thus impact the production of hormones that control appetite, insulin production, body temperature, metabolism, stress levels, and sex drive. Unlike vision and hearing, the sense of smell is fully functional at birth. Newborns can recognize their mothers by smell, and this sensory response is an important part of bonding. In adult relationships, the sense of smell has a significant role in sensual and sexual attraction (Castleman, 1996; Wilson, 1995).

In addition to activating the central nervous system, inhaled oil molecules enter the respiratory system. There the molecules attach to oxygen molecules and circulate through the body, bringing with them the potential for activating self-healing processes. The equivalent in conventional medicine is the use of inhalers in the treatment of asthma. Essential oils can be inhaled directly or mixed with a carrier oil. Electrical and fan-assisted equipment or an aromatherapy light bulb ring may be used to scent a room for therapeutic purposes or to simply make the environment more pleasant. Steam inhalers can be used in the treatment of respiratory infections (Chambers, 1998).

Applied externally, essential oils can calm inflamed or irritated skin, soothe sore muscles, decrease muscular tension, and release muscle spasms. Molecules of essential oils are so tiny they are quickly absorbed through the skin and enter the intercellular fluid and the circulatory system, bringing healing nutrients to the cells. Some oils such as basil, tea tree, and thyme encourage the production of white blood cells, while others such as lavender and eucalyptus fight harmful bacteria, viruses, and fungi. Oils may be applied just about anywhere: neck, face, wrists, over the heart, back, arms, legs, and feet. Massage therapists and acupuncturists often use essential oils in their treatments. Benefits are gained not only from the penetration of the oil through the skin but also from inhalation of the vapor and from direct massage of the skin and muscles. Essential oils do not remain in the body and are excreted in urine, feces, perspiration, and exhalation usually in 3–6 hours (Wilson, 1995).

A diffuser is a special air pump designed to disburse the oils in a microfine vapor into the atmosphere where they stay suspended for several hours. Diffusing releases oxygenating molecules as well as antiviral, antibacterial, and antiseptic properties. Unlike commercial air fresheners, which mask odors, essential oils clean the air by altering the structure of the molecules that create an unpleasant smell. Essential oils help remove dust particles out of the air and, when diffused in the room, can be an effective air filtration system (Wilson, 1995; Young, 1996).

TREATMENT

Essential oils influence health on physical, mental, and emotional levels. They have the ability to penetrate cell walls and transport oxygen and nutrients to the cell. Many have antiviral, antibacterial, antifungal, and antiseptic properties. This property of oils may be significant in the future as microbes continue to mutate and develop resistance to known medications. Aromatherapy can be used for the following purposes:

- Prompt the body and mind to function more efficiently
- Decrease and manage stress
- Refresh or recharge oneself
- Regulate moods—some are energizing and some are sedating
- Aid restful sleep
- Act as a first aid measure
- Reduce weight
- Boost the immune system
- Minimize the discomforts of illness and speed recovery
- Refresh room environment

The purity and authenticity of essential oils is critical to their effectiveness. Oils that are diluted, adulterated, or synthetic should not be used for aromatherapy. Those identified as commercial grade essential oils are likely to be diluted or adulterated in some way. Some are diluted with chemical carriers and passed on to the consumer as "pure essential oils" and are found in bath and cosmetic shops. Those labeled as "infused oils" are also adulterated. "Nature identical" oils are synthetic petrochemical-based products. They have been developed to closely mimic the smell and composition of essential oils. They are not identical, however, and lack many of the healing components of essential oils. Other names for synthetic oils are aroma-chemicals, perfume oils, and fragrance oils. Manufacturers have no restrictions on how essential oils are labeled. In general, those described with terms such as genuine, authentic, or premium are more likely to be pure essential oils. Informed consumers read labels carefully and buy from reputable dealers. The Institute of Aromatherapy can provide information on purchasing essential oils.

Essential oils are quite potent and can irritate the skin, so they should be diluted with a carrier oil before being used on the skin. Carrier oils contain vitamins, proteins, and minerals that provide added nutrients to the body. Some carrier oils can be purchased at supermarkets, while others may be available only at health food stores. Carrier oils include apricot kernel oil, sunflower oil, soy oil, sweet almond oil, grapeseed oil, sesame oil, avocado oil, jojoba, and wheat-germ oil. The fragrance does not have to be intense to be effective. In fact, the more intense the odor, the less pleasant it becomes.

By blending together two or more pure essential oils, a synergy can be created that is more powerful than the individual oils. The interaction of the oils with one another gives an added vibrancy to the blend. Synergistic blends are achieved by combining oils that complement each other. For example, the calming effects of lavender and bergamot or rosemary work well together. Oils with opposite effects, such as a soothing oil and a stimulating oil should not be blended. It is also important that the blend has a pleasing scent. See Box 9.2 for categories of oils to consider when formulating blends.

Box 9.2: Blending Oils According to Effects

Soothing Oils: Chamomile

Uplifting Oils: Black pepper, coriander, jasmine, juniper, eucalyptus, peppermint, tea tree

Balancing Oils: Cypress, lavender

Uplifting and Soothing Oils: Basil, bergamot, frankincense, ginger, neroli, orange, patchpuli, sandalwood

Uplifting and Stimulating Oils: Cedarwood, lemon, lemon grass, myrrh, pine, rose, rosemary, ylang ylang

Uplifting and Balancing Oils: Clary sage, geranium

Box 9.2: Blending Oils According to Effects (*continued*)

Examples of Blends:
  basil, lavender
  bergamot, cypress, jasmine
  chamomile, lavender
  clary sage, lavender, sandalwood
  eucalyptus, chamomile, lavender, bergamot
  geranium, bergamot, lemon, lavender
  ginger, lavender, orange, neroli
  jasmine, rose, lemon, blackpepper
  juniper, bergamot, geranium, frankincense
  lemon, tea tree, ylang ylang
  pine, eucalyptus, lavender
  patchouli, bergamot, geranium
  peppermint, lavender
  sandalwood, ylang ylang, black pepper, neroli

RESEARCH

The research basis for aromatherapy is in its infancy. Much of the research has been performed on animals and isolated tissue cultures. Few trials have been conducted on humans under clinical conditions. Little is known at this time about possible interactions with conventional medications or treatments.

  The antimicrobial aspects of essential oils have been the most widely investigated. The chemical constituents of alcohols, aldehydes, terpenes, and phenyl methyl ethers help to explain this action. Peppermint, commonly known for its benefit in digestive disorders, has been found to inhibit gastrointestinal smooth muscle in tissue models and affects the flow of calcium across the cell wall. A few studies have been conducted on the inhalation of essential oils and a change in brain wave activity. Those oils increasing brain beta wave activity associated with alertness include basil, clove, jasmine, neroli, peppermint, rose, and ylang ylang. Those oils increasing brain alpha wave activity associated with relaxation include bergamot, chamomile, lavender, lemon, and marjoram (Stevensen, 1996).

  For several years, Dr. Susan Schiffman at Duke University has been using apricot oil to help participants at the weight-loss clinic control their eating.

It seems to be helpful for those who eat in response to the feeling of anxiety. Participants inhale whiffs of apricot oil as they do relaxation exercises, thus associating the fragrance with a sense of calmness. Later, when the feeling of anxiety arises, they inhale apricot oil from a vial rather than eat in response to anxiety. At Memorial Sloan-Kettering Cancer Center in New York City, some clients are given heliotropin before having an MRI. This essential oil, a close relative of vanilla, significantly reduces anxiety during the claustrophobic procedure (Castleman, 1996). The Smell and Taste Treatment and Research Foundation of Chicago is conducting many studies on the therapeutic use of essential oils. Researchers at the Foundation have published evidence that aromatherapy with green-apple fragrance may be useful in managing migraine and other chronic headaches. It is hypothesized that the green-apple odor may modify the neurotransmitter involved in the pain pathway (Hirsch, 1998). A copy of all the research articles can be purchased for $200 directly from the Foundation.

Much of the aromatherapy research in conventional health care settings in Britain is being conducted by nurses. A number of studies are being done in intensive care settings and in the fields of midwifery, palliative care, and geriatric care.

INTEGRATED NURSING PRACTICE

Nurses in the United Kingdom are increasingly providing aromatherapy in conventional health care settings, including intensive care areas, renal, burn and neurologic units, cancer wards, HIV/AIDS units, hospices, geriatric areas, and pediatric units. They also use aromatherapy in learning disability settings. This therapy promotes relaxation, relieves stress, anxiety, and pain, stimulates immune function, and treats insomnia, infections, and burns. The active role of nursing in aromatherapy is evidenced by the Royal College of Nursing providing insurance for nurses using aromatherapy within their professional practice (Stevensen, 1996). Those of us practicing in other countries can look to nurses in the United Kingdom as role models for the integration of aromatherapy into nursing practice.

As a nurse in a conventional health care setting, you can promote the use of aromatherapy in a number of ways. Essential oils can be combined with carrier oils and used for back rubs and foot rubs in helping clients relax and decrease their levels of anxiety. Other essential oils can be used as an adjunct to conventional approaches by encouraging the production of white blood cells and for their antibacterial or antiviral action. Acute care and long care settings often have unpleasant smells in rooms and hallways. Essential oils can be diffused into the air to alter the structure of the molecules creating the odor, thus refreshing the environment. Diffusion of essential oils can also help boost the client's immune system, decrease anxiety and stress, aid restful sleep, and speed recovery.

As a nurse, you can teach people a number of things about the use of essential oils. As a general rule, people should purchase essential oils in natural and health food stores rather than stores selling beauty products and perfumes. They should be stored in dark vials, tightly closed and away from heat, light, or dampness. Essential oils should not be ingested, since even modest amounts can be fatal. They must be kept away from children and pets. Pregnant women and persons with epilepsy should consult a knowledgeable health care practitioner or qualified aromatherapist prior to the use of essential oils. Oils other than lavender or tea tree oil must always be diluted before applying on the skin. People who have sensitive skin or allergies should take extra care in massaging the oils into the skin or inhaling the essential oil aromas. Caution people not to rub their eyes if they have any essential oil on their hands. Several oils are photosensitive or phototoxic, causing severe sunburn if people are exposed to the sun within six hours after application. These oils include clove, bergamot, angelica, verbena, bitter/sweet orange, lemon, lime, and mandarin. Certain oils have high toxicity levels, and their use should be limited to qualified aromatherapists. These oils include boldo leaf, calamus, yellow camphor, horseradish, rue, sassafras, savin, tansy, wintergreen, wormseed, and wormwood.

Professional aromatherapists use up to 300 oils. Most people can meet their home needs with fewer than 30 or even just 10: chamomile, clove, eucalyptus, geranium, lavender, lemon, peppermint, rosemary, tea tree, and thyme. Box 9.3 describes helpful oils you can encourage people to have available at home.

Box 9.3: Helpful Oils to Have at Home

Oil	Use
Basil	Decrease sinus congestion; soothe GI tract, aid digestion; decrease headache; decrease anxiety; decrease menstrual cramps
Bergamot	Decrease anxiety, decrease depression; urinary antiseptic; acne, disinfectant for wounds, abscesses, boils
Cedarwood	Decrease respiratory congestion and coughs, expectorant; for pain swelling of arthritis; antifungal for skin rashes

Box 9.3: Helpful Oils to Have at Home (*continued*)

Chamomile	Soothe muscle aches, sprains, swollen joints; GI antispasmodic; rub on abdomen for colic, indigestion, gas; decrease anxiety, stress-related headaches; decrease insomnia; can be used with children
Clary sage	Induce sleep; increase sense of well-being; massage or warm compress for menstrual cramps; do not use in pregnancy until onset of labor
Coriander	Improve digestion, decrease colic, decrease diarrhea; decrease muscle aches and stiffness in joints; decrease mental fatigue and increase memory and mental function
Cypress	Massage or cold compress for rheumatic aches; bruising or varicose veins; respiratory antispasmodic (put couple of drops on hanky and inhale deeply), decrease coughs, asthma, bronchitis
Elemi	Boost immune system; cystitis; speed bone healing (massage in prior to casting); increase healing of cuts, sores, wounds; cool inflammed skin; sedative
Eucalyptus	Feels cool to skin and warm to muscles; decrease fever; relieve pain; anti-inflammatory; antiseptic, antiviral, and expectorant to respiratory system in steam inhalation; boost immune system
Frankincense	Bronchodilatory, acts on mucus enabling sputum to be expelled; infected sores; deepen breathing to induce calmness; incense creates a state conducive to prayer
Geranium	Antibacterial; insecticidal; antidepressant; improve yeast infections; first aid on minor cuts and burns
Ginger	Help ward off colds; calm upset stomach, decrease nausea; soothe sprains, muscle spasms
Green apple	Reduce headache severity; decrease anxiety; aid in weight reduction program; reduce symptoms of claustrophobia
Jasmine	Uplifting and stimulating, antidepressant; massage abdomen and lower back for menstrual cramps

Box 9.3: Helpful Oils to Have at Home (*continued*)

Juniper	Calming, decrease stress; diuretic; muscle aches and pains
Lavender	Calming, sedative, for insomnia; massage around temples for headache; inhale to speed recovery from colds, flu; massage chest to decrease congestion; heal burns
Lemon balm	Calming, sedative, decrease anxiety, decrease depression; antiseptic, antiviral, antifungal, eliminate cold sores
Lemon grass	Sedative; skin antiseptic for acne
Marjoram	Insomnia, decrease tension; muscle and joint pain; inhale to clear sinuses and clear congestion; massage abdomen for menstrual cramps
Neroli	Gentle sedative for insomnia, panic attacks; massage abdomen for irritable bowel syndrome
Orange	General tonic; decrease anxiety; GI antispasmodic for colic and indigestion; massage abdomen for constipation; can be used with children
Peppermint	Increase alertness; GI antispasmodic for colic and indigestion; massage on temples for headache; decongestant for colds, flu
Rose	Antidepressant; increase alertness; compress for eyestrain, headaches; use in massage for PMS
Rosemary	Stimulating; increase circulation to skin; compress on swollen joints; decrease respiratory congestion; antifungal, antibacterial; deodorize the air
Sandalwood	Calm and cool body; decrease inflammation; drops on handkerchief for sore throat, congestion; in bath water for cystitis; improve chapped dry skin; increase sense of peace in meditation or prayer
Tea Tree	First aid kit in a bottle; antifungal, good for athletes foot; soothe insect bites, stings, cuts, wounds; in bath for yeast infection; drops on handkerchief for coughs, congestion

Box 9.3: Helpful Oils to Have at Home (*continued*)

Vetiver	Stimulate production of red blood cells; increase circulation; induce restful sleep; decrease tension
Ylang ylang	Soothe CNS, decrease depression, increase euphoric mood; decrease BP; regulate respiration; calm heart palpitations.

Sources: Castleman, *Nature's Cures* (Emmaus, PA: Rodale Press, 1996); Maxwell-Hudson, *Aromatherapy Message* (Boston: Houghton Mifflin, 1994); Wilson, *Aromatherapy for Vibrant Health and Beauty* (Garden City, NY: Avery Pub. Co., 1995).

TRY THIS: *Soothing Potions*

Rosewater

Instead of using soap, try splashing your face with rosewater, a simple infusion from rose petals that contains some of the flowers' essential oils. Rose oil has mild antiseptic and anti-inflammatory action. It can constrict the tiny blood vessels in your skin to reduce redness, and it's also used in aromatherapy to calm your nerves and elevate your mood. You can buy rosewater in any natural food store but you can also make your own. Put a handful of fresh rose petals into a small saucepan, add enough water to cover the petal completely, simmer for 15 minutes, then remove the pan from the heat. When it's completely cooled, strain away the petals and transfer your rosewater to a clean glass bottle.

Calendula salve

Calendula *(Calendula officinalis)*, is a relative of the common marigold and is an easy-to-grow perennial. Calendula flowers have antibacterial and antifungal properties and also speed up the skin's healing process. The salve is extremely effective for diaper rash and other skin irritations. You can buy the salve or buy dried calendula at herb stores or grow the plant to make your own. Grind one-half cup of dried flowers into a powder in a blender or clean coffee grinder. Combine with one cup of olive oil in a glass canning jar with

TRY THIS: *Soothing Potions (continued)*

a lid. Place the jar in a large pan filled with enough water to cover the bottom half of the jar, and put the pan in the oven. Turn the oven on to the lowest temperature possible and allow the herbs to gently heat in the oil for several hours. Remove from the oven and allow to cool to room temperature. Filter the oil through a strainer lined with several layers of cheesecloth. To make the salve, place one-half cup of the herbal oil in a small heavy saucepan and add one-eighth cup of grated beeswax. Gently heat until the beeswax is completely melted. Test the consistency of the salve by placing a teaspoon of the mixture into the freezer for a minute. If you want a firmer salve, add more beeswax, and if you want a softer salve, add more oil. Pour the salve into small wide-mouth glass jars with lids. If stored in a cool, dark place, the salve will stay fresh for about one year.

Sources: Vukovic, Home Remedies, *Natural Health* (1998), 152–154; Beauty at Home, *Natural Health* (1998), 46.

REFERENCES

Aromatherapy Unlimited. 1997. *Aromatherapy Quarterly.* 55: 23.

Beauty at Home. 1998. *Natural Health.* 1: 46.

CASTLEMAN, M. 1996. *Nature's Cures.* Emmaus, PA: Rodale Press.

CHAMBERS, C. March 9, 1998. Aromatherapy: A complementary therapy. *Nrsg Spectrum.* 11(5): 8.

CRENSHAW, T. L. 1996. *The Alchemy of Love and Lust.* New York: G. P. Putnam's Sons.

HIRSCH, A. R. 1998. Green-apple fragrance may reduce migraine severity. *Headache Q.* 9: 159–163.

MAXWELL-HUDSON, C. 1994. *Aromatherapy Massage.* Boston: Houghton Mifflin.

MEADOWS, J. 1997. Establishing 'True Aromatherapy' in North Amercia. *Aromatherapy Quarterly.* 55: 15.

STEVENSEN, C. J. 1996. Aromatherapy. In M. S. MICOZZI ed. *Fundamentals of Complementary and Alternative Medicine.* New York: Churchill Livingstone, 137–148.

VUKOVIC, L. 1998. Home remedies. *Natural Health.* 1: 152–154.

WILSON, R. 1995. *Aromatherapy for Vibrant Health and Beauty.* Garden City, NY: Avery Pub. Co.

YOUNG, D. G. 1996. *An Introduction to Young Living Essential Oils and Aromatherapy.* Salt Lake City, UT: Essential Press Pub.

RESOURCES

Institute of Aromatherapy
Aromatherapy Consultant Program
3108 Route 10 West
Denville, NJ 07834
973-989-1999
www.aromatherapy4u.com
e-mail: essence@aromatherapy4u.com

National Association for Holistic Aromatherapy (NAHA)
836 Hanley Industrial Court
St. Louis, MO 63144
314-963-2071
www.naha.org
email: info@naha.org

Smell and Taste Treatment and Research Foundation
845 North Michigan Ave.
Chicago, IL 60611
312-938-1047

West Wind School of Aromatherapy
468 Queen St. East, Box 30
Toronto, Ontario, Canada M5A1T7
416-368-1426
www.interlog.com/~westwind
email: westwind@interlog.com

UNIT IV
MANUAL HEALING METHODS

Science becomes dangerous only when it imagines that it has reached its goal.

George Bernard Shaw

10 Chiropractic

It's supposed to be a professional secret,
but I'll tell you anyway. We doctors do
nothing. We only help and encourage the
doctor within.

Albert Schweitzer

Medicus curat, natura sanat.
Medicine treats, but nature heals.

Ambroise Pare, French surgeon,
1517–1590

The word *chiropractic* comes from two Greek words *cheir* (hand) and *prak-tikos* (practical), which were combined to mean "done by hand." Chiropractic, by numbers of practitioners, is the third largest independent health profession in the United States, following conventional medicine and dentistry. Chiropractors are primary health care providers, licensed both for diagnosis and treatment. The practice is limited by procedure (manipulation of the spine) and excludes surgery and prescription medications.

BACKGROUND

Manipulation, as a healing technique, was practiced long before chiropractic. Chinese artifacts as early as 2700 B.C. describe manipulation of the spine. In 1500 B.C., the Greeks gave written instructions on how to manipulate the lumbar spine for back care. Hippocrates, born about 460 B.C. and called the Father of Medicine, used spinal manipulation to reposition vertebrae and cure a variety of dysfunctions. Galen, born about A.D. 130, a Greek physician, anatomist, and physiologist, also used manipulation and reported the cure of a patient's hand weakness and numbness through manipulation of the seventh cervical vertebra. Hippocrates and Galen helped form the foundation of Renaissance medicine during which manipulative healers were known as "bone-setters." The "father of surgery," Ambroise Pare, born about A.D. 1517 incorporated manipulation into his treatment of patients. In the centuries that followed,

171

manipulative techniques were passed down from generation to generation, often within families (Fine, 1997; Redwood, 1996).

Chiropractic was founded in 1895 by Daniel David Palmer, a self-educated American healer. Palmer administered the first chiropractic adjustment to Harvey Lillard, a janitor who had gone deaf 17 years earlier while stooping in a mine. Palmer found what he called a misaligned vertebra, which he manipulated, allowing Lillard to stand up straight, free of back pain, and with his hearing restored. Within two years of this discovery, Palmer founded his Chiropractic School and Cure while at the same time developing the underlying concepts. In 1906, a split in the profession occurred that still exists today. Several faculty members, including John Howard, left Palmer College because of significant differences with Palmer's son, B. J. Palmer. B. J. believed that spinal subluxation or misalignment of the spinal vertebrae, was the cause of all disease whereas Howard believed that additional causes were generally present. Howard opened his National School of Chiropractic around a broad-based and scientific educational curriculum. To this day, those who follow Palmer's path are called "straight" chiropractors, while those who follow the Howard model are called "mixer" chiropractors (*Alternative Medicine,* 1994).

PREPARATION

Chiropractors are licensed in all states of the United States as well as in many other countries. The 16 American chiropractic colleges graduate more than 2,800 chiropractors each year. Colleges also exist in Canada, Australia, England, France, and Japan. Chiropractic education requires at least 60 undergraduate credit hours, including many in the basic sciences. Chiropractic college is a five-year program including courses in anatomy, physiology, pathology, and diagnosis, as well as spinal adjusting, nutrition, physical therapy, and rehabilitation. Educational standards in the United States are supervised by a government-recognized accrediting agency, the Council of Chiropractic Education (*Alternative Medicine,* 1994; Milbank, 1998).

Chiropractors function almost entirely in free-standing private practice. Some continue their education with postdoctoral training in specialty areas such as radiology, orthopedics, neurology, behavioral medicine, family practice, occupational health, and sports medicine.

CONCEPTS

Anatomy

The adult vertebral column is comprised of seven cervical, twelve thoracic, five lumbar, one sacral, and one coccygeal vertebrae. The vertebrae provide attachment for various muscles and protection for the spinal cord and are separated by intervertebral disks. Several curves in the vertebral column increase its strength. The spinal cord, housed in the vertebral canal, conducts sensory and motor impulses to and from the brain and controls many reflexes. Thirty-one pairs of spinal nerves originate from the cord: eight cervical, twelve thoracic, five lumbar, five sacral, and one coccygeal.

The vertebrae, with the exception of the first and second cervical, are much alike and are composed of a body, an arch, and seven projections called processes. See Figure 10.1. The two processes at the top are the superior articular processes, and the two at the bottom are the interior articular processes, and these four are of particular interest to the chiropractic physician. At the end of each of these processes is a facet, which, like the facet of a diamond, is smooth and capped with cartilage to allow for friction-free movement. The two superior articular processes from each vertebrae join with the two inferior articular processes of the vertebra above. The resulting structure is called a facet joint, which is encased in a strong, fibrous joint capsule which prevents the joint from coming apart. The other anatomical feature that is of concern to chiropractic is the sacroiliac joint, which is formed where the sacrum attaches to the ilia.

Assumptions

Chiropractic believes that the body possesses a unique internal wisdom that continually strives to maintain a state of health within the body. This body

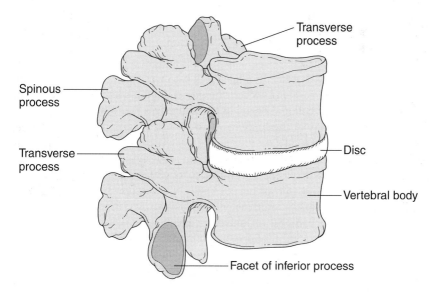

Figure 10.1:   The Vertebrae

wisdom means that every person has an innate healing potential. Accessing this internal healing system is the goal of the healing arts. In addition, it is believed that a balanced, natural diet and regular exercise are essential to proper bodily function and good health. The assumptions of chiropractic are as follows (Redwood, 1996, p. 96):

- Structure and function exist in intimate relation with one another.
- Structural distortions can cause functional abnormalities.
- The vertebral subluxation is a significant form of structural distortion and leads to a variety of functional abnormalities.
- The nervous system plays a prominent role in the restoration and maintenance of proper bodily function.
- Subluxation influences bodily function primarily through neurologic means.
- Chiropractic adjustment is a specific and definitive method for the correction of vertebral subluxation.

Chiropractic addresses the application of this knowledge to diagnose and treat structural dysfunctions that affect the nervous system. Since the nervous system is highly developed in humans, it influences all other systems in the body, thereby playing a significant role in health and disease.

VIEW OF HEALTH AND ILLNESS

Chiropractic believes that health is a state of balance, especially of the nervous and musculoskeletal systems. When the spine is fully aligned, nerve energy flows freely to every cell and organ in the body. This free flow of energy nurtures the innate ability of the body to work effectively and coordinate normal body functions.

Traditionally, chiropractic viewed illness and disease as caused by misalignment of the spinal vertebrae, referred to as vertebral subluxation, leading to irritation and dysfunction of nerves and blood vessels. The disrupted flow of impulses was thought to interfere with normal muscle function, respiration, heartbeat, arterial tone, digestion, and resistance to disease. A more recent theory is that of intervertebral motion dysfunction. This motion theory contends that loss of mobility in the facet joints, rather than misalignment, is the key factor in the concept of subluxation. Subluxation can be caused by just about anything—falls, injuries, genetic spinal weaknesses, improper sleeping habits, poor posture, obesity, stress, and occupational hazards (Redwood, 1996; Salmans 1995).

Although this "one cause" philosophy has been a central concept in chiropractic history, few chiropractors today would endorse this simplistic formulation of illness. They recognize the existence of bacteria and viruses in creating disease, especially in a susceptible person. Susceptibility depends on many factors, one of which is spinal misalignment. Although it now embraces a multifactoral explanation of disease, the chiropractic treatment of choice is spinal adjustment.

DIAGNOSTIC METHODS

Ninety percent of those seeking chiropractic have neuromusculoskeletal symptoms or disorders, primarily back pain, neck pain, and headaches. The central focus of chiropractic diagnosis is the determination of when and where spinal manual therapy (SMT) is appropriate. The diagnostic process also determines what type of adjustment would be most appropriate. Unlike conventional medicine, which typically assumes that the site of a pain is the site of its cause, chiropractors evaluate the site of pain in a regional and whole-body context. Joint pain in the upper extremities, for example, can be caused by injury or pathology in the joint but may also originate from cervical spine dysfunction. Similarly, the source of joint pain in the lower extremities can be in the lumbar spine. The chiropractic assumption is that the source of the pain should be sought along the path of the nerves leading to and from the site of the symptoms. This whole-body approach is a hallmark of chiropractic (Redwood, 1996).

A detailed history is the first step in chiropractic diagnosis. The chiropractor asks about the pattern and quality of the pain and its chronology. Is the pain constant or intermittent? Is the pain a dull ache, a nagging sensation, or a burning sensation? What causes the pain to get worse? What causes the pain to get better? The answers to these types of questions are key to the diagnostic process.

A number of back pain risk factors are critical to diagnosis and for which the physician consistently assesses. Individual factors contributing to back pain include older age, tallness, obesity, smoking, decreased muscle strength, decreased flexibility, lack of physical conditioning, and multiple pregnancies. Other health conditions are considered, such as osteoporosis, multiple myeloma, osteoarthritis, scoliosis, and ruptured disc. Psychological factors include the person's levels of anxiety, stress, and pain tolerance. Occupational risk factors for back pain include heavy physical work; frequent bending, twisting, lifting, pushing, pulling; repetitive strain; and injury or accidents. Recreational risk factors include hockey, football, gymnastics, golf, racquetball, bowling, squash, handball, tennis, backpacking, wrestling, skiing, and other high-impact sports. All applicable risk factors are noted during the history (Whitney, 1997).

The chiropractic physician relies heavily on hands-on procedures using palpation to determine both structural and functional problems. These hands-on procedures are complemented by a neurological physical examination. It is the same neurological assessment done by a conventional physician. Following the neurological evaluation is the motion palpation exam in which the chiropractor physically examines the spine noting how it feels as well as how the client says it feels. The client is gently moved into and out of various postures during this part of the exam. Some postures are done standing while others are done lying down. This process often informs the chiropractor what movements or positions reproduce or aggravate the pain. X-rays to confirm diagnostic findings may or may not be done (Fine, 1997).

Hypermobility of spinal joints is diagnosed by the sound of a repeated click when a joint is moved through its normal range of motion. This unstable type of subluxation is related to flaccid ligaments and is more problematic than the fixated type of subluxation. Hypermobile joints should not be forcibly manipulated since manipulation can move the joint beyond the safe range of motion and increase the degree of hypermobility. Rather, nearby joints that have become fixated to compensate for the unstable joint can be manipulated, and muscle strength and tone can be increased with exercise (Redwood, 1996).

The chiropractor rules out pathologies that are contraindicative to SMT. For example, advanced, degenerative joint disease would rule out all forms of SMT that use significant force on the joint. Chiropractic treatment is not appropriate in the case of spinal infections, fractures, or tumors, which fortunately are fairly rare. In addition, SMT is not done on a woman in late pregnancy or on people whose pain is increased with manipulation. Diagnosis determines appropriate chiropractic treatment, referral for appropriate conventional medical care, or concurrent care.

TREATMENT

Three primary clinical goals guide chiropractic intervention. The first goal is to reduce or eliminate people's pain. Typically this goal is the client's primary, and often only goal. The second clinical goal is to correct the subluxation, thereby restoring biomechanical balance to reestablish shock absorption, leverage, and range of motion. In addition, muscles and ligaments are strengthened by spinal rehabilitative exercises to increase resistance to further injury. The third clinical goal is preventative maintenance to assure the problem does not recur. This goal is comparable to the idea of having teeth cleaned periodically to prevent decay. Maintenance intervals vary from person to person depending on lifestyle.

Back pain is a leading cause of disability and the second most common reason (after the common cold) people visit a doctor. Chiropractors have two times the number of visits for back pain as conventional physicians. Most chiropractors also treat peripheral joints—elbows, knees, and shoulders. In 1994, a panel for the Agency for Health Care Policy and Research of the United States Department of Health and Human Services concluded that spinal manual therapy speeds recovery from acute low back pain and recommended it either in combination with or as a replacement for nonsteroid, anti-inflammatory drugs. At the same time the panel rejected many methods used for years by conventional medicine such as bed rest, traction, and various other physical therapy modalities and cautioned against spinal surgery except in the most severe cases (Redwood, 1996; Whitney, 1997).

Spinal manipulation is an assisted (chiropractor) passive (client) motion applied to the spinal facet joints or the sacroiliac joints. Chiropractors use their hands to apply pressure in specific location and direction. The skill lies in the ability to be specific about which joint is being manipulated, which is especially important in the presence of any unstable joints. A chiropractor has 10–20 different ways of manipulating every movable joint in the body. Chiropractors also practice soft-tissue manipulation to stretch contracted muscles and decrease muscle spasms (Fine, 1997).

High-velocity, low-amplitude (HVLA) thrust adjustment is the most common form of manipulation. It is performed by manually moving a joint to the end-point of its normal range of motion, isolating it by local pressure on bony prominences, and then giving a swift, specific, low-amplitude thrust. Often a series of these thrusts are applied to the back and neck. When the facet joints are forced apart, a small vacuum is created and then released, that creates a popping sound much like people cracking their knuckles. This manipulation does not cause pain, though people may feel a little discomfort the next day due to rebalancing of the contracted muscles. This sensation can be compared to muscular soreness at the beginning of a weight training program. HVLA is absolutely contraindicated in malignancies, bone and joint infections, acute myelopathy, acute fractures and dislocations, acute rheumatoid or rheumatoid-like joint pathology, and unstable joints. Other adjusting methods include low-velocity thrust adjustment with mechanically assisted drop-piece tables, various light touch techniques, ultrasound, and electrical muscle stimulation (Redwood, 1996).

Network chiropractic spinal analysis blends chiropractic and energy field principles. This approach assesses two types of subluxations: structural, involving the joint facets, and soft-tissue involving tension in the muscles and other soft tissue connected to the spine. Network chiropractors treat the soft-tissue subluxations with energy techniques before the structural subluxations are corrected with manipulation (*Alternative Medicine,* 1994).

As holistic practitioners, chiropractors work with many facets of clients' lifestyles. Nutrition education is provided, exercise programs are designed, rehabilitation measures are planned, correct posture and lifting techniques are explained, and activities of daily living are assessed and improved. Conditions commonly seen by a chiropractor include the following:

- Lower back syndromes
- Mid back conditions
- Neck syndromes
- Headaches
- Carpal tunnel syndrome
- Sciatica
- Muscle spasms
- Sports-related injuries
- Whiplash and accident-related injuries
- Arthritic conditions
- Shoulder conditions
- Torticolis
- Extremity trauma

RESEARCH

Procedures have been researched since the early days of chiropractic, though researchers frequently had difficulty in finding a source for publication. Today the *Journal of Manipulative and Physiological Therapeutics* and *Spine* publish much of the chiropractic-related research, and increasingly more chiropractic studies are reported each year in conventional medical journals. The most significant research in the 1980s and 1990s was done outside the United States. The quality and quantity of chiropractic research in the United States is beginning to change, however, as chiropractors become more accepted by biomedical physicians. Professional respect began to improve in the 1990s with the appointment of J. R. Cassidy as the first chiropractic research director of a conventional medical orthopedics department at the University of Saskatchewan in Canada and the appointment of John Triano to the dual role of staff chiropractic physician and clinical research scientist at the Texas Back Institute (*Alternative Medicine,* 1994; Redwood, 1996).

A number of studies have demonstrated the short-term and long-term benefits of chiropractic for treatment of chronic, disabling lower back pain.

- An Australian study showed that people treated by medical doctors lost four times more workdays from low back pain than those treated by chiropractors.

- In 1992 the RAND corporation examined all published literature on the use of manipulation for low back pain and found that manipulation was effective in the following situations: acute low back pain with or without sciatic nerve irritation, subacute low back pain with no neurological involvement or sciatic irritation, and subacute low back pain with minor or major neurological symptoms. Other studies have found similar results for neck pain and pain in other areas of the back.

- Researchers at Northwestern College of Chiropractic in Minnesota are conducting ongoing research on muscle tension headaches. The control group received the tricyclic antidepressant amitriptyline, while the experimental group had spinal manipulation. The chiropractic group maintained their levels of improvement after treatment was discontinued, while those taking medication returned to pretreatment status in an average of four weeks after its discontinuation. Current research is focusing on migraine headaches (*Alternative Medicine,* 1994; Redwood, 1996).

Chiropractic researchers are now looking at the effectiveness in organic or somatovisceral disorders. Continuing studies on hypertension indicate that spinal manipulation lowers blood pressure but, as of now, the changes appear to be relatively transient. A study on spinal manipulation in the treatment of tension headaches found no difference between the manipulation and control groups. A study on dysmenorrhea includes the effect spinal manipulation has on prostaglandins (responsible for uterine contractions) and subjective measures of pain levels and changes in menstrual distress. Another study is looking at the effectiveness of chiropractic treatment and parent education in the treatment of colic in infants. Despite the lack of federal funding and encouragement from government agencies and other health care professionals, chiropractors have made impressive additions to scientific health care knowledge. With the atmosphere of growing medical-chiropractic cooperation and new federal funding of studies comes the anticipation of more widely disseminated research findings (*Alternative Medicine,* 1994; Bove and Nilsson, 1998; Redwood, 1996).

INTEGRATED NURSING PRACTICE

Observing a client's posture and gait is a key component of basic nursing assessment. Normally, people's posture should be erect and at ease with the shoulders level and straight. Movements should be smooth and relaxed. A normal walk is rhythmic, in a straight, upright position with the arms swinging naturally at each side. General nursing assessment data provided by the client includes the following (Sims et al., 1995):

- Description of current mobility, mobility two months ago, and mobility two years ago
- Description of changes in the ability to walk, sit, or stand
- History of injuries and treatments
- Description of daily exercise routine
- List of sport activities
- Description of repetitive movements related to work or other activities

During a nursing assessment, clients are asked to walk across the room and back as you observe for any difficulties with gait or posture that require further evaluation. An older client's gait may include short, shuffling, uncertain, and sometimes unsteady steps with a decreased arm swing. As people age, they often develop slumped shoulders and a more stooped body posture. Pregnant women often experience changes in body posture and gait as their pregnancy advances. The pelvis tips forward, increasing the lumbosacral curve, creating a gradual lordosis—an exaggerated lumbar curve in the spine. The enlarging breasts may pull the shoulders forward, contributing to a stooped body posture. As the pelvic joints relax and the weight and size of the fetus increase, the woman's center of gravity, stance, and gait are altered, contributing to the common complaint of backaches (Sims et al., 1995).

As a nurse, you can intervene with minor difficulties of gait and posture. Teach people to warm up and stretch before exercising and cool down and stretch upon completion. Many people can participate in low-impact aerobic activity that does not stress muscles and joints, such as walking, swimming, dancing, weight training, and bicycling. Other activities you can encourage are yoga, T'ai Chi, and qigong presented in other chapters in this text. Help people become aware of problems they are experiencing in posture and encourage them to walk and sit "straight, tall, and relaxed." Good standing posture is with one's feet facing forward, knees slightly flexed, chest up, shoulders back, and chin parallel to the floor. Good sitting posture includes feet flat on the floor with knees, ankles, and hips at right angles, and chin parallel to the floor.

Nursing practice and chiropractic medicine support the belief that prevention of injuries is preferred over treatment of injuries. Many nursing activities such as lifting, transferring, or positioning clients require muscle exertion by the nurse. To reduce the risk of injury to your clients and yourself, practice proper body mechanics. The coordinated motion of the body depends on the integrated functioning of bones, joints, muscles, and the nervous system. You achieve better body balance from a wide base of support created by separating your feet to a comfortable distance. Your balance will also be improved by bending your knees and flexing your hips, thus bringing the center of gravity closer to your support base. When you are lifting an object or person, use your legs to lift and your arms to support. Facing the direction of movement and pivoting with your feet prevents abnormal twisting of the spine. Balancing activity between arms and legs protects the back from strain.

A referral to chiropractic evaluation and treatment is appropriate for the conditions listed earlier in the chapter. Chiropractors view themselves as contributing members of the health care team and refer to conventional physicians for problems outside their scope of practice. Although chiropractors have clear guidelines for referring to conventional practitioners, biomedical professionals have not developed formal guidelines for referring to chiropractors. It is time that communication and cooperation be broadened between conventional practitioners and chiropractors in an effort to create the most effective health care system for the greatest number of people.

TRY THIS: *Energy Booster*

Poor posture robs your body of energy. You may spend many hours of your day walking incorrectly or slumped in a chair, which interrupts the flow of energy and oxygen through your body and spinal cord. Take a moment to sit up or stand straight. Imagine that a cord is attached to the top of your head, pulling it gently toward the sky. This image helps readjust your posture. Feel your head, neck, shoulders, and spine relax as they realign from a constricting position. This imagery, practiced either sitting or standing, will revive you.

REFERENCES

Alternative Medicine: Expanding Medical Horizons. 1994. A report to the National Institutes of Health on Alternative Medical Systems and Practices in the United States. U.S. Government Printing Office. Washington, DC.

BOVE, G. and N. NILSSON. 1998. Spinal manipulation in the treatment of episodic tension-type headache. *JAMA.* 280(18): 1576–1579.

FINE, J. 1997. *The Ultimate Back Book.* Toronto: Stoddart.

Milbank Memorial Fund. 1998. *Enhancing the Accountability of Alternative Medicine.* New York: Milbank Memorial Fund.

REDWOOD, D. 1996. Chiropractic. In M. S. MICOZZI, ed. *Fundamentals of Complementary and Alternative Medicine.* New York: Churchill Livingstone, 91–110.

SALMANS, S. 1995. *Back Pain.* Allentown, PA: Peoples' Medical Society.

SIMS, L. K. et al. 1995. *Health Assessment in Nursing.* Redwood City, CA: Addison-Wesley.

WHITNEY, W. 1997. *Healthy Back Building.* Antioch, CA: Kat Hill Press.

RESOURCES

American Chiropractic Association
1701 Clarendon Blvd.
Arlington, VA 22209
800-637-6244
www.amerchiro.org

Federation of Chiropractic Licensing Boards
www.fclb.org/fclb

World Chiropractic Alliance
2950 N. Dobson, Suite 1
Chandler, AZ 85224
800-347-1011

11 Massage

> Massage is better than a good tranquilizer
> and serves as a very helpful adjunct to
> other therapies.
>
> *Willibald Nagler, M.D.,*
> *Head of Rehabilitation Medicine,*
> *Cornell Medical Center*
>
> Above all, we need to explore the poten-
> tial of an integrated approach to health
> care where health is much more than sim-
> ply the absence of disease.
>
> *Charles, Prince of Wales*

Massage therapy, the scientific manipulation of the soft tissues of the body, is a healing art, an act of physical caring, and a way of communicating without words. The goal of massage therapy is to achieve or increase health and well-being and to help the body heal itself. Although massage therapists may hold general views of health and well-being, massage therapy has no specific theoretical framework or diagnostic system of disease.

Compared with members of other cultures, people in the United States are generally touch-phobic and touch-deprived. Cross-cultural studies have revealed that people in the United States have one of the lowest rates of casual touch in the world. When psychologist Sidney Jourard observed rates of casual touch among couples in cafes, he reported the highest rates in Puerto Rico (180 times per hour) and Paris (110 times per hour) and one of the lowest in the United States (two times per hour). French parents and children touch each other three times more frequently than their U.S. counterparts. French teens demonstrate significantly more casual touching of friends than U.S. adolescents, who are more likely to fiddle with their rings, crack their knuckles, and demonstrate other forms of self-stimulation. Other studies have found cultures that are more physically affectionate towards infants and children tend to have lower rates of adult violence. In spite of advertising pleas to "reach out and touch someone," the majority of North Americans have precious little physical contact with family members, friends, and co-workers (Castleman, 1996; Colt, 1997).

Concerns have been escalating about "inappropriate" touch, sexual abuse, and sexual harassment in schools and workplaces in the United States. Some schools have instituted "teach, but don't touch" policies. It is rare to see teachers put their hands on the shoulder of a child who is crying. Sadly, to protect themselves from being accused of inappropriate touch, many people are not touching at all. While concern for protecting children from those who would touch inappropriately is valid, the implications of a "hands-off" barrier have significant negative effects on growth, development, and emotional well-being.

Massage, a hands-on touch therapy, has reached out to an ever-widening U.S. audience. Massage is now the third most common form of alternative treatment in the United States, after relaxation techniques and chiropractic. The power of touch has people in the United States spending almost $4 billion yearly on professional massages as 25 million individuals make 60 million visits each year. These numbers do not include institutions that offer massage in the workplace or the children of thousands of parents who learn baby massage (Colt, 1997; Meyer, 1997).

BACKGROUND

The idea that touch can heal is an old one. Cave paintings in the Pyrenees show that 15,000 years ago people treated injuries with what looks like massage. References to massage are found in 4,000-year-old Chinese medical texts. Hippocrates, in the fourth century B.C. wrote, "The physician must be acquainted with many things and assuredly with rubbing" (the ancient Greek and Roman term for massage). Some of the greatest physicians in history advocated massage, including Celsus (25 B.C.–A.D. 50), Galen (131–200), and Avicenna (980–1037). Ambroise Pare (1517–1590) the "father of surgery," William Harvey (1578–1657), who demonstrated the circulation of blood, and Herman Boerhaave (1668–1738), who introduced the clinical method of teaching medicine, all utilized massage as a healing technique. Roman gladiators were massaged before entering the arenas and eighteenth century Swedish cavalrymen were rubbed down between battles. In the Middle Ages, Christians viewed massage as the work of the devil and many therapists were burned at the stake as witches. Remnants of this attitude have continued into the twentieth century as massage is sometimes assumed to be a front for prostitution (*Alternative Medicine,* 1994; Colt, 1997).

The German emperor Frederick II (thirteenth century) was curious to know what language children would speak if they were raised without hearing any words at all. Stealing a number of newborns from their parents, he gave them to nurses who physically cared for the infants but were forbidden to cuddle or talk to them. All the children died before they could talk. The discovery that was made was important: tactile stimulation can be a matter of life and death. Most recently a similar situation occurred in the early 1990s in Romania when thousands of infants were stockpiled into orphanages. Some were virtually left alone in their cribs for two years and were discovered to be severely impaired from this isolation (Colt, 1997).

Infant massage dates to ancient times. An Indian medical text from 1800 B.C. recommends diet, exercise, and massage as healing techniques. The practice spread to the United States in the 1980s after the publication of *Infant Massage* by Vimala Schneider McClure, and *Baby Massage* by Amelia Auckett. Both women received their massage training in India.

Massage was introduced into the United States in the mid-nineteenth century by two New York physicians who were trained in Sweden. The first massage therapy clinics were opened by Swedish physicians after the Civil War and had among their clients, members of congress and Presidents Harrison and Grant. At first physicians performed massage, but they eventually delegated the technique to nurses and physical therapists and by the mid-twentieth century, massage therapy was virtually abandoned by most health care professionals except nurses. For many years, during the time of relatively little technology, it was standard nursing practice to give back rubs after bathing clients, and back rubs were also a routine part of Hour of Sleep Care. Advanced medical technology, sophisticated equipment, and nurses assuming more of a management role left little time for hands-on nursing care. An upsurge of interest in the field began in the 1970s with Dr. Dolores Kreiger and Dr. Martha Rogers, two nurse pioneers who advocated the art and caring form of touch in nursing practice. At the turn of the new century, nurses are returning to their tradition in providing comfort and care through the use of touch and massage (*Alternative Medicine,* 1994; Milbank, 1998; Mower, 1997).

In many areas of the world, massage continues as an integral part of health systems. In the former Soviet Union, Germany, China, and Japan, massage therapists work along with physicians in the hospital setting as important members of the health care team. In Germany today, doctors will write a prescription for 10 massage treatments as readily as for a bottle of tranquilizers, and massage is covered by Germany's national health insurance plan.

PREPARATION

Twenty-five states, the District of Columbia, and some cities require massage therapists to have 500 or more hours of education from a recognized school and some states also require the passing of a licensing exam. The curriculum consists of 300 hours of massage theory and technique, 100 hours of anatomy and physiology, and 100 hours of additional courses to meet the school's specific program objectives. Additional states are expected to adopt licensing acts in the near future. The American Massage Therapy Association accredits 60 programs throughout the United States. Curriculums must consist of 500 or more hours and include specified hours of anatomy, physiology, massage theory and practice, and ethics. The National Certification Exam was first administered in 1992, and by 1997, 27,000 therapists were certified. The International Association of Infant Massage certifies instructors who take four days of training, read course material, and pass a take-home exam.

CONCEPTS

Skin

In many ways, human beings are wired for touch. The skin is the body's largest organ, covering almost 20 square feet and accounting for nearly one-quarter of the body's total weight. As many as five million touch receptors in the skin—3,000 in a fingertip—send messages via the spinal cord to the brain. The sense of touch is the earliest to develop in the human embryo and at less than eight weeks of gestation, a light stroking of the face will cause bending of the neck and trunk away from the source of stimulation. The skin has four main functions: protection from mechanical and radiation injuries, and from invasion by foreign substances; as a sense organ; as a temperature regulator; and as a metabolic organ. Of all the sensory organs, the skin is the most important. People can survive without the senses of sight, sound, smell, and taste, but would find it difficult to survive without the functions performed by the skin (Colt, 1997; Montagu, 1971).

Touch

Touch is a primal need, as necessary for growth and development as food, clothing, or shelter. Touch can be thought of as a nutrient transmitted through the skin in many different ways: holding, cuddling, nuzzling, caressing, and massage. From the bonding of parent and newborn to the holding the hand of a dying loved one, touch is the most intimate and powerful form of communication between people. It can be aggressive as in the spanking of a child or a punch in the face. It can be tender as in the hug that comforts a crying friend or the touch of a lover. Even casual touch has an effect. Waitresses who touched their customers on the hand or shoulder as they returned change, for example, received larger tips than those who did not. Politicians act on this knowledge when they reach out to touch potential voters (Colt, 1997).

The importance of the sense of touch is evident in many English expressions. Some people have to be "handled" carefully because they are "thin-skinned" while others are "thick-skinned." "Touchy" people are overly sensitive or easily angered. Some people are "soft touches" and other have "the human touch." Some people "rub" others the wrong way. "Feeling" for another person is a description of empathy. A "touching" experience is something that is deeply felt (Montagu, 1971). As biomedicine continues to make incredible advances in technology, it leaves behind one of the most valuable senses of a human being—that of touch. This sense of isolation may explain, in part, the increasing interest in healing practices, most of which include the experience of touch.

Trigger Points

When a person is injured or bodily systems are malfunctioning, trigger points or pain reflexes appear throughout the body. A trigger point is a "knot" of tensed muscles, which, when stimulated, triggers a referred pain response in other parts of the body. Some of the trigger points are in the area of the injury or problem, while others are at a distance. Rubbing and exerting pressure on these points have been found to have a positive effect on the healing process (Jahnke, 1997; Segen, 1998).

Fascia and Fascial Restrictions

The fascia is the tough connective tissue that exists in the body almost like a three-dimensional web from head to foot. If somehow every structure of the body were removed except the fascia, the body would retain its shape. Every muscle, bone, organ, nerve, and blood vessel of the body is covered with fascia like a continuous saran wrapping. It varies in thickness and density and in the amount of collagenous fiber, elastic fiber, and tissue fluid it contains. The function of the fascia is to support cells, muscles, groups of muscles and organs and act as a shock absorber. At the cellular level, fascia creates the interstitial spaces and is important in cellular respiration, elimination, metabolism, fluid, and lymphatic flow.

Each time a person experiences a trauma, undergoes an inflammatory process, or suffers from poor postures over time, the fascial system becomes restricted and the person loses flexibility and spontaneity of motion. As the fascia continue to slowly tighten, an abnormal pressure develops on the nerves, muscles, bones, or organs, resulting in poor cellular efficiency, necrosis, pain, and dysfunction throughout the body (Ramsey, 1997).

VIEW OF HEALTH AND ILLNESS

It is believed that massage aids the ability of the body to heal itself and is aimed at achieving or increasing health and well-being. Only now is science beginning to catch up with people when it comes to appreciating the importance—and the power—of touch. The Touch Research Institute (TRI) at the University of Miami School of Medicine brings together researchers from Duke, Harvard, Princeton, and other universities to study touch and how it might be used to promote health and treat disease.

Stronger, sustained touch in massage can have an even greater effect than other forms of touch. A skilled massage therapist not only stretches and loosens muscle and connective tissue, but also greatly improves blood flow and the movement of lymph fluid throughout the body. Massage speeds the removal of metabolic waste products resulting from exercise or inactivity, allowing more oxygen and nutrients to reach the cells and tissues. The release of muscular tension also helps to unblock and balance the overall flow of life energy throughout the body known as qi, ki, prana, or subtle energy. In addition, massage can stimulate the release of endorphins and serotonin in the brain and nervous system. The benefits of massage are described in Box 11.1.

As an adjunct to medical treatment, massage may be helpful in relieving backaches, headaches, muscle spasm and pain, hypertension, swelling and pain from injuries or after surgery, grand mal epileptic seizures, insomnia, anxiety, and depression. It can be a palliative treatment for the comfort of those with terminal conditions, and can help maintain circulation and muscle tone for bedridden people. Even people in deep comas may show improved heart rates when their hands are held. Most newer comprehensive cancer treatment programs offer massage as a standard component of care. Massage can reduce agitation in people with Alzheimer's Disease, and it has been used to relieve stress at disaster sites. After the Oklahoma City bombing, volunteer therapists gave massages to exhausted rescue workers, numbed survivors, and overworked pathologists. The state medical examiner observed that the massage therapists were accomplishing more in 15 minutes than psychologists could in an hour or two (*Alternative Medicine,* 1994; Colt, 1997; Jahnke, 1997).

Massage has been used with psychiatrically disabled individuals as an adjunct to conventional psychiatric interventions. Clients are given an executive massage, done with the client fully dressed and seated on a massage chair.

Box 11.1: The Benefits of Massage

Physical Level

- relieves muscle tension and stiffness
- reduces muscle spasm and tension
- speeds recovery from exertion
- improves joint flexibility and range of motion
- increases ease and efficiency of movement
- improves posture
- stimulates lymphatic circulation, which decreases edema
- improves local circulation, which increases healing of injured tissues
- lowers blood pressure, slows heart rate
- eases tension headaches

Mental Level

- induces a relaxed state of alertness
- reduces mental stress thus clearing the mind
- increases capacity for clearer thinking

Emotional Level

- satisfies the need for caring and nurturing touch
- increases feelings of well-being, decreases mild depression
- enhances self-image
- reduces levels of anxiety
- increases awareness of mind-body connection

Sources: *Alternative Medicine* (Washington, DC: U.S. Government Printing Office, 1994); Castleman, *Nature's Cures* (Emmaus, PA: Rodale Press, 1996); Ramsey, "Holistic manula therapy techniques," *Primary Care: Clinics in Office Practice* (Philadelphia: W. B. Saunders, 1997), 759–784.

The head, neck, back, arms, and legs are massaged for 10 to 20 minutes per session. Hilliard's study (1995) found that massage was an effective stress reducer for inpatient and outpatient clients who sought safe touch and relaxation resulting in a sense of emotional well-being.

For some situations, massage is contraindicated:

- Phlebitis/thrombosis
- Severe varicose veins
- Any acute inflammation of the skin, soft tissue, or joints
- Areas of hemorrhage or heavy tissue damage
- Unregulated blood pressure
- Febrile state
- Herniated disc
- Recent fractures or sprains
- Some types of cancer

TREATMENT

Touch is the fundamental medium of massage therapy. It is, however, more than just mechanical manipulation. Touch is a form of communication, thus one of the most significant benefits is the comfort of human care conveyed by the therapist. Massage communicates gentleness and connection, trust and receiving, and peace and alertness.

The first massage therapy appointment usually begins with questions about one's physical condition, medical history, and current aches and pains. The therapist determines what a client hopes to gain from the massage. The client undresses in private and uses a sheet or blanket for draping. The individual decides whether underwear is on or off. The client lies on a cushioned table and the therapist uncovers only that part of the body being massaged, using oil or lotion to help the hands move smoothly. It is recommended that clients not eat just before a massage and drink extra water afterward to clear the body of toxins released from deep tissues. At home, clients are encouraged to enjoy a salt bath as another aid in detoxifying the body. One-half cup each of sea salt, epson salt, and baking soda are added to a tub of warm water for the salt bath.

From hour-long massages in therapists' offices to 10-minute massages at the workplace, a massage is available for practically every body and budget. Massage therapists offer their services in a wide variety of settings such as private practice clinics, health clubs and fitness centers, chiropractic offices, nursing homes and hospitals, salons and resorts, on-site in the workplace, and even in clients' homes. There are almost as many styles of massage as there are practitioners. Most therapists combine a variety of methods in their work, which allows them to tailor each session to the specific needs of the client.

Swedish Massage

Swedish massage was developed about 150 years ago by Peter Ling of Sweden, who integrated ancient Asian massage with a Western understanding of anatomy and physiology. It is the most common form of massage in the United States. Swedish massage uses a system of long gliding strokes, as well as kneading and friction techniques on the more superficial layers of the muscles, combined with active and passive movements of the joints. It is used primarily for a full-body massage to promote general relaxation, improve circulation and range of motion, and relieve muscle tension.

Swedish massage uses five basic strokes. *Effleurage,* French for "touching," is the introductory stroke. The therapist uses the whole hand providing long, gliding strokes relaxing the central nervous system and preparing the local area for the other strokes. *Petrissage* involves grasping muscle groups and lifting them, stretching them away from the bones and then kneading or rolling them. This technique is the closest in imitating exercise because it makes the muscles contract. This stroke is used mostly on flaccid muscles that need to have their contractile ability increased. Petrissage also stimulates the central nervous system and therefore is not used with clients who have cerebral vascular dysfunctions. *Friction* involves using the fingers and thumbs to press on small areas and move in a circular motion around the area. *Vibration* involves placing the hands on a muscle group and moving them back and forth quickly in a shaking motion. *Tapotement* involves striking the skin with the outside edges of the hands, fingers, or cupped palms to stimulate circulation (Castleman, 1996; Wine, 1997).

Shiatsu Massage

In Japanese, *shi* means "finger" and *atsu* means "pressure." Shiatsu massage is the Japanese adaptation of acupressure. Like Chinese acupuncture and acupressure, shiatsu is based on the idea that life energy, *ki,* flows along invisible pathways called meridians. Health is related to a free flow of energy, and illness is caused by blockages to the flow. Blocked energy can cause physical discomforts, so the aim is to release the blocks associated with the discomfort or disease and rebalance the energy flow. Therapists use their hands, elbows, and even their feet to press for about 30 seconds on each point. Depending on the way it is done, Shiatsu can be gentle or quite forceful. Done on a floor mat rather than a massage table, a typical Shiatsu session lasts about an hour (Castleman, 1996).

Trigger Point Massage

Trigger point massage is a type of deep massage, in which the fingers are used to release knots and tender spots in muscles. Rubbing and exerting pressure on these points has been found to have a positive effect on the healing process by interrupting the cycle of spasm and pain. Techniques are similar to those used in shiatsu but are based on Western anatomy and physiology. Trigger point massage is typically a technique incorporated into Swedish or sports massage.

Sports Massage

Sports massage uses techniques of Swedish massage and Shiatsu massage but focuses on parts of the body that are likely to be stressed by a particular sport. It takes less time than Swedish or Shiatsu and is usually more vigorous. For example, runners might need to have their hamstrings worked extensively. This technique also concentrates on reducing or eliminating factors that interfere with human performance such as muscle spasms, tendonitis, and muscle fatigue.

Prior to the athletic event, massage loosens, warms, and readies the muscle for intensive use, especially when combined with stretching. Besides helping prevent injury, it can improve performance and endurance. Post-event massage relieves pain, prevents stiffness, and returns the muscles to their normal state more rapidly. The use of massage in sports health care is increasing rapidly in both training and competition. Recreational athletes have also discovered the benefits of sports massage as a regular part of their workouts.

Myofascial Release

Myofascial release is a whole body therapy preceded by a comprehensive evaluation and diagnostic workup. The therapist evaluates the fascial system through visual analysis and palpation of tissue and fascial layers. Normal tissue is soft and mobile in all directions. Abnormal tissue may feel hot, hard, sensitive, or somewhat stringy or crunchy. When the therapist has determined where the fascial restrictions lie, gentle pressure is applied in the direction of the restriction, which is designed to break up the collagen of the fascia. Myofascial release is effective in strains and sprains, headaches, chronic pain, tempomandibular pain (TMJ), and adhesions. Myofascial release is contraindicated in malignancy, open wounds, cellulitis, febrile state, hematoma, infection, advanced degenerative changes, acute circulatory conditions, and acute rheumatoid arthritis (Barnes, 1987).

Rolfing

Developed by the late biochemist Ida P. Rolf, Rolfing (also known as structural integration) is a system of whole-body manipulation in which the rolfer uses the fingers, knuckles, and elbows to stretch the fascia, which tends to bind up because of injury, bad posture, emotional problems, or genetic weaknesses. The fascia is stretched to release patterns of tension and rigidity and return the body to a state of correct alignment. Other massage therapists work by applying smooth strokes over muscles; rolfers press deeply into muscle tissue and fascia to release them. Clients are asked to breathe deeply during the session and visualize the muscle lengthening. The new Rolfing method is more gentle and far less painful than the original style of treatment. Practitioners use a broad range of touch and pressure from feather-light to deep massage. When performed with the right sensitivity, even deep and heavy pressure may not be painful (*Alternative Medicine,* 1994; Stolzoff, 1997).

Executive Massage

Executive massage is done with the client fully dressed, seated on a portable massage chair. The person's face is supported by a doughnut-shaped pillow to allow for easy breathing. The sessions, which last 10–20 minutes, involve massage of the head, neck, back, arms, and hands. This type of massage is often provided in the workplace or in shopping malls. The purpose of the massage is to decrease tension, reduce stress, and enhance people's adaptive capabilities (Hillard, 1995).

Thai Massage

Some people call Thai massage passive yoga, as the receiver is fully clothed, lies on a futon, and is deeply stretched, compressed, and gently rocked. The whole body of the therapist is used to treat the whole body of the receiver. The experience feels like a combination of yoga, shiatsu, and meditation. Point pressure and kneading of the tissues is similar to massage techniques. Yoga techniques involve positioning the client in numerous stretches similar to yoga poses, then gently rocking the person to deepen the stretch and open the joints. The gentle rocking creates an energy flow through the different stretches. Thai massage gives the person the flexibility, inner organ massage, oxygenation of the blood, and quieting of the mind that comes with yoga, but because the receiver is passive the session becomes meditative. Sometimes the therapist stands on the recipient and gently rolls one foot on and off the body. This compression can be gentle to deep and can energize or relax the recipient (Mann, 1993).

Infant Massage

Infant massage is gaining in popularity in the United States. Researchers have found infant massage produces weight gains in premature infants, reduces complications in cocaine babies, and helps depressed mothers soothe their babies. In healthy babies it improves parent-infant bonding, eases painful procedures such as inoculations, reduces pain from teething and constipation, reduces colic, induces sleep, and makes parents feel good.

Self-Massage

Self-massage is a wonderful way for people to better acquaint themselves with their entire bodies. It is a process in which they learn to be aware of and release tensions and inhibitions, to reclaim parts of themselves that have been neglected, and to accept themselves as they are. Getting to know and appreciate one's body through touch is an important part of self-acceptance. The more in touch people are with themselves, the more they come in touch with the reality and experience of the world around them. Heightened awareness of the unity of body, mind, and spirit often leads to an increased perception of the unity of all nature. As it builds self-confidence and self-acceptance, this awareness enables people to respond with more compassion and caring to others.

Self-massage is done in a warm, comfortable, and quiet environment. Breath work and relaxation techniques are utilized to ground and center before the experience. Self-massage often begins with gazing at oneself naked in a mirror withholding judgment and criticism. Then the person finds a position that is relaxing and comfortable. Without a set route or sequence, individual senses guide self-massage. At times the whole body may be explored and massaged and at other times people may feel like spending the time on one part, such as the face and head. Self-massage is done slowly and rhythmically with the eyes closed so that all one's attention can be focused on the sensation.

RESEARCH

During the past half-century, numerous reports on clinical trials have been published in health care literature. These reports have documented the benefits of massage therapy for the treatment of pain, inflammation, lymphedema, nausea, muscle spasm, various soft-tissue dysfunctions, grand mal seizures, anxiety, depression, and insomnia. A large number of studies have also been reported in China and Europe (*Alternative Medicine,* 1994).

The following studies have been conducted at the Touch Research Institute at the University of Miami School of Medicine:

- Premature infants who were massaged 15 minutes three times a day gained 47 percent more weight in their first 10 days than those who were not touched. They were discharged from the hospital six days sooner, at a savings of $10,000 each (Colt, 1997).
- Cocaine-exposed preterm infants given massages three times a day for a 10-day period showed fewer postnatal complications, less stress behaviors, more mature motor behaviors, and a 28 percent greater daily weight gain (Field et al., 1986).
- Fifty-two depressed adolescent inpatients received a 30-minute back massage every day for five days while the control group viewed relaxing videos. The massaged group showed less depression and anxiety and more normal sleep patterns (Field et al., 1992).
- Forty HIV-positive men had 45-minute massages once a day, five days a week for one month. They demonstrated an increase in serotonin levels and in natural killer (NK) cells, a key component of the immune system. This study was the first time anyone ever boosted NK cells without drugs (Castleman, 1996).
- Workers who received a 15-minute chair massage twice weekly for one month performed math problems in half the time and with half the errors. In addition, their levels of cortisol, a stress hormone, dropped 24 percent (Castleman, 1996).

Other studies indicate the following benefits:

- Massage therapy was effective in reducing the frequency of episodes and disability in persons suffering from chronic inflammatory bowel disease (Joachim, 1983).
- Older persons who received massage therapy demonstrated physiological signs of relaxation such as decreased blood pressure and heart rate, and increased skin temperature (Fakouri and Jones, 1987).

Other studies have demonstrated increased leg strength in cyclists who received a 10-minute massage compared to those who simply rested following extreme exercise. Studies have also measured increased levels of endorphins following a 30-minute massage. Lymph drainage massage has been shown to be more effective than mechanized methods or diuretic drugs to control lymphedema secondary to radical mastectomy. Saliva samples in elderly people who were massaged demonstrated a significant increase in IgA, a protein produced by the immune system that acts as the body's first line of defense against the common cold (Castleman, 1996). Oleson and Flocco (1993) found that massage of the ears, hands, and feet of women with premenstrual syndrome experienced a 62 percent reduction in symptoms. Studies under way at the Touch Research Institute include HIV-exposed infants, depressed infants, infant colic, children with asthma, children neglected and abused, children with diabetes or rheumatoid arthritis, depressed adolescent mothers, adolescents with eating disorders, HIV-positive adults, adults with hypertension, fibromyalgia, or spinal cord injuries, and domestic violence victims (*Alternative Medicine,* 1994).

INTEGRATED NURSING PRACTICE

Massage provides a valuable tactile approach, which, when combined with verbal approaches, communicates nurses' care and compassion. Back rubs, lasting three to five minutes, offer physiological and mechanical benefits to clients in a variety of settings. A back rub is usually given after the bath, but you may also find that one given in the evening will help clients to relax and fall asleep. Massage the back in a slow, rhythmical, and relaxed manner. Tightness through the shoulder and neck muscles from an uncomfortable resting position can be relieved with friction or petrissage. Gently rubbing the skin over bony areas increases circulation and helps prevent skin breakdown. If you are caring for someone who is in bed a great deal of the time, offer massage each time the person's position is changed. Observe for areas of redness, especially over the sacrum and the back of the heels, elbows, and knees. Stroking toward the pressure areas encourages capillary dilatation.

Some people, self-conscious about full-body or even back massage, may accept and benefit from hand and foot massage. See Figure 11.1 for the procedure for a hand massage. These same steps can be adapted for a foot massage. By stimulating the circulation, massage eases stiffness and pain in persons with arthritis and helps drain lymph and decrease fluid retention in persons with dependent edema.

Childbirth nurses and nurse midwives have long advocated massage during pregnancy. A light natural oil such as tangerine, almond, or safflower is used, avoiding the addition of any essential oils, which may have ill effects on the fetus. The benefits of massage during pregnancy are (Arcier, 1990):

- Relaxing. Massage helps reduce tension in the neck and shoulders and, in the later stages of pregnancy, in the lower back.
- Uplifting. Massage minimizes fatigue and improves the flow of energy and induces a general feeling of well-being.

While holding the client's hand, place massage oil or lotion on the hand. Gently bend the hand backward and forward to limber the wrist. Grasp each finger and do range of motion exercises.

A

With the client's elbow resting on the table, hold the hand upright and massage the palm of the hand with the cushions of your thumbs, using circular movements in opposite directions.

B

Figure 11.1:   Procedure for Hand Massage

C

Massage each finger from the base to the tip, along all surfaces of the finger.

D

Use your thumbs to massage the wrist and top of the
hand, using circular movements. Repeat three times.
Repeat the entire procedure on the other hand.

Figure 11.1:   (*continued*)

- Improves circulation. Massage may help prevent varicose veins that may
  accompany pregnancy.
- Stimulates lymphatic drainage. Massage helps reduce fluid retention in
  the ankles and feet that often occurs during the later stages of pregnancy.
- Tones muscles. Massage helps relieve the pain of distended ligaments
  and decrease the tendency to cramp that may occur toward the fifth
  month of pregnancy.
- Maintains skin tone. Massage increases the skin's suppleness and elasticity and may help prevent stretch marks.

Midwives and maternal child nurses incorporate massage during labor and delivery. During contractions, deep massage of the lower back and hips provides counterpressure that many women find helpful. In between contractions, you can massage the shoulders, back, hands, and feet to increase comfort and relaxation. If contractions are lagging, a light massage of the breasts may stimulate activity. After delivery, gentle heat may be applied to the breasts followed by a firm massage around the breast toward the nipple to assist in milk letdown.

If you practice nursing in newborn nurseries and neonatal intensive care units, you should advocate infant massage and incorporate it as a basic nursing intervention. Most premature and drug-exposed infants given three massages a day are more alert, active, and responsive than nonmassaged infants. Massaged infants are also able to calm themselves, sleep more deeply, and have fewer episodes of apnea. Dr. Ruth Diane Rice (1975), a nurse and specialist in early child development, has conducted research on massage with premature infants. She believes that revolutionary changes are necessary in the care of newborns if the high incidence of learning disabilities, hyperactivity, emotional disturbances, and other disorders which have their origins in infancy are to be prevented.

Whether you are massaging a newborn or teaching parents infant massage, the process lasts for as little as a few minutes or as long as a half hour but should be performed only when a baby is willing. If a baby is crying, hiccuping, turning his head to the side, the massage should be discontinued and tried another time. The oil for infant massage should be a light-textured, unscented oil such as almond, coconut, or safflower oil. Infants should not be massaged with synthetic, petroleum-based products because they have no nutritional value and are not absorbed into the skin. The following are some gentle massage strokes for infants:

- Foot: press all over the bottom of the foot using the thumbs
- Leg: hold the leg like a baseball bat and move the hands up the leg squeezing slightly and turning in opposite directions
- Stomach: make scooping strokes, one hand following the other
- Chest: begin with both hands at the center and gently push out to the sides along the rib cage
- Back: with fingers spread apart, "comb" the back from the neck to the buttocks
- Hand: roll each finger between one's finger and thumb; press gently all over the palm, using the thumbs
- Face: make small circles around the jaw using the fingertips

In the psychiatric setting, you may integrate executive massages for those clients who wish to use massage as a stress reducer. Debbie Hilliard (1995), a Clinical Nurse Specialist and a Certified Massage Practitioner, has utilized massage for several years with people experiencing persistent mental illness. She found that, while massage was not suitable for all clients, the majority who sought the treatment reported subjective relief from tension, anxiety, and muscle pain. Massage also provides an appropriate way to meet people's basic need for touch.

You may wish to expand your expertise in massage by becoming a massage therapist and combining that practice with your practice of nursing. Box 11.2 lists some massage programs specifically designed for nurses.

Box 11.2: Massage Programs for Nurses

Bonnie Mackey, A.R.N.P., M.S.N.
Mackey Health Institute, Inc.
1900 S. Olive
W. Palm Beach, FL 33401
888-200-0496

New Center College for Wholistic Education and Research
Syosset, NY

Royal College of Nursing
London, England

TRY THIS: *Massage*

One-Minute Massage

Revive your hair and your spirits with a simple scalp massage you can do anytime and almost anywhere. With your fingertips, rub entire scalp using small circular motions. Massage stimulates the scalp oils that bring out the natural shine in hair. It is also an all-over energy booster.

TRY THIS: *Massage* (*continued*)

Two-Minute Massage

Mix a tablespoon each of wheat germ, olive oil, and sunflower oil. Rub on your shoulders and neckline. After two minutes, rinse and pat dry. Lavish damp skin with lotion.

Partner Massage

- Set the mood with scented candles and soft music in a dimly lit room.
- Lay folded quilts on the floor rather than using your bed so you can easily move around your partner.
- Remove jewelry to avoid catching hairs as you work.
- Comfort your partner by covering her/him with a sheet and placing a pillow under the knees when lying on the back and under the ankles when lying on the front.
- Massage works best when strokes are lubricated. Any vegetable oil will work, but scented massage oils can add to the sense of relaxation and sensuality.
- Begin with both of you doing slow deep breathing to center and ground.
- Warm up the oil by rubbing it between your hands before applying it.
- Begin with light strokes and proceed to deeper pressure only after the muscles in the area have relaxed and warmed up.
- Your partner should tell you if any strokes feel uncomfortable: too light, too deep, or on a tender spot.
- Take your time: ideally 2–3 minutes per foot, 10 minutes per leg, 15–20 minutes for the back, and 15 minutes for the front including 5 minutes on the face.
- Stroke toward the heart instead of against the flow of blood returning to the heart.
- Never press directly on the spinal column, just on the muscles on either side of it.
- The best massage comes from using your whole body, not just your arms.

Sources: Castleman, *Nature's Cures* (Emmaus, PA: Rodale Press, 1996); Meyer, "A touching experience," *Cooking Light* (1997) 6: 84–88.

REFERENCES

Alternative Medicine: Expanding Medical Horizons. 1994. A report to the National Institutes of Health on Alternative Medical Systems and Practices in the United States. U.S. Government Printing Office. Washington, D.C.

ARCIER, M. 1990. *Aromatherapy.* London: Hamlyn.

BARNES, J. F. September 16, 1987. Myofascial release. *Physical Therapy Forum.* 30–32.

CASTLEMAN, M. 1996. *Nature's Cures.* Emmaus, PA: Rodale Press.

COLT, G. H. 1997. The magic of touch. *Life.* 52–62.

FAKOURI, C., and JONES, P. 1987. Relaxation Rx: Slow stroke back rub. *J Gerontological Nursing.* 13: 32–35.

FIELD, T. et al. 1992. Massage reduces anxiety in child and adolescent psychiatric patients. *J Am Acad Child Adoles Psychiatry.* 31: 125–131.

FIELD, T. et al. 1986. Tactile/kinesthetic stimulation effects on preterm neonates. *Pediatrics.* 77: 654–658.

HILLARD, D. 1995. Massage for the seriously mentally ill. *J Psychosoc Nurs.* 33(7): 29–30.

JAHNKE, R. 1997. *The Healer Within.* San Francisco: Harper.

JOACHIM, G. 1983. The effects of two stress management techniques on feelings of well-being in patients with inflammatory bowel disease. *Nursing Papers.* 15: 5–18.

MANN, C. M. 1993. Thai massage. *Massage Magazine.* 66: 32–38.

MEYER, M. 1997. A touching experience. *Cooking Light.* 6: 84–88.

Milbank Memorial Fund. 1998. *Enhancing the Accountability of Alternative Medicine.* New York: Milbank Memorial Fund.

MONTAGU, A. 1971. *Touching: The Human Significance of the Skin.* New York: Perennial Library.

MOWER, M. B. 1997. Massage returns to nursing. *Massage Magazine.* 69: 47–55.

OLESON, T. and W. FLOCCO. 1993. Randomized controlled study of premenstrual syndrome treated with ear, hand, and foot reflexology. *J Obstetrics and Gynecology.* 82: 906–911.

RAMSEY, S. M. 1997. Holistic manula therapy techniques. *Primary Care: Clinics in Office Practice.* Philadelphia: W. B. Saunders. 24(4): 759–784.

RICE, R. D. 1975. Premature infants respond to sensory stimulation. *APA Monitor.* 6(11): 8–9.

SEGEN, J. C. 1998. *Dictionary of Alternative Medicine.* Stamford, CT: Appleton & Lange.

STOLZOFF, R. 1997. The Rolfing method. *Massage Magazine.* 70: 34–38.

WINE, A. K. 1997. Petrissage and Vibration. *Massage Magazine.* 70: 105–107.

RESOURCES

American Massage Therapy Association
820 Davis Street, Suite 100
Evanston, IL 60201
847-864-0123
www.amtamassage.org

American Oriental Bodywork Therapy Association
609-782-1616

Associated Bodywork and Massage Professionals
800-458-2267
www.abmp.com

Hospital-Based Massage Network Newsletter
5 Old Town Square, Suite 205
Fort Collins, CO 80524
970-407-9232

International Association of Infant Massage
1720 Willow Creek Circle, Suite 516
Eugene, OR 97402
800-248-5432

International Massage Association
202-387-6555
www.imagroup.com

International Nursing Touch Therapy Association
email: intta@aol.com

Nursing Touch Massage Therapy Association
email: ntmta@aol.com

National Certification Board of Therapeutic Massage and Bodywork
8201 Greensboro Dr., Suite 300
McLean, VA 22102
800-296-0664
www.ncbtm.com

Rolf Institute
205 Canyon Blvd.
Boulder, CO 80302
800-530-8875

Shiatsu Academy of Tokyo
320 Danforth Ave., Suite 206
Toronto, Ontario Canada, M4K 1N8
416-466-8780

12 Pressure Point Therapies

Our deepest fear is not that we are inadequate. Our deepest fear is that we are powerful beyond measure. It is our Light, not our darkness, that most frightens us. We ask ourselves, who am I to be brilliant, gorgeous, talented and fabulous? Actually, who are you not to be? You are a child of God. Your playing small doesn't serve the world. There's nothing enlightened about shrinking so that other people won't feel insecure around you. We were born to make manifest the Glory of God that is within us. It's not just in some of us; it's in everyone. And as we let our own Light shine, we unconsciously give other people permission to do the same. As we are liberated from our own fear, our presence automatically liberates others.

Marianne Williamson, A Return to Love

Acupuncture, acupressure, Jin Shin Jyutsu, Jin Shin Do, and reflexology are different forms of the same practice of stimulating points on the body to balance the body's life energy. Jin Shin Jyutsu, Jin Shin Do, and reflexology are forms of acupressure and in this chapter the term *acupressure* includes all the forms. Acupuncture and acupressure are based on the theory that applying pressure or stimulation to specific points on the body known as acupuncture points, can relieve pain, cure certain illnesses, and promote wellness. Acupuncture uses needles while acupressure uses finger pressure. Although the older of the two techniques, acupressure is not as powerful and could be considered the over-the-counter version of acupuncture. Acupressure is easy to learn and convenient for self-care whereas acupuncture requires training to use the needles. Frequently, these practices are part of a holistic approach to wellness and are combined with diet, herbs, mind-body techniques, and spiritual therapies.

Consumers in the United States have increasingly turned to acupuncture and acupressure to maintain their health and treat various disorders. They spend $500 million a year on acupuncture for complaints ranging from low-back pain to migraines to gallstones (Thompson, 1997). Used with great success on humans for thousands of years, acupuncture and acupressure are now available for cats, dogs, and horses through veterinarians trained in Traditional Chinese Medicine (Schwartz, 1996).

BACKGROUND

Acupuncture and acupressure started in China several thousand years ago. The practice spread to Korea around 300 A.D. and to Japan in the seventeenth century. In the late nineteenth century a Canadian physician, Sir William Osler, became interested in acupressure techniques, but they remained largely unknown in North America until the 1970s. Accompanying President Richard Nixon on his trip to China in 1972, James Reston, a reporter for the *New York Times,* wrote about his experience with acupuncture for relief of pain following abdominal surgery in China. This article began the upsurge of interest in these therapies in the United States. At the present time, acupuncture and acupressure are practiced widely in Asia, the former Soviet Union, and Europe and are gaining in popularity in North America (Milbank, 1998).

Jin Shin Jyutsu (pronounced jin-shin, JIT-soo) and Jin Shin Do are Japanese phrases meaning The Way of the Compassionate Spirit. They are ancient practices that fell into relative obscurity until they were dramatically revived in the early 1900s by Master Jiro Murai in Japan. Dying from a terminal illness, he turned in desperation to Jin Shin Jyutsu and meditation. Within a week he was completely well. He spent the remaining 50 years of his life researching and sharing his knowledge of this healing art, which he referred to as the art of happiness, the art of longevity, and the art of benevolence. After World War II, a Japanese American, Mary Burmeister, studied with Master Murai for many years and eventually returned to the United States with the "gift" of Jin Shin Jyutsu and Jin Shin Do. Today, thousands of students throughout the United States and around the world study and practice Jin Shin Jyutsu and Jin Shin Do (Worldworks, 1996).

Reflexology, an associated ancient practice, limits the use of acupressure points, or reflexes, to the feet, hands, and ears. William Fitzgerald, an American physician, introduced reflexology to the West in 1913. He noted that postoperative pain was less when pressure was applied to people's feet and hands just before surgery. In spite of Fitzgerald's work, it was the efforts of Eunice Ingham, a physical therapist, who expanded and refined Fitzgerald's observations and found that reflexology not only reduced pain but provided other health benefits as well. Ingham mapped the specific reflex zones on the feet, hands, and ears that reflexologists use today. This work gave her the distinction of being the founder of modern reflexology in the West (Rosenfeld, 1996).

PREPARATION

The United States has more than 40 schools and colleges of acupuncture, 20 of which have either been approved or are currently being reviewed for approval by the National Accreditation Commission for Schools and Colleges of Acupuncture and Oriental Medicine. Thirty-two states regulate the practice of acupuncture, and of the 6,500 acupuncturists practicing in the United States, about 3,300 have taken the examination administered by the National Commission for the Certification of Acupuncturists (NCCA). To take the exam, candidates must have completed three years of full-time training and apprenticed with a certified acupuncturist for three years. Immigrant acupuncturists trained abroad must have practiced acupuncture for four years in lieu of apprenticeship (Castleman, 1996; Milbank, 1998).

An estimated 5,000 American doctors now include acupuncture in their practices. Most are family physicians, anesthesiologists, orthopedists, and pain specialists. Few physicians are NCCA-certified but most are certified by the American Academy of Medical Acupuncture instead. Even though acupuncture is used in China to treat many conditions, in the United States conventional physicians have taken the technique out of context, using it most often to relieve acute and chronic pain. Nationally, an estimated 12,000 nonmedical doctors practice acupuncture, including nurses, naturopathic physicians, and chiropractors (Weil, 1995).

Professionals using acupressure are usually physical therapists or massage therapists with special training in this field. Some nurses are trained in acupressure and use it to help clients sleep and to reduce levels of anxiety. Midwives may use acupressure techniques to promote relaxation during labor and reduce breast engorgement after delivery. No specific license or certification is needed to practice any of the forms of acupressure.

CONCEPTS

Meridians

Acupuncture, acupressure, Jin Shin Jyutsu, Jin Shin Do, and reflexology are treatments rooted in the traditional Eastern philosophy that qi, or life energy, flows through the body along pathways known as meridians. Like major power lines, the meridians connect all parts of the body. As vital energy flows through the meridians, it forms tiny whirlpools close to the skin's surface at places called *hsueh,* which means cave or hollow. In Traditional Chinese Medicine, these are acupuncture points; in India, *marma* points. These pressure points function somewhat like gates to moderate the flow of qi. Acupuncture needles inserted into these points or pressure on these points releases blocked energy and improves the circulation of qi in the body (Collinge, 1998).

The body has 14 major meridians and 360 to 365 classic points through which qi can be accessed. Most practitioners, however, focus on 150 points. The points themselves are metaphors for a person's journey through life with names such as "Spirit Gate," "Great Esteem," "Joining the Valleys," and "Inner Frontier Gate." Each meridian is also associated with an internal organ after which it is named: stomach, spleen, heart, small intestine, bladder, kidney, circulation–sex, gall bladder, liver, lung, and large intestine. The triple-warmer meridian is associated with the thyroid and adrenal glands, the governing meridian with the spine, and the central meridian with the brain. Chapters 2 and 3 present more detailed information regarding energy and meridians.

Microsystems

At many points in the body the meridians converge. These points are reflexes to distant parts of the body and are called microsystems. Microsystems are areas of the body that are small, local representations of the whole body and are located on the feet, hands, and ears. In other words, each individual part of the body has an associated reflex on the ear, the hand, and the foot. The reflexes are symmetrical in that organs on the right side of the body are in the right foot, and the left organs on the left foot. The reflexes also correspond in descending order: the brain reflexes are in the tips of the toes, the eyes and ears under the toes, the shoulders and lungs on the ball of the foot, the stomach and pancreas on the instep, the intestines and colon towards the heel, and the hips on the heel. See Figures 12.1 a, b, c for reflexology maps.

Mind-Body Connections

In the pressure point tradition, the mind, body, spirit, and emotions are never separated. Thus, the heart is not just a blood pump; the heart also influences one's capacity for joy, one's sense of purpose in life, and one's connectedness with others. The kidneys filtrate fluids but they also manage one's capacity for fear, one's will and motivation, and one's faith in life. The lungs breathe in air and breathe out waste products, but they also regulate one's capacity to grieve, as well as one's acknowledgment of self and others. The liver cleanses the body, and it also influences one's feeling of anger as well as that of vision

Figure 12.1(a): Foot Reflexology Points

1. Head and brain
2. Pituitary and pineal glands
3. Throat and thyroid gland
4. Sinus
5. Eyes and ears
6. Shoulder
7. Heart
8. Lungs and thymus gland
9. Diaphragm and solar plexus
10. Stomach

11. Liver
12. Gall bladder
13. Kidney
14. Adrenal gland
15. Spleen
16. Pancreas
17. Small intestine
18. Large intestine
19. Bladder
20. Sacrum and sciatic nerve

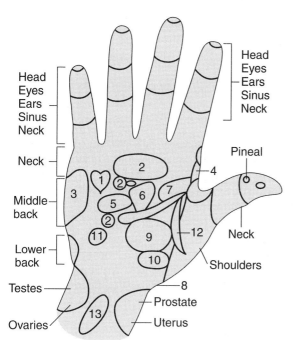

Head
Eyes
Ears
Sinus
Neck

Head
Eyes
Ears
Sinus
Neck

Neck

Middle back

Lower back

Testes

Ovaries

Pineal

Neck

Shoulders

Prostate

Uterus

Figure 12.1(b):
Hand Reflexology Points

1. Heart (left hand) and thymus gland
2. Lungs
3. Liver (right hand) and shoulders
4. Solar plexus
5. Pancreas
6. Kidneys and adrenals
7. Stomach
8. Large intestine
9. Small intestine
10. Bladder
11. Appendix
12. Thyroid
13. Sacrum and pelvis

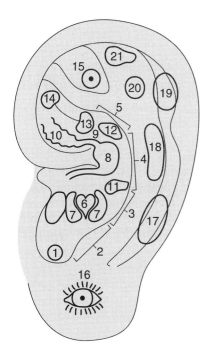

Figure 12.1(c): Ear Reflexology Points

1. Endocrine glands and hormones
2. Head and brain
3. Neck
4. Upper and middle back
5. Lower back
6. Heart and thymus gland
7. Lungs
8. Stomach
9. Small intestine
10. Large intestine
11. Spleen
12. Liver
13. Kidney
14. Bladder
15. Nervous system and spirit
16. Eyes and face
17. Shoulders
18. Arm and elbow
19. Hand
20. Leg and knee
21. Foot

and creativity. The stomach has a part in digestion of food and influences one's ability to be thoughtful, kind, and nurturing as well. These are just a few of the mind-body connections that pressure point practitioners recognize (Grissmer, 1996).

VIEW OF HEALTH AND ILLNESS

Health is viewed as a state of harmony, or balance, of the opposing forces of nature, both internal and environmental. The body requires balanced yin and yang energy to function properly and utilize its natural ability to resist disease. It is believed that everything needed to maintain and restore health already exists in nature and that pressure point therapies free up energy and restore balance, thus enabling individuals to maintain or regain their health.

Symptoms are caused by an imbalance of yin and yang in some part of the body leading to excesses or deficiencies of life energy throughout the body. When the flow of energy becomes blocked or congested, people experience discomfort or pain on a physical level, may feel frustrated or irritable on an emotional level, and may experience a sense of vulnerability or lack of purpose in life on a spiritual level. When the flow of energy is interrupted, the area cannot nourish or cleanse. If not corrected, these blocks and imbalances in energy channels can result in dis-ease and eventually illness.

The goal of care is to recognize and manage the disruption before illness or disease occurs. Qi can be thrown out of balance in a number of ways, including genetic vulnerability, accident or trauma, diet, lifestyle, emotional upset, spiritual distress, climate, or noxious agents. Pressure point practitioners bring balance to the body's energies, which promotes optimal health and well-being, and facilitates people's own healing capacity.

DIAGNOSTIC METHODS

The initial consultation involves a holistic assessment, because no part of the self is considered a neutral bystander when the body is in a state of imbalance. A detailed medical history is an important part of the diagnostic process. Special attention is paid to the connection between body, mind, emotions, and spirit.

If pressure point therapies are done within the context of Traditional Chinese Medicine, palpation is the major diagnostic method. Reading the pulses provides a remarkable amount of information about the person's condition. Imbalances in the body can be detected through palpating microsystems on the feet, hands, and ears. If something feels different in the microsystems, the corresponding organ is examined in more detail. Chapter 3 discusses the diagnostic process of Traditional Chinese Medicine in greater detail.

TREATMENT

Pressure point therapies consider symptoms to be an expression of the condition of the person as a whole. Thus, sessions focus not only on relieving pain and discomfort, but also on responding to disruptions before they develop into illnesses.

Acupuncture

To restore the flow of energy, acupuncturists insert sterile, hair-thin needles at points along the meridians. The needles are rotated, twirled, or accompanied by a weak electrical current, and are often left in several minutes or longer. Acupuncturists also may apply heat or use finger pressure to alter the flow of qi. Clients feel little, if any, pain. Some people experience sensations of warmth, tingling, heaviness, or a dull ache.

Evidence now indicates that, in addition to restoring the flow of energy within the meridians, acupuncture reduces pain by triggering the release of endorphins. Acupuncture also stimulates the nervous system to release ACTH, a chemical that aids in fighting inflammation, prostaglandins which help wounds heal more quickly, and other substances that may promote nerve regeneration. Unlike drugs and surgery, acupuncture has virtually no side effects (Castleman, 1996).

Jin Shin Jyutsu, Jin Shin Do

Jin Shin Jyutsu/Jin Shin Do can be applied as self-help and also by a trained practitioner. It is practiced by placing the fingertips over clothing on designated pressure points, to harmonize and restore the energy flow. Rather than doing something to the body, Jin Shin encourages the body to "let go," which is seen as the path to awakening one's awareness of harmony within the self and the universe.

A session generally lasts about an hour with the client lying on a table fully clothed. The practitioner's hands act as "jumper cables" to "kick start" the correct flow of energy. A spot on the shoulder may be held at the same time as a spot on the knee. The practitioner uses special sequences of hand positions to stimulate the circulation of energy. The touch is gentle, steady, and never involves force. It is generally pain-free; any tenderness in a particular area is caused by a blockage and tends to dissipate as the area is held. Some people may feel hot or cold or feel a sensation in another part of the body than the one where the practitioner is working. Most people experience a sense of deep relaxation with Jin Shin Jyutsu/Jin Shin Do (*Alternative Medicine,* 1992).

Reflexology

Reflexologists manipulate the reflex zones most commonly on the feet but the hands or ears may also be manipulated. A session usually lasts about 45 minutes with the client sitting comfortably in a chair with the practitioner using thumb and fingers in small, creeping movements over the sole of the foot. This manipulation prompts the nervous system to speed up the body's response to an afflicted area by stimulating the flushing of toxins from the area.

Uses

According to the World Health Organization, pressure point therapies are widely used around the world to treat many conditions including allergies, bronchitis, cerebral palsy, diabetes, hemorrhoids, hepatitis, herpes, infertility, premenstrual syndrome, stroke, and ulcers. In the United States, reduction of pain is a major therapeutic use including pain from dental work, temporomandibular joint syndrome (TMJ), migraine headaches, osteoarthritis, low back pain, sciatica, carpal tunnel syndrome, and sports injuries. Acupuncture can provide symptomatic relief of the pain of bursitis and is much safer than anti-inflammatory drugs and injections of steroids. Researchers are investigating the use of acupuncture to ease withdrawal symptoms of smokers, alcoholics, and drug addicts who are trying to manage their addictions. Some studies have reported that acupuncture increases uterine contractions in pregnant women who are past their delivery dates (Castleman, 1996; Milbank, 1998; Weil, 1995).

Contraindications

Pressure point therapy is not appropriate for every ailment. It is not indicated for an acute or infectious illness, fever, or if surgery is needed. Foot injuries need to heal before the use of reflexology. If someone has a pacemaker, practitioners avoid stimulating the left chest zone. If someone has gallstones or kidney stones, the gallbladder and kidney points are avoided. During pregnancy, since pressure point therapy may induce uterine contractions, it is not recommended (Rosenfeld, 1996).

RESEARCH

In 1997 the National Institutes of Health assembled a panel of experts in a scientific court known officially as a consensus conference. A panel of 12 experts was drawn from a variety of backgrounds, including biomedical research scientists, physicians, and others. The panel's task was to listen to as much evidence as the acupuncture/pressure point research community could present in the first half of the three-day conference. The panel's judgment included the following statement: "There is sufficient evidence of acupuncture's value to expand its use into conventional medicine and to encourage further studies of its physiology and clinical value" (NIH, 1997). The panel determined that acupuncture was clearly effective for nausea and vomiting from pregnancy, sea sickness, chemotherapy, and anesthesia and for postoperative pain from dental surgery. The panel also noted "other situations such as addiction, stroke rehabilitation, headache, menstrual cramps, tennis elbow, fibromyalgia, myofascial pain, osteoarthritis, low back pain, carpal tunnel syndrome, and asthma where acupuncture may be useful as an adjunct treatment or an acceptable alternative or be included in a comprehensive management program" (NIH, 1997). This panel focused only on data collected by means of randomized controlled clinical trials and, as such, did not review data on technique, cost-benefit, patient preference, or practitioner education. The National Institutes of Health's Office of Alternative Medicine has awarded grants to continue research on acupuncture for chronic sinusitis in HIV infection, postoperative oral surgery pain, premenstrual syndrome, osteoarthritis, and depression. It is anticipated that further research results in pressure point therapies will be available in the not-too-distant future.

- In a recent national survey of acupuncture users, the research team at the Traditional Acupuncture Institute found that 90 percent of clients reported that their symptoms disappeared or improved after treatment. Of those who said they still had a condition, many said they now found it easier to live with. The improvements people experienced were physical, emotional, mental, spiritual, and social. Seventy-nine percent said they used fewer prescription drugs and 71 percent said they avoided surgery that had been recommended. According to reports of these clients, acupuncture costs about 60 percent as much as care by conventional physicians. Respondents repeatedly praised their practitioners for paying attention to all aspects of themselves and for teaching them self-care (Cassidy, 1997).
- An important study was conducted on women experiencing symptoms of premenstrual syndrome. Ear, hand, and foot reflexology treatments resulted in 62 percent of the women reporting a decrease in symptoms (Oleson and Flocco, 1993).

INTEGRATED NURSING PRACTICE

If you are interested in incorporating pressure point therapies into your nursing practice, you may want to attend a weekend or week-long program on reflexology, Jin Shin Jyutsu, or Jin Shin Do. Even without further education, you can incorporate hand, foot, or ear massages into your practice. This type of massage is easy to learn and nonintrusive. The procedure for a hand massage is in Figure 11.1 in the chapter on massage therapy. These procedures can be modified for an ear massage. The hands, feet, and ears are fairly small. If you simply massage them, focusing on any tender spots you find, you are bound to send qi or energy to all parts of the body. Few people object to this type of massage. Even if the recipient has no particular physical complaints, this type of massage is wonderfully relaxing.

You can teach clients about a number of pressure points as you advocate self-help. Box 12.1 describes this process for headaches, hiccups, and carpal tunnel syndrome. To ease tension and restore energy, try this pressure point: hold your left palm in front of you, fingers together. The fleshy spot between your thumb and index finger is a key pressure point. Using your right thumb, massage this spot in a circular motion for a slow count of 15. Then switch hands, and repeat the process. You can also teach clients several finger holds to improve their general level of well-being. Explain that they should gently hold the appropriate finger on either hand while imaging the negative emotions melting away and an easing of the physical symptoms:

- Thumb. Corresponds to worrying, depression, anxiety. Physical symptoms may be stomachaches, headaches, skin problems, and nervousness.
- Index finger. Corresponds to fear, mental confusion, frustration. Physical symptoms are digestive problems and muscle problems such as backaches.
- Middle finger. Corresponds with anger, irritability, indecisiveness. Physical symptoms are eye or vision problems, fatigue, and circulation problems.
- Ring finger. Corresponds with sadness, fear of rejection, grief, negativity. Physical symptoms are digestive, breathing, or serious skin problems.
- Little finger. Corresponds with insecurity, effort, overdoing it, nervousness. Physical symptoms are sore throat and bone or nerve problems.

Some nurses have furthered their education by completing advanced degrees in acupuncture. Two nurses are on the faculty at The Traditional Acupuncture Institute in Columbia, Maryland. Patricia Mahone, R.N., M.Ac., has a 20-year background in medical-surgical, orthopedic rehabilitation, outpatient, and home care nursing. In her quest for providing more holistic care, she explored guided imagery and Healing Touch therapy. As a client, she experienced relief from asthma, fatigue, and headaches through acupuncture and went on to earn a masters degree in acupuncture (Marghi, 1996). Ann Bailey R.N., M.S., M.Ac., has been a nurse since the 1960s and has been successfully practicing acupuncture since 1985. She holds a masters degree in nursing as well as in acupuncture. She is recognized in her field as an expert in bridging conventional health care practices with alternative therapies. She has written and narrated tapes explaining exactly how, when, and for whom acupuncture is helpful. See the Resource section for information on the tapes.

Box 12.1: Self-Help: Pressure Points

The following are several examples of how people can use pressure points to relieve discomfort or pain. Once you think you have located one of the appropriate points, probe the area with a fingertip or pencil eraser in a tight circular motion in the general location. Points often feel tender, sore, or tingling. Press the point for one minute, then stop for a few seconds, and press again. Work the point for 5 to 20 minutes. If you are experiencing a headache, hiccups, or symptoms of carpal tunnel syndrome, experiment for yourself and find which points work best for you. Remember, only some of the points need to be worked to achieve relief.

Headache

Point 1.   Hold your hand open, palm down, and find the point in the center of the fleshy webbing between the thumb and index finger.

Point 2.   Find the point on the top of the foot in the valley between the big toe and second toe.

Point 3.   Point number three is at the base of the back of the skull in the hollow above the two large vertical neck muscles.

Point 4.   This point is in the hollow above the inner eyes, where the bridge of the nose meets the ridge of the eyebrows.

Point 5.   Find the point between the eyebrows in the indentation where the bridge of the nose meets the forehead.

Point 6.   This point is two finger-widths above the webbing of the fourth and fifth toes in the groove between the bones.

Hiccups

Point 1.   Find the point in the indentation behind each earlobe.

Point 2.   This point is located at the base of the throat in the center of the collarbone.

Box 12.1: Self-Help: Pressure Points (*continued*)

Point 3.	Find this point on the center of the breastbone three thumb-widths up from the base of the bone.
Point 4.	This point is located three finger-widths below the base of the breastbone in the pit of the abdomen. If you are healthy, do not press this point for more than two minutes. If you are not healthy, do not press this point at all.

Carpal Tunnel Syndrome

Point 1.	Find the point in the middle of the inner side of the forearm, two and a half finger widths below the wrist crease.
Point 2.	This point is located in the middle of the inside of the wrist crease.
Point 3.	Find the point on the outside of the forearm, midway between the radius and ulna, two and a half finger widths below the wrist crease.

Sources: Castleman, *Nature's Cures* (Emmaus, PA: Rodale Press, 1996); Gach, *Acupressure's Potent Points* (New York: Bantam Books, 1990).

TRY THIS: *Foot Massage*

When your feet ache, your whole body suffers. Here are instructions for a 10–15 minute foot massage to relax and soothe your feet and perhaps your entire body.

- Sit in a comfortable, quiet place where you will not be disturbed. You may want to have soothing music in the background.

- Pour a small amount of nongreasy lotion or massage oil into your hands and rub them together.

- Begin massaging one foot, stroking each toe in an up-and-down motion. Then massage the entire foot using kneading, wringing motions until the lotion is absorbed.

TRY THIS: *Foot Massage* (*continued*)

- Holding your foot firmly in one hand, press the thumb of the other hand (slightly bent) on the sole of the foot near the heel. Apply even pressure with the thumb and "walk it" forward, little by little. Press one spot, move forward, press again, move forward, and so on.

- When you get to the toes, go back to the heel and trace another line from heel to toe. Continue this process until the entire sole of the foot has been worked.

- Repeat the entire process with the other foot.

Sources: Gach, *Acupressure's Potent Points* (New York: Bantam Books, 1990); Norman, *A Guide to Foot Reflexology* (New York: Simon & Schuster, 1988).

REFERENCES

CASSIDY, C. M. 1997. Patients point to what makes acupuncture care special. *Meridians.* 4(2): 30–36.

CASTLEMAN, M. 1996. *Nature's Cures.* Emmaus, PA: Rodale Press.

COLLINGE, W. 1998. *Subtle Energy.* New York: Warner Books.

GACH, M. R. 1990. *Acupressure's Potent Points.* New York: Bantam Books.

GRISSMER, J. 1996. *Meridians.* 4(1): 37–38.

MARGHI, J. R. April 22, 1996. Needles of a different gauge. *Nursing Spectrum.* 5.

Milbank Memorial Fund. 1998. *Enhancing the Accountability of Alternative Medicine.* New York: Milbank Memorial Fund.

NIH. November 1997. *Consensus Development Conference Statement of Acupuncture.* Office of the Director of the National Institutes of Health.

NORMAN, L. 1988. *A Guide to Foot Reflexology.* New York: Simon & Schuster.

OLESON, T. and W. FLOCCO. 1993. Randomized controlled study of premenstrual syndome treated with ear, hand, and foot reflexology. *J Obstetrics and Gynecology.* 82: 906–911.

ROSENFELD, I. 1996. *Dr. Rosenfeld's Guide to Alternative Medicine.* New York: Random House.

SCHWARTZ, C. 1996. *Four Paws Five Directions.* Berkeley, CA: Celestial Arts.

THOMPSON, D. November 17, 1997. Acupuncture works. *Time.* 150(2): 84.

WEIL, A. 1995. *Natural Health, Natural Medicine.* Boston: Houghton Mifflin Co.

Worldworks. 1996. History of Jin Shin Jyutsu. worldworks@lifematters.com

RESOURCES

American Academy of Medical Acupuncture
5820 Wilshire Blvd., Suite 500
Los Angeles, CA 90036
800-721-2177
800-521-2262
www.medicalacupuncture.org

American Association of Acupuncture and Oriental Medicine
4101 Lake Boone Trail, Suite 201
Raleigh, NC 27607
919-787-5181

British Columbia Acupressure Therapists Association
718 Wallace Cresent
Comox, BC, Canada V9M 3V8
250-383-2404

Canadian Acupressure Institute Inc.
733 Johnson St.
Victoria, BC, Canada
250-388-7475
email: caii@tnet.net

International Institute of Reflexology
P.O. Box 12642
St. Petersburg, FL 33733
813-343-4811

Jin Shin Institute
Santa Rosa, CA
707-525-0412

Jin Shin Foundation for Bodymind Acupressure
1084G San Maiguel Canyon Rd.
Watsonville, CA 95076
408-763-7702
fax: 408-763-1551

National Commission for the Certification of Acupuncturists
P.O. Box 97075
Washington, DC 20090

Traditional Acupuncture Institute
10227 Wincopin Circle, Suite 100
Columbia, MD 21044
410-728-2080
www.acupuncture.com
www.ampsc.com/~acupressure/JinShinDo.htm

Ann Bailey
Acupuncture Explained.
Four cassettes/5 hours $39.95 ($55.95 Canada)
ISBN 1-889643-07-6
800-748-5804
www.pentonoverseas.com

13 Hand-Mediated Biofield Therapies

Healing energy is a beneficent power available to all living things.

Dora Kunz

The more high technology around us, the more the need for human touch.

John Naisbitt, Megatrends

A wide variety of alternative healing practices emerging in popularity are designed to balance the body's biofield, or energy field, and increase the flow of energy. Richard Gerber, M.D., author of *Vibrational Medicine,* defines biofield therapy or energy medicine as the emerging science of using various forms of energy for diagnosis and healing. Reviewing hundreds of research studies, Gerber hypothesizes that conscious and unconscious thoughts exist as energy that surrounds and permeates the body. While these studies are in their early stages, validation of the existence of the human energy field is beginning to emerge. More detailed discussion of the concept of body energy is found in chapter 2.

The three most prominent therapies using the hands to alter the biofield and impact the healing process are Therapeutic Touch (TT), Healing Touch (HT), and Reiki. All three approaches could be simply defined as the use of the hands on or near the body with the intention to help or to heal (Quinn, 1998). Actually, the word *touch* is a misnomer in TT and HT, because the practitioner need not touch the recipient to achieve the desired effects during a healing session. Techniques are usually performed inches and sometimes feet from the recipient's body. These therapies are modern interpretations of several ancient healing practices, traditionally known as the "laying on of hands." TT, HT, and Reiki, however, must not be confused with faith healing, as the context in which they are practiced is not religious but scientific.

The goals of these hand-mediated therapies are to accelerate the person's own healing process and to facilitate healing at all levels of body, mind, emotions, and spirit. All three are forms of treatment and are not designed to diagnose physical conditions. Nor are they meant to replace conventional surgery, medicine, or drugs in treating organic disease (Quinn, 1998).

BACKGROUND

Therapeutic Touch is the brainchild of a nurse, which some suggest is part of its one-of-our-own appeal to the estimated 40,000 to 50,000 American nurses who practice TT. Dolores Krieger, R.N., Ph.D., Professor Emeritus, New York University, launched the TT movement in 1970 after studying with Dora Kunz, a past president of the Theosophical Society of America and a natural healer. TT refers to the Krieger-Kunz Method of Therapeutic Touch (Krieger, 1979; Kunz, 1991) and was originally developed as an energy field interaction between nurse and client. Dr. Krieger, along with Janet Quinn, R.N., Ph.D., from the University of Colorado School of Nursing, have devoted their careers to the research, study, and teaching of TT. TT has been taught in more than 80 universities and colleges in the United States and in more than 70 other countries, primarily in schools of nursing.

TT theory further developed within Rogers's (1990) nursing theory of unitary human beings. Rogers's perspective is that energy fields are the fundamental units of people and their environment. Understanding the human-environmental process is linked to energy field concepts such as openness, mutual process, dynamic unity, and capacity to establish pattern. Basic principles include the belief that human and environmental fields are a continuous mutual process, that change in these fields is expressed in continuously higher frequency wave patterning, and that change is continuously innovative, to some extent unpredictable, and increasingly diverse. Rogers states that the human and environmental fields cannot, in fact, be separated. Thus the nurse's energy field is unified with the client's energy field. Nursing interventions are viewed as the knowledgeable and purposeful patterning of the nurse's and client's energy fields to maximize healing and well-being (Rogers, 1990).

In the 1980s, scientists in the emerging field of psychoneuroimmunology (PNI) or mind-body medicine began to study energy medicine. Among them were Herbert Benson, M.D., and Joan Borysenko, Ph.D., who discovered and studied the body's innate "relaxation response" as it relates to self-healing. Many of the PNI researchers were influenced by Eastern traditions that view the mind, body, spirit, and health as one and energy as something that people can deliberately nurture within themselves. Today, the field of mind-body medicine is well established and recognized with scientific breakthroughs occurring regularly.

Healing Touch refers to approaches taught in the American Holistic Nurses Association's (AHNA) Certificate Program in Healing Touch for

Health Care Professionals. HT was developed by Janet Mentgen, R.N., B.S.N., a Colorado nurse, who has been practicing energy-based care since 1980. When Mentgen was introduced to TT, she added it to her extensive healing repertoire and created the Healing Touch approach. In 1990, her five-course sequence in HT became the first certified program offered by the AHNA.

Reiki is a Tibetan/Japanese technique for stress reduction, relaxation, and promotion of healing. The word *Reiki* is made of two Japanese words: *rei,* which means "God's Wisdom or the Higher Power," and *ki,* which is "life force energy." Thus Reiki means "spiritually guided life force energy." Reiki is an ancient Buddhist practice rediscovered by a Japanese physician, Dr. Usui, using ancient Tibetan texts. He first used Reiki on himself and his family and then began to share his knowledge with the larger public. He opened a clinic in Tokyo in 1922 and his fame for healing spread quickly all over Japan. Reiki was introduced in the United States by Hawayo Takata, a Japanese-American woman who studied with Dr. Usui (Van Sell, 1996).

PREPARATION

Therapeutic Touch does not require extensive formal training. It can be learned by most anyone who is motivated by compassion and committed to helping others. Family members can be taught how to use it effectively with their loved ones. In fact, one of the leading researchers and teachers of this method, Janet Quinn, Ph.D., R.N., has created a videotape home-study course for family caregivers as well as a series of three videotapes for nurses who wish to incorporate TT in their practice. (See the Resource section.) TT was developed by nurses, and all nurses, regardless of clinical speciality, can use it in any setting. It is an independent nursing intervention and as such does not need a physician's order.

Nurses who seek certification as Healing Touch practitioners from the AHNA are expected to do extensive reading, including books about techniques, healing traditions, self-healing, and possible theoretical explanations. The preparation may take two to three years of study. Most programs strongly emphasize "healer, heal thyself," and practitioners are encouraged to process their own issues.

Reiki is usually learned from a Reiki Master. There are two degrees in Reiki healing, as well as a Master degree that prepares one to teach others. Most people can complete the first degree in a weekend course. The content includes historical information, the concept of energy healing, how to transfer energy from oneself to another person, and the hand positions used in healing. The second degree, also done over a weekend, includes learning how to do distant healing and further enhancement of one's physical, mental, emotional, and spiritual healing abilities. The Master degree takes years of additional study and a training mentorship with a Master Reiki practitioner. AHNA often approves Reiki programs for continuing education units.

CONCEPTS

By any name—qi, ki, prana, subtle energy—a life force energy is universally recognized in biofield therapies as the core of life and the driving force in healing. The belief is that all living beings are complex networks of interwoven vibratory fields, are surrounded by an energy field, and that energy centers control the energy flow into and out of the body. It is at this level of the subtle energy system that both health and illness originate. Energy field theory is based on quantum physics law, which assumes that matter is energy and that all living things generate vibratory fields interconnected by mathematical laws.

At this time no adequate Western scientific evidence supports the existence of this human energy field, but that it exists is the working hypothesis of TT. Many of the most sophisticated instruments widely used in conventional medicine for diagnosis and treatment are energy-medicine devices. The electrocardiogram, electroencephalogram, electromyogram, ultrasound, and magnetic resonance imaging all measure the electromagnetic frequencies emitted by various parts of the body. The use of electromagnetic fields to heal bone fractures, relieve pain, reduce inflammation, and improve circulation are examples of energy medicine in treatment (Null, 1998). Chapter 23 covers electromagnetic healing in greater detail. As scientists learn to recognize the subtler expressions of energy, old and new energy therapies will continue to complement the practice of conventional medicine.

People can detect a far greater spectrum of energies than can scientific measuring devices. Elmer Green (1989) of the Menninger Foundation believes that people's ability to sense and work with subtle energies is based in a communication system in the body that links the endocrine glands, nervous system, and the biofield. William Collinge, author of *Subtle Energy* (1998), believes that many phenomena that are dismissed as coincidences are examples of extrasensory perception, deja vu, and precognition that are part of a subtle perceptual system outside usual perception. He believes that everyone has the ability to sense energies that are not detectable technologically, but that many Western individuals reject their intuitive experiences because of a belief that anything that cannot be measured does not exist.

It is this energy field that skilled biofield practitioners can literally feel and modulate. The working hypotheses of TT are as follows (Quinn, 1998):

- Human beings are energy fields.
- These energy fields are receptive to intentional repatterning.
- Trained practitioners may assist in the intentional repatterning of a recipient's energy field.

Researchers and proponents of TT believe an intent or strong wish to help the receiver is necessary as well as a conscious use of self as a link between the universal life energy and the other individual. Prior to the actual intervention, practitioners focus completely on the well-being of the recipient in an act of unconditional love and compassion. Compassion, basic to all nursing intervention, involves two things: intention and action. TT practitioners always set their intention in mind first before entering and intervening in others' energy fields (Quinn, 1993).

In the early days, most biofield therapists thought they acted solely as a conduit or a channel for environmental energy. Because people are open systems, the transfer of energy is a natural, continuous event. Therefore, it is conceivable that one person could transfer energy to another through conscious intent. That view has since been modified to include repatterning the recipients' energy systems by providing a template of sorts upon which the repatterning occurs (Quinn, 1992; Slater, 1996). When two people are in close proximity to one another, their energy fields overlap. As they intermingle, each energy field influences the other. Through close proximity or actual touch, two people create a larger, joint energy field by connecting their individual energy fields. In intentional healing situations, practitioners regulate their own internal energy frequencies, allowing recipients to draw upon the healers' resources and energy patterns. Fahrion, Wirakis, and Pooley (1992) found that in an intentional healing situation, with or without physical contact, a state of coherence and synchrony between the brain waves of the healer and the recipient develops and they literally become unified in one energetic field.

VIEW OF HEALTH AND ILLNESS

Within individuals, energy flows like a river. If it encounters no obstructions, it is smooth, gliding, and barely perceptible. People whose energy flows smoothly usually report good health and a feeling of peace with themselves and with others. Health, then, is defined as an abundance of qi and a balance or harmony of body, mind, and spirit. In addition, healthy people experience an equilibrium between their own energy systems and those of the environment. If obstructions or imbalance in energy occur, such as trauma, pain, rage, sadness, or any physical, mental, emotional, or spiritual problem, the balanced stream of energy is disrupted and illness or disease may result.

The locus of healing is within each person and cannot be "given" to a client by a biofield therapist. People must, and do, heal themselves. Healing environments are created when nurses enter into caring moments with clients. This moment provides a spirit-to-spirit connection in which the nurse becomes a resource for clients to heal themselves. As recipients become engaged in the healing process, they often find new ways of coping with their illness.

TREATMENT

Sessions of TT last up to 30 minutes and can be done with the client sitting or lying down, fully clothed. Practitioners often combine both physical and non-physical contact during the course of treatment. It is not necessary, however, to touch the physical body, which makes this technique especially helpful in situations where the person may not be able to tolerate contact, such as with burn victims or in the case of acute rheumatoid arthritis. Clients do not have to believe in the efficacy of TT to receive benefit. The one absolutely essential ingredient in TT, however, is the goodwill and compassion of the practitioner.

The first step in the TT process is centering, which is performed by the practitioner before beginning the actual treatment. Centering is a general term for any method that people use to quiet themselves physically, mentally, and emotionally. Centering can be achieved by many methods, such as deep breathing, visualization, and focusing, which allow the practitioner to relax and focus on the intent of the healing session. Being centered allows healers to operate intuitively, with awareness, and to channel energy throughout their bodies. Box 13.1 describes one centering method.

Once centered, nurses use their hands to assess the recipient's energy field. The hands are positioned two to six inches from the body and, beginning at the head, are smoothed over the face, side and back of the head, and shoulders as if smoothing out a piece of fabric. The assessment continues down the body and over both legs. Some nurses are able to feel the energy field when they first learn TT, while for others it takes months of practice to experience the sensations. Different people describe different sensations commonly characterized as heat, cold, tingling, buzzing, emptiness, or pressure. The energy field is assessed for bilateral similarities or differences in the flow of energy. A healthy energy field is symmetrical with a smooth, flowing texture.

The next step in TT is clearing and balancing the energy field. Again, the hands are moved in a flowing motion two to six inches from the body. Blocked areas of energy are moved by using slow brushing motions from the top down and away from the body. This motion is repeated until the nurse no longer feels the blockage and the energy is moving freely and easily. This step typically lasts for five to fifteen minutes.

Direction of energy is the next step in TT. Nurses redirect energy through their own intentionality. Depending on the particular problem, nurses consciously focus their attention and intention on slowing the energy flow, stimulating the energy flow, or reestablishing the rhythm of the energy flow in problem areas. This redirection is done by placing one hand on the recipient's middle back at the level of the kidneys while holding the other hand two to three inches in front of the corresponding area on the abdomen. Practitioners visualize universal energy entering their bodies through their feet or their crown chakras. This

---

Box 13.1: How to Center

- Sit or stand comfortably and close your eyes or focus on one spot on the floor.
- Breathe in and out, slowly and deeply, concentrating on how the breath feels as it goes in and out.
- Breathe in relaxation and peace while breathing out stress and tension.
- Imagine a fairly large tree: really sense the tree as it sounds, as it smells, and according to the season.
- Get close to the tree and put your hands on the tree; lean up against the tree and put your full weight on the tree.
- Look up through the branches and feel the sun shining down; feel the sun traveling down through the tree and coming in through your head, down through your body, and out your legs.
- Focus once again on your breathing and know that you can come back to this place at any time.

With practice and experience, you will be able to center yourself within one or two deep breaths.

Source: Therapeutic Touch Video Courses from the National League for Nursing by Janet Quinn, R.N., Ph.D.

---

healing energy then moves through the nurse's body, pouring out through the hand that is on the recipient's back, and flowing through the recipient's body to the hand on the front of the abdomen. This process lasts as long as it is comfortable or effective, typically for five to fifteen minutes. The ending phase of TT is similar to the beginning phase as the hands are swept over the body from head to toe, smoothing out the energy field. The treatment session often ends in helping clients "ground" or become aware of their current physical experience. Often it is accomplished by the nurse gently holding the tops of both feet for a minute or two (Mackey, 1995; Macrae, 1988; Schmidt, 1995).

The process of an HT session may be similar to TT. Practitioners generally use their hands to assess the recipient's energetic state. The goal is to smooth the flow of energy, to mobilize it if stuck, and to leave the client with an energy flow that feels smooth, powerful, and unobstructed. HT techniques are developed intuitively and derived from various approaches such as TT, Native American medicine, and other energy healing modalities. HT treatments might last five minutes or as long as necessary, depending on the problem, the technique chosen, the practitioner's skill, and the recipient's response (Slater, 1996).

A Reiki session typically lasts one hour and consists of practitioners channeling universal life-force energy through themselves to the client. The goal is to restore balance in the client's energy field. During sessions, practitioners lay their hands on or above a specific problem area while transferring universal life energy to the recipient. A series of fifteen hand positions are designed to cover all body systems. Each hand position is held for five minutes or until the flow of energy is reestablished (Van Sell, 1996).

TT, HT, and Reiki are used only as forms of treatment, not to diagnose physical conditions. They work in conjunction with other medical or therapeutic techniques to promote healing and relieve side effects of conventional therapies. Indications include irritability and anxiety; lethargy, fatigue, and depression; premenstrual syndrome; nausea and vomiting; chemotherapy and radiation sickness; wound and bone healing; and acute musculoskeletal problems such as sprains and muscle spasms. These healing practices are often effective in many types of pain (Quinn, 1998). The only possible side effects of biofield therapies are temporary light headedness and/or a temporary sensation of heat. The primary contraindication to TT, HT, and Reiki is someone who does not want it, which falls under the doctrine of informed consent.

Practitioners believe that when they work with energy fields, they are dealing with that person as a whole and healing may occur at many levels. Recipients may experience emotional and spiritual growth as well as physical improvement, while in some cases the therapy may seem not to work at all. Even when these methods do not help people to resolve a particular problem, the session is soothing and relaxing.

RESEARCH

Most published research on hand-mediated biofield therapies is on TT, which is now being validated scientifically. Often the assumption is made that the research on TT can be applied to all biofield approaches. Such an assumption may be efficient, but not necessarily correct. Each modality must be studied for its own efficacy.

Substantial research on Therapeutic Touch demonstrates the effectiveness as follows:

- TT has statistically been shown to significantly reduce "state anxiety" in clients on a cardiovascular unit ($p < .001$) (Heidt, 1981; Quinn, 1984), and in oncology clients receiving chemotherapy ($p < .05$) (Guerrero, 1986). Olson and colleagues (1997) found that anxiety decreased in the expected direction but that the sample size of 9 was too small to achieve significant difference.
- TT has relieved tension headache pain ($p < .0001$) (Keller and Bzdek, 1986).

- TT has been found to be effective in decreasing pain and distress in elders with degenerative arthritis ($p < .001$) (Peck, 1997).
- Hospitalized psychiatric clients showed behavior changes with the use of TT as compared to relaxation groups. Those who received TT were assessed to be more amenable to talking, calmer, more self-disclosing, and more cooperative than usual (Gagne and Toye, 1994; Hughes et al., 1996).
- A study of stress reduction in 30 hospitalized children ages 2 weeks to 2 years found that children in the group given TT were calmer and had decreased pulse rate and peripheral skin temperature compared with control subjects (Kramer, 1990).
- Wright (1991) explored whether disturbances in energy field could be verified independently by different TT practitioners. Practitioners assessed 52 people with chronic pain to determine the location of energy field disturbances. A highly significant level of agreement was established among the experts as to the location of pain conditions, solely on the basis of assessing the energy field with their hands.

Interestingly, the studies in which results have been statistically insignificant used healthy volunteers as subjects; those in which results were significant used actual clients in real-life situations of illness and disease. This apparent discrepancy may indicate that TT relieves unhealthy stress levels but does not affect appropriate ones (Quinn, 1988). In 1989, Quinn analyzed published TT research and discovered methodological problems. She found a time discrepancy between TT research and TT practice. In research, five minutes were allotted for treatment, while in actual practice, TT treatments ranged from 9 to 32 minutes. Her recommendation was that in future research, TT treatments should be longer and follow standard practice more closely. Her second finding was that mock or control treatments should be done by nurses who have no experience with TT, because skilled practitioners may not be able to eliminate their healing intentions.

INTEGRATED NURSING PRACTICE

Hand-mediated biofield therapies of TT and HT have been pioneered by nurses and are easily learned by nurses. Although many nursing curricula currently include TT, most of us did not receive information about the use of hand-mediated biofield therapies in nursing school. If you have not been taught either of these therapies, you may want to learn from Dr. Janet Quinn's "A Video Course for Health Care Professionals," attend weekend or week-long continuing education conferences, or participate in the Healing Touch certification program sponsored by the American Holistic Nurses Association. You may find Dr. Krieger's book *Therapeutic Touch Inner Workbook* helpful in your course of study.

You can use TT, HT, and Reiki in almost any clinical setting including hospitals, nursing homes, home health care, hospice, and private practice. TT, HT, and Reiki are used in Lamaze classes, labor rooms, newborn nurseries, neonatal intensive care units, pediatric units, medical-surgical units, recovery rooms, and in behavioral medicine. These therapies are helpful for people with a variety of medical and nursing diagnoses. TT is supported by the National League of Nurses and the American Nurses Association. "Energy-field disturbance," defined as a state in which a disruption of the flow of energy surrounding a person's being results in a disharmony of the body, mind, or spirit, is listed as a nursing diagnosis by the North American Nursing Diagnostic Association. This diagnosis specifies that additional training is required before using TT as a nursing intervention and states that the diagnosis may not be considered conventional by some (Carpenito, 1994). TT has been the subject of numerous doctoral dissertations and masters theses, and in early 1994, the National Institutes of Health awarded a research grant to study TT.

In the current health care environment, people with acute and chronic disorders are rapidly discharged back to the community. Family and friends are often overwhelmed by caregiver responsibilities. Often they feel helpless in the face of their loved one's obvious suffering or pain. Teaching caregivers TT can be a powerful nursing intervention that counteracts the sense of helplessness many of them experience. As caregivers discover that TT can minimize the experience of pain and increase the sense of relaxation, they often feel they have something "worthwhile" to offer. In addition, the use of TT can be helpful to the caregiver, who is most likely exhausted from trying to carry on the normal daily routine, as well as care for the sick or injured person. Because the first step of TT is centering, the process demands that caregivers take a few minutes for themselves as they concentrate on their well-being and sense of peace. As caregivers increase their self-awareness, they are quicker to recognize tension and stress in their bodies, which, hopefully, encourages them to develop stress management skills. Dr. Janet Quinn has also made a TT video tape for caregivers, which is straightforward and easy to learn.

TT, HT, and Reiki produce a sense of well-being and relaxation for both the nurse and the recipient. For some nurses, it is the first time they have been given permission to be quiet, take a breath, and center during working hours. When you walk into a client's room or home in a peaceful state of mind, that gentleness, that kindness permeates the environment. Recipients react positively to the treatments, but also to the individual attention from nurses as they build relationships with clients, offer noninvasive nurturing touch, and reduce

TRY THIS: *Experience Your Energy Field*

- Vigorously rub your hands together for 20–30 seconds.
- Hold your palms together, parallel but not touching.
- Slowly separate them a couple of inches.
- Slowly bring them close together again.
- Repeat this process several more times, each time separating your palms by an additional two inches, until they are eight inches apart.
- You should be able to detect your energy field as you bring your palms together; you may feel a sense of bounciness, sponginess, or elasticity; some people describe it as the feeling of two magnets repelling each other.

clients' stress and anxiety. As Dr. Janet Quinn (1992, p. 28) has said, "We can participate in creating environments that will support healing. We can become midwives to this process of healing, creating and being safe, a sacred space into which the healing might emerge. We can, literally, become the healing environment." TT is one of the ways we, as nurses, create healing environments.

REFERENCES

CARPENITO, L. J. 1994. *Handbook of Nursing Diagnosis.* Philadelphia: JB Lippincott.

COLLINGE, W. 1998. *Subtle Energy.* New York: Warner Books.

FAHRION, S. L., M. WIRAKIS, and P. POOLEY. 1992. EEG amplitude, brain mapping, and synchrony in and between a bioenergy practitioner and client during healing. *Subtle Energies.* 3(1): 143–157.

GAGNE, D. and R. C. TOYE. 1994. The effects of therapeutic touch and relaxation therapy in reducing anxiety. *Archives of Psychiatric Nursing.* 8(3): 184–189.

GERBER, R. 1996. *Vibrational Medicine.* Santa Fe: Bear & Co.

GREEN, E. and A. GREEN. 1989. *Beyond Biofeedback.* New York: Knoll Pub.

GUERRERO, M. A. 1986. The effects of Therapeutic Touch on state-trait anxiety level of oncology patients. *Masters Abstracts International.* 24(03): 252. (University Microfilms No. 1326756.)

HEIDT, P. 1981. Effect of therapeutic touch on the anxiety level of hospitalized patients. *Nursing Research.* 30(1): 32–37.

HUGHES, P. P., R. MAIZE-GROCHOWSKI, and C. N. D. HARRIS. 1996. Therapeutic Touch with adolescent psychiatric patients. *J Holistic Nursing.* 14(1): 6–23.

KELLER, E. and V. M. BZDEK. 1986. Effects of therapeutic touch on tension headache pain. *Nursing Research* 35(2): 101–106.

KRAMER, N. A. 1990. Comparison of therapeutic touch and casual touch in stress reduction of hospitalized children. *Pediatric Nursing.* 16: 483–485.

KRIEGER, D. 1996. *Therapeutic Touch Inner Workbook: Ventures in Transpersonal Healing.* Santa Fe: Bear & Co.

KRIEGER, D. 1979. *The Therapeutic Touch. How to Use Your Hands to Help or to Heal.* New York: Prentice Hall.

KUNZ, D. 1991. *The Personal Aura.* Wheaton, IL: Quest.

MACKEY, R. B. 1995. Discover the healing power of Therapeutic Touch. *AJN.* 95(4): 27–32.

MACRAE, J. 1988. *Therapeutic Touch: A Practical Guide.* New York: Knopf.

NULL, G. 1998. *Healing with Magnets.* New York: Carroll & Graf Pub.

OLSON, M. et al. 1997. Stress-induced immunosuppression and Therapeutic Touch. *Alternative Therapies.* 3(2): 68–74.

PECK, S. D. E. 1997. The effectiveness of Therapeutic Touch for decreasing pain in elders with degenerative arthritis. *Journal of Holistic Nursing* 15(2): 176–198.

QUINN, J. F. 1998. *Foundations of Healing Praxis.* Denver, CO: University of Colorado Health Sciences Center.

QUINN, J. F. 1993. Psychoimmunologic effects of Therapeutic Touch on practitioners and recently bereaved recipients: A pilot study. *Advances in Nursing Science.* 15(4): 13–26.

QUINN, J. F. 1992. Holding sacred space. The nurse as healing environment. *Holistic Nursing Practice.* 6(4): 26–36.

QUINN, J. F. 1989. Therapeutic Touch as energy exchange: Replication and extension. *Nursing Science Quarterly.* 2(2): 79–87.

QUINN, J. F. 1988. Building a body of knowledge: Research on Therapeutic Touch, 1974–1986. *J Holistic Nursing.* 6(1): 37–45.

QUINN, J. F. 1984. *An investigation of the effects of Therapeutic Touch on anxiety of preoperative open heart surgery patients.* National Institutes of Health, Center for Nursing Research, Grant number R23 NU 01067.

ROGERS, M. E. 1990. Nursing: Science of unitary, irreducible, human beings: Update 1990. In E. A. M. Barrett, ed. *Visions of Rogers' Science-Based Nursing.* New York: National League for Nursing, 5–11.

SCHMIDT, C. M. 1995. The basics of therapeutic touch. *RN.* 58: 50–54.

SLATER, V. E. 1996. Healing Touch. In M. S. MICOZZI, ed. *Fundamentals of Complementary and Alternative Medicine.* New York: Churchill Livingstone.

VAN SELL, S. L. 1996. Reiki: An ancient touch therapy. *RN.* 59: 57–59.

WRIGHT, S. M. 1991. Validity of the human field assessment form. *Western J of Nursing Research.* 13(5): 635–647.

RESOURCES

Nursing

American Holistic Nurses Association
P.O. Box 2130
Flagstaff, AZ 86003
800-278-2462
www.ahna.org

Colorado Center for Healing Touch
198 Union Blvd., Suite 204
Lakewood, CO 80228
303-989-0581
www.healingtouch.net

Haelan Works
3080 Third St.
Boulder, CO 80304
303-449-5790
email: janetquinn@aol.com

Nurse Healers Professional Associates
1211 Locust St.
Philadelphia, PA 19107
215-545-8079

General

International Society for the Study of Subtle Energies and
     Energy Medicine (ISSSEEM)
356 Goldco Circle
Golden, CO 80401
303-278-2228
email: 74040.1273@compuserve.com
www.vitalenergy.com/ISSSEEM

Reiki Training International
P.O. Box 2765
Indianapolis, IN 46206
800-506-1144
email: dcisme@indy.net
www.w3w.com/all.html

14 Combined Physical and Biofield Therapies

> We surely owe it to ourselves, as well as
> to patients, to explore the potential of
> such treatments to alleviate pain, suffer-
> ing, and disability.
>
> *Charles, Prince of Wales*

> There are two ways to live your life.
> One is as though nothing is a miracle.
> The other is as though everything is a
> miracle.
>
> *Albert Einstein*

The two methods described in this chapter, Applied Kinesiology and Polarity
Therapy, are a combination of physical and biofield interventions. Applied
Kinesiology is both a diagnostic method and treatment modality using energy, lymphatic, neurovascular, and muscle systems. Polarity Therapy, a non-
diagnostic healing system, is based on the theories of Traditional Chinese
Medicine and Ayurvedic medicine and combines bodywork, diet, exercise, and
counseling in the treatment of clients.

BACKGROUND

Applied Kinesiology was developed in the 1960s by George Goodheart and
Alan G. Beardell, American chiropractic physicians. In the 1970s, John Thie,
also a chiropractor, took their work, simplified it for the general public, and
called this modified approach "Touch for Health." Polarity Therapy is a system
of health care developed in the 1920s by an Austrian-American holistic physician, Randolph Stone, who was a chiropractor, osteopath, and naturopath. He
studied and tested health theories from around the world, combining ancient

and modern techniques. His first work was published in 1947 and by 1954 he had completed the seven books which contain his findings.

PREPARATION

Health care professionals may go on to study Applied Kinesiology only after completion of their basic professional education. Applied Kinesiology is practiced by chiropractors, nurses, osteopaths, naturopaths, dentists, or physicians. Interested professionals take the training in a post-graduate setting, usually in weekend classes. The basic course takes more than 100 hours of classroom study and numerous hours of practice in the clinical setting after which students can test for basic proficiency. Another 200 hours of classes and the writing of at least two research papers are taken to reach the next step where a diplomate written and oral exam is given. Organized courses in Applied Kinesiology are taught in Europe, Canada, the United States, and Australia. There is no licensure per se, and providers of Applied Kinesiology practice on their professional license.

Polarity Therapy is practiced by a variety of health care professionals who have completed their basic education. To achieve the level of Associate Polarity Practitioner, the applicant must take 155 classroom and clinical hours of study. Those wishing to become Registered Polarity Practitioners must take an additional 460 hours of study for cumulative hours totaling 615. No licensure is available at the present time. Some states, however, are considering licensing polarity therapists under massage therapists, even though they are distinct therapeutic practices (American Polarity Therapy Association, 1997).

CONCEPTS

As in many alternative practices, the concept of energy is at the heart of Applied Kinesiology and Polarity Therapy. The belief is in a life force of subtle energy that surrounds and permeates all living things, often referred to as a biofield. It is unclear at this time whether the biofield is electromagnetic or the biofield is a field in physics other than an already known field. The present hypotheses are that the biofield is a form of bioelectricity, biomagnetism, or bioelectromagnetism. The exact nature is not yet established and some researches deny the reality of a biofield (*Alternative Medicine,* 1994).

Meridians

Applied Kinesiology works closely with the meridian system and pressure points. Meridians are a network of energy circuits that run vertically through the body. Each meridian passes close to the skin's surface at places called pressure points. Since each meridian is associated with an internal organ, the points offer surface access to the internal organ system. Each of the 14 meridians has related specific neurovascular points and neurolymphatic points.

Neurovascular Points

Neurovascular points are located mainly on the head. A few seconds after placing one's fingers on these points, a slight pulse can be felt at a steady rate of 70–74 beats per minute. This pulse is not related to the heart beat, but is believed to be the primitive pulsation of the microscopic capillary bed in the skin (Thie, 1996).

Neurolymphatic Points

The lymphatic system in the body flows only in one direction and acts as a drainage system of the body. It produces antibodies, makes white blood cells, and transports fats, proteins, and other substances to the blood system. The energy to the lymphatic system is regulated by neurolymphatic reflexes, located mainly on the chest and back. These reflex points act like switches that get turned off when the system is overloaded. They are usually tender spots and those which are the most sore are in greatest need of massage.

Polarity

The term *polarity* refers to the universal pulsation of expansion/contraction or attraction/repulsion known as yin and yang energy in Traditional Chinese Medicine. These polarized forces together make up the whole of anything. For example, all tissues in one's body can be understood in terms of charged energy categorized as positive, negative, or neutral. These three are in constant dynamic tension with each other, creating the basis for health or illness. Polarity between different body parts appears to be equivalent to polar differences in electromagnetic fields. Polarity therapists think of the right hand as the giving energy hand and the left as the receiving energy hand. It is believed that energy is affected and possibly distorted by life experiences and that these distortions may be corrected by a variety of healing methods.

VIEW OF HEALTH AND ILLNESS

Well-being and health are determined by the nature of the flow of energy within and without the body. When energy flows smoothly without significant blockage or fixation, the person experiences health in an ongoing and dynamic way. Disease and pain occur when energy is blocked, fixed, or unbalanced.

When someone's physical body, thoughts, and emotions are out of alignment with the energy necessary to meet a life challenge, an energy imbalance results. Within the Applied Kinesiology framework, one of the signs of an imbalance is a weakening of the muscles and a change in the posture. If these minor problems are not corrected, the imbalances may develop into physical, mental, and emotional discomfort or pain. Pain and discomfort are seen as signals to people to learn, change, and realign their lives.

DIAGNOSTIC METHODS

An Applied Kinesiology exam depends on knowledge of functional neurology, anatomy, physiology, biomechanics, and biochemistry. It is combined with standard procedures, laboratory findings, and x-rays and history taking. Generally, problems can be related to chemical imbalance, structural imbalance, mental stress, or any combination of these states. General examination procedures are used to assess the health of the client and are followed by specific examination procedures such as testing reflexes or assessing clients' balance.

Every muscle in the body is related to a specific organ or gland through the sharing of lymphatic vessels or meridians. Because organs and glands have few pain and sensory fibers, people are largely unaware of energetic imbalances in these parts. Unbalanced organs or glands, however, refer pain externally to the corresponding surface meridians and muscles indicating the cause of the problem. For example, the deltoid muscle in the shoulder shares a relationship with the lungs. If a person has abnormal lung function, such as bronchitis, pneumonia, congestion, or the flu, the problem may exhibit as a weakness in one or both deltoid muscles. When the lung problem is cleared up, the deltoid muscle returns to a normal state (Levy and Lehr, 1996).

Manual muscle testing is done to augment the other examination procedures. Goodheart and Beardall designed specific methods for testing the function of the 576 muscles of the body. Muscle weaknesses are often so subtle that physical therapists would consider the muscle strength to be within normal limits. No more than 15 percent difference should be discernable between the right and left sides. The testing positions are intended to isolate the muscle from the group with which it normally works, making it less strong than if it were used in the usual way. Small children, the elderly, and the frail will not be as strong as a healthy adult. It is more difficult to test a person who has great strength, such as an athlete, because the weakness cannot be distinguished by the tester.

A number of causes result in weak muscles including immobility, lack of exercise, poor posture, gland/organ dysfunction, dysfunction of the nerve supply, impairment of lymphatic drainage, decreased blood supply, blockage of meridians, and chemical imbalance. Testing of individual muscles is combined with knowledge of the basic mechanics and physiological functioning of the body to provide practitioners with information necessary to formulate a diagnosis.

TREATMENT

Applied Kinesiology and Polarity Therapy practitioners believe that the body, mind, emotions, and spirit are interdependent. It is believed that people are responsible for their own health and that they can take simple steps to improve and maintain their level of wellness. The practitioner's role is to facilitate and support clients' self-healing capabilities.

Applied Kinesiology uses various methods to strengthen those muscles and related organs that were found to be weak during the diagnostic phase. Improvement in the flow of energy can be measured by increased muscle strength, which is assumed to lead to an increase in energy to the corresponding organs.

Neurovascular holding points are located mainly on the head. The practitioner makes simple contact with the pads of the fingers for anywhere from 20 seconds to 10 minutes, depending on the severity of the problem. This method appears to improve the blood circulation to both the muscle and the related organ, and the weak muscle will have increased strength when retested (Thie, 1996).

Neurolymphatic points are located mainly on the chest and back. Practitioners work on the points that are related to a specific weakened muscle by a deep massage of the points for 20–30 seconds. This massage is believed to turn on the blocked reflexes, allowing the lymph flow to return to normal. The weak muscle will have improved in strength when retested (Thie, 1996). Figure 14.1 illustrates the neurolymphatic points for the lungs.

Meridians are traced in the designated direction using both sides of the body. Practitioners use the flat of their hands to give better coverage. It can be done over clothing without actually touching the client. Tracing the meridian adds the practitioner's flow of energy to the recipient's energy in a blocked meridian and may restore the normal flow of energy (Thie, 1996). Figure 14.1 also illustrates the lung meridian.

Acupressure points are held on the same side of the body as the muscle that is weak. The first arm and leg points are held at the same time, one with each hand. Light pressure is maintained for about 30 seconds or until a pulse is felt in the leg. The hands are then moved to the second acupressure points and held, again waiting for the pulse in the leg (Thie, 1996). Figure 14.2 illustrates the pressure points for the lungs.

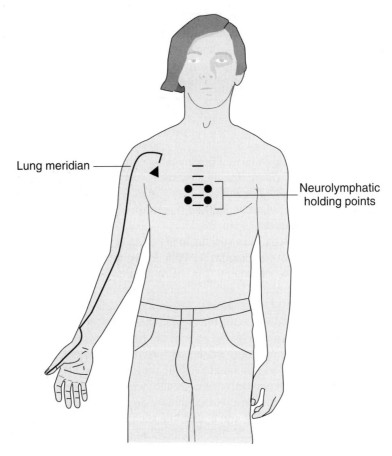

Figure 14.1:　Lung Meridian and Neurolymphatic Holding Points

In a typical Polarity Therapy session, the practitioner assesses energy flow using palpation, observation, and interview with the recipient clothed for the entire session. Sessions usually take 60–90 minutes and involve both touch and verbal interaction. Touch contact may be light, medium, or firm and is used to stimulate and balance the body's biofield. During the session, the practitioner supports the client in increasing self-awareness of subtle energy sensations, which may be experienced as tingling, warmth, or wavelike movement. Clients are also helped to process feelings and develop specific strategies for reducing stress and increasing wellness. Clients are encouraged to take responsibility for their lives and create positive thinking that is the cornerstone of good health (American Polarity Therapy Association, 1997).

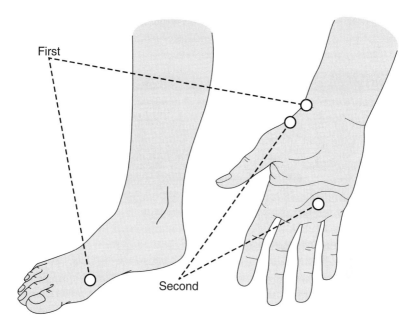

First

Second

Figure 14.2: Pressure Points for Lungs

Both Applied Kinesiology and Polarity Therapy believe that nutrition plays a major role in health and well-being. Kinesiology assesses people's nutritional status, including food intolerances, vitamin and mineral deficiencies, and other chemical sensitivities. Polarity nutrition views food as energy and develops an ongoing, changing nutritional awareness rather than a rigid set of rules. Many practitioners support the value of a vegetarian diet with no meat, fish, fowl, or eggs. They also advocate periodic use of a "cleansing diet," consisting of fresh and cooked vegetables, as well as herbal cleansing practices and formulas (American Polarity Therapy Association, 1997).

Exercise is an important part of these therapies. Applied Kinesiology practitioners encourage clients to walk for exercise. Walking is one of the few exercises that benefits all parts of the body. All of the muscles are flowing when people walk with their arms swinging. Polarity yoga is a series of simple self-help energy techniques that create relaxation and balance. This body work includes gentle rocking and stretching postures combining breath and self-massage, both of which affect the flow of energy.

Applied Kinesiology can relieve pain, stress, and muscular disorders. It is used to detect allergies, nutritional deficiencies, back or neck pain, fatigue, headache, tension, and the common cold and is believed to have some benefit for those with learning disorders. Polarity Therapy induces profound relaxation, new insight into energy flow patterns, and relief from some physical problems.

RESEARCH

Although many anecdotes recount improvement and cures with Applied Kinesiology and Polarity Therapy, little research is available as a basis for judging the usefulness of these methods. In general, rigorous research has been hindered by the disbelief of the concept of a biofield. This belief has affected funding, publishing, and status of researchers. Applied Kinesiology and Polarity Therapy would benefit from research on their efficacy and their scientific bases (*Alternative Medicine,* 1994).

INTEGRATED NURSING PRACTICE

As a nurse, you need advanced study to apply the specific techniques of Applied Kinesiology and Polarity Therapy. As a practitioner in Applied Kinesiology, you may actively intervene or make suggested changes to address food allergies, chemical imbalances, or nutritional deficiencies as determined by

TRY THIS: *Emotional First Aid*

The next time you are upset try this procedure to decrease your stress.

- Hold your frontal eminences on your forehead either with the first two fingers of your hands—the right and left at the same time—or place the palm of your hand flat on your forehead.

- While applying light pressure, in your mind go over exactly what you are thinking and how you are feeling about the problem. Continue holding these points and going over what is bothering you for a few minutes or until you feel the emotions becoming less strong.

- Let go with your hands and look around you. Mentally review the issue again. If stressful feelings are still there or have changed to other stressful feelings (fear changed to anger, for example) go back and begin the process again. After a further few minutes, release the pressure and check your feelings about the situation again.

- Hopefully your mind feels clearer and the same emotions no longer have the same stressful impact.

TRY THIS: *Redirecting the Flow of Energy*

Sit facing a partner and, placing both hands in the air, move your hands close to your partner's hands without touching. Experiment with distance and where you can feel the energy pulsating between your hands. Imagine that your partner's energy is coming in your left hand from your partner's right hand and your energy is flowing out your right hand into your partner's left hand. Imagine the circular circuit between the two of you as the energy flows up the left arm, across the heart, and down the right arm. Imagine how connected you feel at this given moment.

your clinical assessment. If appropriate, clients are encouraged to take care of their physical body with moderate exercise such as walking or swimming.

As a Polarity Therapist, you may suggest dietary changes which help balance the body. You may also suggest specific cleansing diets, herbs, and procedures to rid the body of toxic accumulations of waste products. Clients who have restricted breathing patterns may be given breathing exercises. Bodywork in Polarity Therapy involves many techniques, most of which are gentle, such as cranial holds, rocking movements, or reflexology movements. As a Polarity Therapist, you also pay close attention to people's thoughts and feelings. Negative thoughts and feelings can be detrimental to a state of well-being.

REFERENCES

Alternative Medicine: Expanding Medical Horizons. 1994. A report to the National Institutes of Health on Alternative Medical Systems and Practices in the United States. U.S. Government Printing Office. Washington, DC.

American Polarity Therapy Association. 1997. *Understanding Energy in the Healing Arts.* Boulder, CO: APTA.

LEVY, S. L. and C. LEHR. 1996. *Your Body Can Talk.* Prescott, AZ: Hohm Press.

THIE, J. F. 1996. *Touch for Health.* Marina del Rey, CA: DeVorss & Co.

RESOURCES

American Polarity Therapy Association
2888 Bluff Street, #149
Boulder, CO 80301
303-545-2080
email: SatvaHQ@aol.com
www.polaritytherapy.org

Touch for Health Kinesiology Association
11262 Washington Blvd.
Culver City, CA 90230
800-466-8342
email: admin@tfh.org

UNIT V
MIND-BODY TECHNIQUES

Peace comes within the souls of men
When they realize their oneness with the universe.

Black Elk

15   Yoga

> Yoga is a technique ideally suited to pre-
> vent physical and mental illness and to
> protect the body generally, developing
> an inevitable sense of self-reliance and
> assurance.
>
> *Sir Yehudi Menuhin,*
> *world-famous violinist*

Yoga has been practiced for thousands of years in India, where it is a way of life that includes ethical models for behavior and mental and physical exercises aimed at producing spiritual enlightenment. Although yoga developed from Hinduism, it is not a religion, but rather a journey of the body, mind, and spirit on a path toward unity. It is a method for life that can complement and enhance any system of religion, or it can be practiced completely apart from religion.

The Western approach to yoga tends to be more fitness-oriented, while the Eastern approach to yoga is to prepare people for the experience of self-realization. Most Westerners begin yoga with the goal of managing their stress, learning to relax, and increasing their vitality and well-being. After learning yoga, many become more interested in the underlying principles of physical fitness and keeping the mind focused, calm, and clear. Yoga is meant to prepare the body and mind for a useful, dedicated life (Budilovsky and Adamson, 1998).

BACKGROUND

The word *yoga* means to direct and concentrate one's attention and comes from the Sanskrit word *yuj,* to yoke or to join. Yoga was first described by Patanjali, an Indian sage who, thousands of years ago, wrote the *Yoga Sutra,* which recorded information that had been passed down orally for many years. This text has helped to define and shape the modern practice of yoga. Yoga first came to the United States in the 1890s, when Swami Vivekananda became a popular teacher and guide. In the 1960s, the Maharishi Mahesh Yoga, the creator of Transcendental Meditation, became a popular figure for America's "hippie generation," and the vogue has continued to grow since then.

The various methods of yoga all have the same goal: to attain a state of pure bliss and oneness with the universe. Raja Yoga emphasizes control of the intellect to attain enlightenment, accomplished through meditation, concentration, and breath control. Kriya Yoga is the practice of quieting the mind through scriptural study, breath control, mantras, and meditation. Karma Yoga focuses on service to all beings as the path to enlightenment. Bhakti Yoga emphasizes devotion to the divine. Inana Yoga's goal is wisdom and the direct knowledge of the divine. Tantra Yoga involves the study of sacred writings and rituals. Mantra Yoga is the study of sacred sounds. Kundalini Yoga is the study of energy movement along the spine (Budilovsky and Adamson, 1998).

   Although these many branches of yoga exist, this chapter focuses on Hatha Yoga as the form of yoga most frequently practiced by Westerners. In this particular type of yoga, the path to enlightenment is through control over the physical body as the key to control of the mind and freedom of the spirit. Physical exercises, breath control, and meditation tone and strengthen the whole person—body, mind, and spirit.

CONCEPTS

Classical yoga incorporates eight limbs or paths that provide structure for one's daily life. These physical and psychological practices are believed to contribute to a higher level of personal development. The outer aspect of yoga consists of right living (abstinence and personal discipline), right care of the body (body control), and enhancement of vital energy (breath control). Yoga also has an inner dimension that is the key purpose of yoga. Detachment, concentration, and meditation together form a single process toward the development of pure consciousness (Frawley, 1997). Box 15.1 lists the eight limbs of yoga.

Abstinences

Abstinences are about what not to do in life. The first abstinence is about nonviolence. Nonviolence not only means not physically hurting others but also having nonviolent words and nonviolent thoughts. Truthfulness, the second abstinence, results in personal integrity and strength of character. Nonstealing, the third abstinence, includes not stealing other's material belongings as well as not taking credit for things one has not done, not stealing the center of attention, and so forth. The fourth abstinence, chastity or nonlust, means holding people in high esteem and loving and respecting others. The fifth abstinence is nongreed, which means living simply and viewing possessions as tools to use in life. Nongreed leads to the avoidance of jealousy and envy (Budilovsky and Adamson, 1998).

Personal Disciplines

Personal disciplines are about what to do in life. Purity, the first discipline, is achieved through the practice of the five abstinences. The abstinences clear

Box 15.1: The Eight Limbs of Yoga: Guidelines for Living

1. Abstinences (yamas)
   Nonviolence (ahimsa)
   Truthfulness (satya)
   Nonstealing (asteya)
   Chastity or nonlust (brahmacharya)
   Nongreed (aparigraha)
2. Personal Disciplines (niyamas)
   Purity (shauca)
   Contentment (santosha)
   Self-discipline (tapas)
   Self-study (svadhyaya)
   Centering on the divine (ishvara-pranidhana)
3. Body Control (asanas)
4. Breath Control (pranayama)
5. Detachment (pratyahara)
6. Concentration (dharana)
7. Meditation (dhyana)
8. Pure Consciousness (samadhi)

away negative ways of being, leading one straight to purity. Purity also relates to cleanliness and respect for all life. Contentment, the second discipline, means finding happiness with who one is and with what one has. The third discipline, self-discipline, means being able to make a commitment and adhere to it. The fourth discipline, self-study, means studying oneself through introspection. Centering on the divine, the fifth discipline, involves devotion. These disciplines work with any religion because individuals are encouraged to focus on how the divine is in them, part of them, and all around them (Budilovsky and Adamson, 1998).

Body Control

Body control, an important part of Hatha Yoga, is attained through a number of poses or asanas. These body positions are what most Western people think of when they hear the word *yoga*. These poses help people learn to control their bodies, making them stronger, more flexible, better functioning, and more resistant to disease and other problems. Poses are also meant to facilitate meditation. The poses are frequently classified into the following groups: standing poses, inverted poses, twists, backward bending poses, forward bends, and poses for restoration. Another way of classifying poses is: balance, strength, flexibility, and relaxation. The belief in nonviolence also applies to the poses, which means that physical exercise is never done to the point of pain, because pain is indicative of doing violence to the body (Johnsen, 1998).

Breath Control

Breath control teaches people to direct energy or prana for optimal physical and mental benefit. When air is inhaled, so is vital energy that flows into the body to nourish and enliven. The purpose of balancing the breath is to make respiratory rhythm more regular, which in turn has a soothing effect on the entire nervous system. It is the best antecedent to meditation, because it focuses attention inward and reduces scattered thinking (Chopra, 1991).

Detachment

The practice of detachment is related to the senses. It is the withdrawal of the senses from everything that stimulates them. The goal of detachment is to gain mastery over external influences. This detachment can happen during breathing exercises, during meditation, and while doing the poses. The process of detachment can also be an effective technique for pain control (Frawley, 1997).

Concentration

Teaching the mind to focus on one thing instead of many is the goal of concentration. Concentration is sustaining attention while at the same time quieting the mind and relaxing the breathing. Frequently people focus on one object such as a candle flame, the figure of a circle, or a single sound. The purpose is to learn to push away the many thoughts that usually float around in one's mind. Concentration works directly on the body, allowing each yoga pose to accomplish the maximum possible benefit (Taylor, 1997).

Meditation

Breath control, detachment, and concentration lead to the state of meditation. Meditation occurs when people become absorbed into the object upon which they are concentrating. At this point, nothing else exists. It is through the process of meditation that people are able to clear their minds of clutter and thus think more quickly and see things more clearly in daily life (Budilovsky and Adamson, 1998). Meditation is covered as a separate topic in chapter 16.

Pure Consciousness

The other seven limbs of yoga lead to pure consciousness. It means a total merging with the object of meditation and, in such a way, becoming one with the universe. Generally speaking, it is "mind without thought." Many religions throughout history have pure consciousness as part of their tradition. Christianity refers to it as "pure love" and Judaism as the "divine nothingness" or "the naught." It is more than a mental or emotional experience. Physically, breathing slows drastically, the heart rate drops, and EEGs demonstrate unique patterns unlike any of the other three common states of consciousness—waking, sleeping, or dreaming. It is an ideal state, a state of pure bliss, that is elusive for most people. A few rare and diligent yogis have been able to maintain this state for extended periods of time. Most others get occasional glimpses of it while meditating (Budilovsky and Adamson, 1998; Dossey, 1989).

VIEW OF HEALTH AND ILLNESS

In yoga, health is related to the Five Sheaths of Existence. The first sheath is the physical body; the second is the vital body, life force, or prana; the third sheath is the mind, including thoughts and emotions; the fourth sheath is the higher intellect; and the fifth sheath is bliss, filled with positive energy and inner peace. It is believed that imbalances in any of these sheaths can result in illness. For example, intense anger, a disturbance in the third sheath, disrupts one's breathing pattern, which leads to an imbalance in prana or life force. The disrupted breathing allows the invasion of a virus leading to a disruption in the first sheath, manifesting as a cold. Living one's life in moderation is thought to keep all five sheaths in balance, which contributes to health and well-being.

Yogic thought places food or ahara on three levels. The first is the physical food that nourishes the body. The second is impressions or the sensations of sound, touch, sight, taste, and smell that nourish the mind. The third level is associations or the people who nourish the soul. Health and well-being are withdrawal from wrong food, wrong impressions, and wrong associations, while simultaneously opening up to the right food, right impressions, and right associations. Just as a healthy body resists toxins and pathogens, a healthy mind resists the negative influences around it (Frawley, 1997).

The yogic perspective of health and illness is related to internal and external balance. Although it is recognized that viruses, bacteria, genetics, and accidents can cause illness, disorders can also be brought on by:

- Insufficient prana, or life force
- Blocked prana
- Inappropriate diet
- Lack of cleanliness
- Unhappiness
- Pessimism and negativity.

Healthy habits, maintenance of the body, peacefulness of mind, and calmness of spirit protect people from ill health. Yoga is a great preventive medicine. It helps the body cleanse itself of toxins by removing obstacles to the proper flow of the lymphatic system. Lymph is pumped through the body by movement—musculoskeletal movement, respiratory movement, circulatory movement, gastrointestinal movement, and so forth, all of which are part of yoga. Yoga also increases the flow of vital energy throughout the body by opening up and increasing the flexibility of body joints, considered to be minor chakras. Yoga poses and breathing techniques allow energy and lymph to flow freely through the entire body, resulting in a body that works better, feels better, and fights disease more effectively. Health, from a yogic perspective, can be described as the body easeful, the mind peaceful, and the life useful (Collinge, 1998; Johnsen, 1998).

TREATMENT

People can do as much or as little yoga as they wish. Some start with all three practices—poses, breath control, and meditation. Others start with the poses and may or may not develop interest in breathing and meditation.

As practiced in the United States, a typical yoga session lasts 20 minutes to an hour. Some spend 30 minutes doing poses and another 30 minutes doing breathing practices and meditation. Others spend the majority of the time doing poses and end with a short meditation or relaxation procedure. Some people practice one to three times a week in a class, while others practice daily at home. Yoga should not be done within one to two hours after a heavy meal for sake of abdominal comfort when doing the poses. Caffeine, and other stimulants, should be avoided because they may interfere with the goal of relaxation. Yoga should never be done under the influence of alcohol or recreational drugs, as they may decrease concentration, coordination, and strength, thus increasing the risk of physical injury. Yoga is best done in comfortable, loose clothing using a nonslippery surface such as a rug, mat, or blanket. Since it is important that the process have one's full attention, the room should be void of all extraneous noise, even soft background music.

Yoga is tailored to the individual and can be done with great benefit at the beginner level as well as at the most advanced level. Participants must remember that yoga is not a competitive sport and thus a person's level does not matter. If people are stiff and out of shape, sick, or weak, sets of easy exercises help to loosen the joints and stimulate circulation. If practiced regularly, these simple exercises alone make a great difference in people's health and well-being.

Poses can be slow and careful or more vigorous. Beginning poses are used to relax tension in the muscles and joints and center the mind. Attention is paid to how the body feels and what it is doing. Every movement is made gently and slowly. Strain or force is to be avoided because yoga is a nonviolent approach that is done comfortably. Strength training is isometric as the muscles are tensed in opposition to each other. After one assumes the pose, it is held for as long as it can be done comfortably, usually about six breaths. Each pose, in a well-structured workout, includes a pose and its opposite, such as a forward bend and a backward bend, so the body stays physically balanced. Breathing should be easy, fluid, and continuous and used to facilitate the poses (Christensen, 1996).

Every yoga session should end with a few minutes of complete and total relaxation. This period is an important part of bringing the mind and body together to maximize the benefits. Some people end the session with chanting to reach a deeper state of relaxation.

Yoga offers a number of health benefits with virtually no risk of injury. The physical and psychological benefits include the following (*Alternative Medicine,* 1994; Dworkis, 1997):

- Increases flexibility of muscles and joints
- Tones and strengthens muscles
- Improves endurance
- Increases circulation
- Lowers blood pressure
- Increases lymph circulation
- Improves digestion and elimination
- Promotes deeper breathing
- Increases brain endorphins, enkephalins, and serotonin
- Increases mental acuity

- Augments alpha and theta brain wave activity
- Promotes relaxation
- Manages stress

Yoga is not a cure-all for disease. It can help, however, to relieve symptoms, decrease pain, and improve the quality of life. It helps prevent disease by reinforcing lifestyle changes such as positive health habits and attitudes.

RESEARCH

A tremendous amount of scientific research documents the benefits of yoga. Monroe and colleagues (1989) listed some 1,600 studies and many more have been conducted since then. Some of those studies indicated the following:

- People practicing yogic meditation show significantly less stress as measured by skin resistance within 10 minutes of beginning to meditate. The anxiety level remains reduced for long periods of time following the session (Benson, 1972).
- Yoga decreases the respiratory rate and increases the efficiency of the heart (Bakker, 1976; Ornish et al., 1983).
- Blood pressure and carbon dioxide levels are lowered and the brain waves reflect a more relaxed state (Blacknell et al., 1975; Fenwick et al., 1977).
- With regular practice, the right and left brain demonstrate improved communication on EEG synchronicity (Banquet, 1976).
- Physical fitness improves (Therrien, 1968).
- When used in conjunction with dietary changes, cholesterol levels have been shown to drop an average of 14 points in three weeks (Ornish et al., 1983).
- Yoga increases chest expansion, vital capacity, and tidal volume (Maris and Maris, 1979; Shivarpita, 1981).
- Blood sugar levels in those with diabetes are better controlled (Monroe and Fitzgerald, 1986).
- Yoga has been used successfully in drug treatment programs (Benson, 1969).
- Yoga is an effective adjunct for people with asthma, heart disease, migraine headaches, cancer, and arthritis (Gore, 1982; Ornish et al., 1983; Benson et al., 1977; Frank, 1975).
- People with osteoarthritis who followed a supervised program of yoga showed significant improvement in range of motion, decreased tenderness, and decreased hand pain during activity (Garfinkel et al., 1994).

- Individuals experiencing carpal tunnel syndrome had statistically significant improvement in grip strength and pain reduction through a program in yoga (Garfinkel et al., 1998).

INTEGRATED NURSING PRACTICE

The regular practice of yoga builds and tones muscles, increases flexibility, improves endurance, and promotes a state of relaxation. The physiologic responses are the opposite of the fight-or-flight stress response. Stretching and deep breathing bring on a profound sense of relaxation. Gentle stretching and range of motion joint exercises decrease muscle tension and joint stiffness. The mindful focus on awareness of self, breath, and energy minimizes anxiety associated with stress. Just getting your body down on the floor tends to clear the mind. Perhaps it is because being on the floor is so unusual to us that it changes our attitude toward and our awareness of our body (Kabat-Zinn, 1994).

Hatha yoga is designed by and for healthy, flexible people. Even when experiencing a serious illness, however, most people can work on breath control even if they do not feel up to doing the poses. The breathing exercises and relaxation response nourish the body, quiet the mind, and contribute to a more balanced state. Encourage individuals to check with their primary care practitioner if they have recently had surgery, have a debilitating physical handicap, or have cancer, diabetes, epilepsy, heart disease, high blood pressure, HIV, multiple sclerosis, or any other serious condition. Yoga, combined with a low-fat diet and moderate aerobic exercise, can significantly reduce blockages in coronary arteries (Ornish, 1990). Other studies have shown yoga to be effective in treating arthritis, diabetes, mood disorders, asthma, hypertension, menstrual cramps, back pain, and chronic fatigue.

Yoga can benefit people of any age, from children to older adults. Children take naturally to yoga and usually find it to be much fun. Getting the whole family involved is one way to maintain the routine. Some adults find yoga complements their aerobic routine, while others engage in yoga as a great nonaerobic conditioner. It is possible to learn yoga from books or video tapes, but it is easier to learn from a teacher. Yoga classes are available in many places such as health clubs, community centers, universities, and hospitals.

As a nurse, you can encourage people to utilize yoga as a way to start on the path of taking responsibility for their well being. Consistent practice of yoga changes people's attitudes about their body and their beliefs about what they can do to take care of themselves, both of which are crucial to well-being. For some, the physical exercise may be a way to attain a specific goal such as improving flexibility, improving muscle tone, or losing weight. Others have no specific goal other than the exercise itself and becoming aware of their self, breath, and energy. The relaxation that accompanies yoga can stimulate self-healing and contribute to a sense of inner peace (Dworkis, 1997).

Almost anyone can be taught the Mountain Pose, which is a standing position of postural awareness. When this pose is practiced well, the body is prepared for almost all daily movement: standing, sitting, walking, and running. Like the mountain poised between heaven and earth, this pose establishes a grounding through the legs and feet and encourages the lift of the spine. Instruct people to stand sideways near a full-length mirror so they can check their alignment, which may feel strange at first. (See Figure 15.1.) Once people are in alignment, they should notice their physical sensations. Is weight balanced evenly between the feet? Are the legs firm but not tight? Are shoulders relaxed? Does the spinal cord feel light and the head feel balanced on the torso? Is breathing comfortable and easy? Encourage people to practice the Mountain Pose several times a day. Standing well reduces strain on the joints, ligaments, and muscles, especially on those of the spinal column and lower

Figure 15.1:   Mountain Pose (Tadasana)

extremities. It also aids respiration, digestion, and elimination. The Mountain Pose conveys a sense of poise and self-esteem.

Benefits from any fitness program, including yoga, can occur only with continued practice. Try some of these suggestions to help people develop a regular pattern:

- Encourage them to make time for their practice every day, to give themselves permission to take care of themselves and take time to relax. They may find that doing a few poses before bedtime or early in the morning works best. Even if they practice for only five minutes, a daily practice is the foundation on which to build.
- To maintain their practice, many people find it helps to go to a yoga class at least once a week. The support of practicing with others and the information they get from teachers helps strengthen their commitment to yoga.
- Suggest that they may want to create a dedicated yoga space. They may have to temporarily push things aside to have enough space for their practice. Or they may simply choose a place to spread their yoga mat on the floor. Having a regular space for practice helps people focus in on the poses without being distracted by their surroundings.
- Have people start with the poses they like. If they like a pose, they will do it even if it is difficult. You may suggest that they take one pose they like from each class and practice it at least once a day, which takes only a few moments. Gradually they can begin to combine the poses to form their own yoga session.

One of many applications of yoga is in pregnancy and childbirth. In fact, many of the techniques taught in childbirth classes, such as focus, relaxation, and systematic breathing have their roots in yoga. The gentle stretching of the poses helps ease the muscle aches of pregnancy and strengthens the muscles that will be used during delivery. The breathing techniques may lessen the shortness of breath that often accompanies advanced pregnancy (Collins, 1998).

Yoga practiced while pregnant is slightly different from regular yoga in that some poses are contraindicated. These poses are the extreme stretching positions and any position that puts pressure on the uterus. Full forward bends will probably be uncomfortable for both woman and baby. Remind the woman that her center of balance has shifted completely, and thus she must be careful with balance poses. Pregnant women should never lie on the stomach for any pose. After the twentieth week, they should lie on their left side rather than their back. If any pose feels uncomfortable, the woman should stop at once. If they experience dizziness, sudden swelling, extreme shortness of breath, or vaginal bleeding, they should see their midwife or doctor immediately (Budilovsky and Adamson, 1998).

TRY THIS: *Heart Breathing*

- Sit comfortably and close your eyes.
- Simply notice your breathing without trying to change it. Pay attention to your in-breath and your out-breath.
- Now imagine that the breath is pouring into your heart with each inhalation and flowing out of your heart with each exhalation. Just feel the breath flowing in and out of your heart. Imagine the breath is pure love.
- Do this breath awareness for 5–10 minutes.
- Now let your attention return to your environment, slowly open your eyes, get up, and move on.
- Think about the feeling throughout the day.

Source: Budilovsky and Adamson, *The Complete Idiot's Guide to Yoga* (New York: Alpha Books, 1998).

With midwife or doctor approval, most women can usually start gentle yoga poses two weeks after delivery, a few weeks longer if they have had a cesarean section. They should start with a few poses and gradually work back to their regular routine. If their postpartum bleeding gets heavier or brighter red, they need to stop and call their midwife or doctor. Filling their body with energy through breathing exercises may promote self-healing after childbirth.

As people learn yoga, they will find that each sequence of poses helps them focus on something specific; for example, one sequence can improve balance, while another may release anger and negative feelings; some sequences will tone internal organs, increase lung capacity, or build upper-body strength. People choose the sequences that are right for them. It is most important to remind people that it is not a matter of being a beginning, intermediate, or advanced student but rather that they keep practicing, doing as much as they can whenever they can. Yoga moves at their pace, in the time they have (Budilovsky and Adamson, 1998).

REFERENCES

Alternative Medicine: Expanding Medical Horizons. 1994. A report to the National Institutes of Health on Alternative Medical Systems and Practices in the United States. U.S. Government Printing Office. Washington, DC.

BAKKER, R. 1976. Decreased respiratory rate during the TM technique: A replication. In T. ORME-JOHNSON and J. FARROW, eds. *Scientific Research in Transcendental Meditation Programme,* Vol 1, 140–141. Geneva, Switzerland: Marharishi European Research University Press.

BANQUET, J. P. 1976. EEG and meditation. *JAMA.* 224: 791–799.

BENSON, H. 1969. Yoga and drug abuse (letter). *N Engl J Med.* 281: 1133.

BENSON, H. 1972. The physiology of meditation. *Sci Am.* 226: 84–90.

BENSON, H. et al. 1977. Relaxation response: Bridge between psychiatry and medicine. *Med Clin North Am.* 61: 929–938.

BLACKNELL, B. et al. 1975. Effects of transcendental meditation on blood pressure: A controlled pilot experiment (abstract). *Psychosom Med.* 37: 86.

BUDILOVSKY, J. and E. ADAMSON. 1998. *The Complete Idiot's Guide to Yoga.* New York: Alpha Books.

CHOPRA, D. 1991. *Perfect Health.* New York: Harmony Books.

CHRISTENSEN, A. 1996. *The American Yoga Association Wellness Book.* New York: Kensington Books.

COLLINGE, W. 1998. *Subtle Energy.* New York: Warner Books.

COLLINS, C. 1998. Yoga: Intuition, preventive medicine, and treatment. *JOGNN.* 27(5): 563–568.

DOSSEY, L. 1989. *Recovering the Soul.* New York: Bantam Books.

DWORKIS, S. 1997. *Recovery Yoga.* New York: Three Rivers Press.

FENWICK, P. B., et al. 1977. Metabolic and EEG changes during TM: An explanation. *Biol Psychol.* 5:101–118.

FRANK, J. D. 1975. The faith that heals. *Johns Hopkins Med J.* 137: 127–131.

FRAWLEY, D. 1997. Pratyahara: Yoga's forgotten limb. *Yoga International.* 33: 32–37.

GARFINKEL, M. S., et al. 1998. Yoga-based intervention for carpal tunnel sydrome. *JAMA.* 280(18): 1601–1603.

GARFINKEL, M. S., et al. 1994. Evaluation of a yoga-based regimen for treatment of osteoarthritis of the hands. *J Rheumatol.* 21: 2341–2343.

GORE, M. M. 1982. Effect of yogic treatment on some pulmonary functions in asthmatics. *Yoga Mimamsa.* 20: 51–58.

JOHNSEN, L. 1998. Hatha traditions. *1998 Guide to Yoga Teachers & Classes.* 4: 39–45.

KABAT-ZINN, J. 1994. *Wherever You Go, There You Are: Mindfulness Meditation in Everyday Life.* New York: Hyperion.

MARIS, L. and M. MARIS. 1979. Mechanics of stress release: The TM program and occupational stress. *Police Stress.* 1: 29–36.

MONROE, R. and L. FITZGERALD. 1986. Follow-up survey on yoga and diabetes. *Yoga Biomedical Bulletin.* 1: 4, 61.

MONROE, R., A. K. GOSH, and D. KALISH. 1989. *Yoga Research Bibliography, Scientific Studies on Yoga and Meditation.* Cambridge, England: Yoga Biomedical Trust.

ORNISH, D. 1990. *Dr. Dean Ornish's Program for Reversing Heart Disease.* New York: Random House.

ORNISH, D. et al. 1983. Effects of stress management training and dietary changes in treating ischemic heart disease. *JAMA.* 249: 54–59.

SHIVARPITA, J. H. 1981. The effects of Hatha Yoga postures and breathing. *Research Bulletin of Himalayan International Institute.* 3: 4–10.

TAYLOR, E. 1997. *A Psychology of Spiritual Healing.* West Chester, PA: Chrysalis Books.

THERRIEN, R. 1968. Influence of a 5BX and a Hatha Yoga training programme of selected fitness measures. *Completed Research in HPER.* 11: 125.

RESOURCES

American Yoga Association
513 South Orange Ave.
Sarasota, FL 34236
800-226-5859
email: AmYogaAssn@aol.com

Yoga International
R.R. 1, Box 407
Honesdale, PA 18431
800-253-6243
email: yimag@epix.com

Yoga Research Center
P.O. Box 1386
Lower Lake, CA 95457
707-928-9898

Yogic Science Research Foundation
1228 Daisy Lane
East Lansing, MI 48823
517-351-3056

www.yogaclass.com/central.html
www.yogasite.com

16   Meditation

What lies behind us and what lies before us are tiny matters compared to what lies within us.

Oliver Wendell Holmes

In prayer we talk with God, in meditation we listen.

Edgar Cayce, 1877–1915

Meditation is a general term for a wide range of practices that involve relaxing the body and stilling the mind. The root word, *meditari,* means to consider, or one could say, to pay attention to something. As the founder and director of the Stress Reduction Clinic at the University of Massachusetts Medical Center, Jon Kabat-Zinn (1994, pp. xvi–xvii) states, "Meditation is simply about being yourself and knowing something about who that is. It is about coming to realize that you are on a path whether you like it or not, namely, the path that is your life. . . . Meditation is the process by which we go about deepening our attention and awareness, refining them, and putting them to greater practical use in our lives."

In 1975, Dr. Herbert Benson wrote the book *The Relaxation Response,* which drew the attention of Western health care practitioners to the physical and psychological benefits of relaxation. As Benson pointed out, the components of relaxation are quite simple: a quiet space, a comfortable position, a receptive attitude, and a focus of attention. The relaxation response involves physiological and psychological effects that appear common to many forms of focused attention in addition to meditation: prayer, yoga, biofeedback, and the presuggestion phase of hypnosis. These practices are covered in other chapters in this text. Benson (1975) described meditation as a process that anyone can use to calm down, cope with stress, and, for those with spiritual inclinations, feel as one with God or the universe. Meditation can be practiced individually or in groups and is easy to learn. It requires no change in belief system and is compatible with most religious practices.

BACKGROUND

Most meditative practices have come to the West from Eastern practices, particularly those of India, China, Japan, and Tibet. Meditative techniques, however, can be found in most cultures of the world where prayer, meditation, ritual, or contemplation are all initiated by shifting into a relaxed state. Nearly all major religions include some form of meditative practice. Christianity, Judaism, Buddhism, and Islam all use repetitive prayers, chants, or movements as part of their worship rituals. Although religious practices in the West are not typically labeled "meditative," they in fact are. The Catholic practice of using rosary beads while saying the "Hail Mary" is a familiar example. The repetition of the words combined with the movement of the beads induces a state of relaxation and a quieting of the mind.

Until recently, the primary purpose of meditation has been spiritual or religious. Since the 1970s, it has been explored as a way of reducing stress on both body and mind. Many conventional health care practitioners recommend it for widely diverse situations from natural childbirth to managing hypertension to pain control. For many years, nurses have taught clients progressive relaxation in a wide variety of clinical settings.

PREPARATION

Practicing meditation does not require a teacher and many people learn the process through instruction from books or audiotapes. Some people, however, find that the structure of a meditation class is helpful. Many varieties of teachers and classes are available. Currently no certification process is available for a meditation teacher. The general standard is some years of daily meditation practice before one teaches others. Both Christian and Buddhist traditions offer regular classes and retreats designed to teach meditative practices and the process of being a spiritual being in a material world. In the Hindu tradition, people learn meditation from a guru who is a spiritual teacher or guide. Whatever the tradition, teachers encourage self-responsibility and the practice of mindfulness in everyday life (Kahn, 1996).

CONCEPTS

Meditative State

Meditation is about being aware of who one is in the here-and-now rather than about feeling a particular way. It means letting go of any expectations of the process and simply observing what happens as it unfolds. People are sometimes concerned that they do not have the skills to meditate. As Dr. Jon Kabat-Zinn (1994, p. 33) states, "Thinking you are unable to meditate is a little like thinking you are unable to breathe, or to concentrate or relax. Pretty much everybody can breathe easily. And under the right circumstances, pretty much anybody can concentrate, anybody can relax." All forms of meditation require regular, daily practice over a period of time to experience the many benefits.

Attention and Concentration

Basic to all meditative techniques is the intentional focus of attention on one thought, word, sound, image, or physical sensation for a sustained period of time. The mind is fully alert but not focused on the external world or events. The normal rapid series of thoughts and feelings are replaced with inner awareness and attention. Rather than the mind jumping around between the past and the future, attention is in the present reality. It is impossible to make the mind empty, but it is possible to focus on one thing which helps the mind let go of the tendency to worry, plan, think, analyze, remember, or solve problems. A passive, nonjudgmental attitude is necessary during meditation. When thoughts intrude, they are noticed, and then let go as the attention returns to the original focus.

In some types of meditation, the focus is on the breath, the primary purpose being to calm the mind and body. It is a process of keeping the attention on the breath while breathing deeply, slowly, and regularly. The awareness is on the breath moving in and the breath moving out and allowing all other thoughts, feelings, or sensations to pass by as this focus is maintained. Through regular meditation practice, it becomes a habit to breathe more consciously and deeply throughout the day, so that in the long run, the breath becomes a calming force in daily life (Collinge, 1998).

Some people use a mantra as their focus of attention. A mantra is a sound or sounds that resonate in the body and evoke certain energies. Mantras, such as OM, soothe the mind and awaken the senses. Another beginning mantra is OM SHANTI SHANTI SHANTI. Shanti means peace, and when repeated three times, it balances the body, mind, and spirit.

A mandala meditation uses an object to focus the mind through sight. A mandala is a circular geometric design that draws the eye to the center and is meant to suggest the universe's circular patterns from atoms to solar systems. Mandalas appear as labyrinths in the floors of some cathedrals in Europe. The faithful follow the course of the labyrinth into the center as penitence or in spiritual contemplation. Mandalas have recently become popular in the United States among some Christian religious groups who are renewing the contemplative aspects of their faith. Using mantras and mandalas together is an effective focus for meditation (Dahlke, 1992). Figure 16.1 is the mandala that appears in the floor of Chartres Cathedral in France. Using a pencil, trace the walking path to the center and then back to the outer world again.

Meditation is both simple and difficult: simple because it is nothing more than maintaining focused attention, difficult because of the habitual, lifelong

Figure 16.1:   Mandala in the Floor of Chartres Cathedral

pattern of letting the mind wander wherever it wants. With extended practice, the mind tends to become better and better at staying focused. The stability and calmness that come with focused attention are the foundation of meditation.

VIEW OF HEALTH AND ILLNESS

Many disorders or diseases are aggravated or caused by stress. Everly and Benson (1989) have labeled these as disorders of arousal, in which the limbic system of the brain has become over stimulated. In addition, overactivity of the sympathetic nervous system and exhaustion of the adrenal glands are related to stress. It is thought that excessive limbic activity may inhibit immune function, which may account for the association of chronic stress and increased susceptibility to infection.

A relaxed state is the opposite of the aroused state of fight or flight. The fight-or-flight reflex increases blood pressure, heart rate, breathing, metabolism, and blood flow to the muscles. The response triggered by all the relaxing practices does the opposite and results in a lower blood pressure and slower heart rate, breathing, metabolism, and blood flow. Relaxation and meditation also decrease the production of adrenergic catecholamines, thereby decreasing limbic activity. Since the state of mind, the emotional, attitudinal, and intellectual components of oneself, initiates activities in the nervous system, people can consciously choose to trigger the benefits of meditation. Some relief can be found from simply taking a deep breath, relaxing, and repeating the words: "My body, mind, and spirit are always working to keep me supremely well" (Jahnke, 1997).

As stated in the report from the National Institutes of Health, "Meditation techniques offer the potential of learning how to live in an increasingly complex and stressful society while helping to preserve health in the process. Given their low cost and demonstrated health benefits, these simple mental technologies may be some of the best candidates among the alternative therapies for widespread inclusion in medical practice and for investment of medical resources" (*Alternative Medicine,* 1994. p. 16).

TREATMENT

The relaxation response can be evoked by any number of techniques, including progressive relaxation, meditation, prayer, jogging, swimming, Lamaze breathing exercises, yoga, T'ai Chi, and Qigong. The beauty of these techniques is their simplicity. They allow the mind to have a focus while enhancing one's vitality and well-being.

The varieties of meditation have many different names. Some are religious practices and some are not. Some are complicated while some are simple. Each type of meditative practice involves a form of mental focusing and the adoption of a nonjudgmental attitude toward intruding thoughts. All types appear to produce similar physical and psychological changes. People beginning the practice of meditation should look around for a form that seems comfortable, that suits them, and that does not conflict with their belief system (*Alternative Medicine,* 1994; Weil, 1995).

Transcendental Meditation (TM) was developed by the Indian leader Maharishi Mahesh Yogi in an effort to make the ancient practice of meditation more attainable to Westerners. TM is a sound-focused form of meditation and is simple and easy to learn. To prevent distracting thoughts, a person is given a mantra (a word or sound) to repeat silently over and over again while sitting in a comfortable position. When thoughts other than the mantra come to mind, the person is to notice them and then gently return the focus to the mantra. It is expected that people will practice TM for 20 minutes, once or twice a day. The trademarked Transcendental Meditation is a commercial enterprise that is a fairly expensive undertaking. Classes are typically found in Ayurveda schools and health care centers. Local centers may be found on the internet at www.tm.org/

The essence of Buddhist meditation is training the mind in compassion and in wisdom. The goal is to develop compassion for all living things. Meditation begins with a time of contemplation, which typically includes such points as (Drubwang, 1998):

- Just as I wish to be free from suffering and experience only happiness, so do all other beings.
- I am no different from any other being; we are all equal.
- My happiness and suffering are insignificant when compared with the happiness and suffering of all other living beings.

The next step is a process of meditating on any determinations that might have been made during contemplation. The practice is concluded by dedicating one's life and purpose to the welfare of all living beings. It is believed that many of the daily problems people experience will disappear, because most of them arise from regarding oneself as more important than others.

Mindfulness, an ancient Buddhist practice, is both a philosophy as well as a meditation practice. Its primary principle is "being in the moment." Most often people go through daily routines with little awareness or attention. People read while they eat, exercise while watching TV, or cook while talking to their children, and the nuances of these experiences are lost. This situation might be called living mindlessly by ignoring present moments. Mindfulness is the opposite of living on "automatic pilot." It is the art of conscious living through focusing full attention on the activity at hand. While it may be simple to practice mindfulness, it is not necessarily easy. Habitual unawareness is persistent and mindfulness requires effort and discipline. Thus, to eat a peach mindfully would involve being actively aware of every sensation, every smell, every taste, noticing its texture, its color, its weight, and how it feels on the tongue. This technique can be practiced with any activity (Kabat-Zinn, 1994).

Mindfulness meditation is a daily practice that encourages living in the moment. It begins by sitting quietly with eyes closed and focusing on breathing. The flow of thought during the meditation is observed as thoughts come and go.

The key to mindfulness meditation is the ability to accept rather than judge the wandering thoughts, bringing attention back to the breathing as needed.

Tibetan meditation is a breath-focused form of meditation. The person simply focuses attention on each in-breath and out-breath. When thoughts about anything other than the breath intrude, they are noted by silently saying "thinking," and then attention is returned to the breath. It is recognized that thought cannot be completely halted and that thoughts are a natural process and are simply to be noted in a nonjudgmental way.

Forms of moving meditation include the Chinese martial art T'ai Chi, the Japanese martial art Aikido, the Indian practice of yoga, and the walking meditation in Zen Buddhism. Instead of focusing on a word or on breathing, movement meditations use physical sensations as the focus of concentration. In walking meditation, for example, attention is given to the feeling of each step as it is taken. Intruding thoughts are simply noticed and attention is returned to the step. Research has found that focused walking, in contrast to unfocused walking, is associated with reduced anxiety and fewer negative thoughts (Benson, 1997).

If practiced regularly, even 15 minutes twice a day, meditation produces widespread positive effects on physical and psychological functioning. The autonomic nervous system responds with a decrease in heart rate, lower blood pressure, decreased respiratory rate and oxygen consumption, and a lower arousal threshold. People who meditate say that they have clearer minds and sharper thoughts. The brain seems to clear itself so that new ideas and beliefs become available. This clearer mind may be accompanied by a cognitive restructuring in which people interpret life events in a more positive, more realistic fashion. Meditation's residual effects—improved stress-coping abilities—are a protection against daily stress and anxiety. All other self-healing methods are improved with the practice of meditation (Benson, 1997; Jahnke, 1997).

Some adverse effects of meditation are possible. Relaxation exercises should not be practiced while driving or operating potentially dangerous machinery. Some people have been stressed so long that they are unfamiliar with deep relaxation and therefore feel threatened by it. In meditation, people are taught to accept nonjudgmentally whatever thoughts occur. Sometimes, however, extremely upsetting thoughts arise and it is impossible to remain nonjudgmental, which could lead to disparaging thoughts about one's abilities. The adverse effects for more experienced meditators are temporary fear, anxiety, confusion, depression, or self-doubt. For an unknown reason, these kinds of thoughts are more likely to arise during the first 10 minutes of meditation. In rare instances, relaxation exercises may trigger seizures in people with sleep onset seizure disorders. People with schizophrenia may experience an acute episode following intensive meditation. Meditation may also be inappropriate for people with extreme anger, hostility, or obsessive thoughts, because they may be unable to quiet their minds adequately and therefore may not perceive the experience as relaxing (*Alternative Medicine,* 1994).

RESEARCH

Since the 1960s a large body of research has been documented regarding meditation and the relaxation response. Research has demonstrated a wide range of effects including the following:

- Subjects experienced a reduction in chronic pain, with more activity, less anxiety, and less depression (Caudill et al., 1991; Kabat-Zinn et al., 1986).
- Subjects in a stress reduction and relaxation program demonstrated statistically significant improvement in physical and psychological health and self-esteem. In addition, subjects reported personal changes such as greater peace of mind, less anger, better relationships with family members, etc., that are difficult to quantify or measure directly (Roth and Creaser, 1997).
- People with hypertension experienced a reduction in blood pressure (Schneider et al.,1992; Stuart et al., 1987).
- Cortisol levels were reduced during meditation in individuals who have elevated blood cortisol levels brought on by stress (MacLean et al., 1992).
- Thirty-six percent of women with unexplained infertility became pregnant within six months of meditation practice (Domar et al., 1992).
- One study showed a 57 percent decrease in symptoms of premenstrual syndrome (Goodale et al., 1990).
- Fewer respiratory crises occurred in people with asthma, emphysema, and chronic obstructive pulmonary disease (Kabat-Zinn et al., 1986).
- Oxygen consumption rapidly decreased—10–17 percent within the first three minutes of the relaxation exercise (Benson, 1997).
- Less pain and anxiety resulted with femoral angiography procedure (Mandle et al., 1990).
- Seventy-five percent of people with sleep-onset insomnia were cured (Jacobs et al., 1993).
- Panic attacks were reduced (Kabat-Zinn et al., 1986).
- Meditation has been useful in the treatment of posttraumatic stress syndrome in Vietnam veterans (Brooks and Scarano, 1985).

- Those individuals using meditation experienced a significantly larger decrease in tobacco, alcohol, and illicit drug use than standard substance abuse treatment programs or preventive programs (Sharma et al., 1991).
- Slowed brain waves led to improved moods and increased feelings of pleasure (Benson, 1997).
- Cerebral blood flow increased and heart rate decreased (Jevning et al., 1996; Telles et al., 1995).
- Intelligence-related measures showed longitudinal increase (Cranson et al., 1991).
- High school sophomores experienced increased self-esteem (Benson, 1994).

When a group of 2,000 meditators were compared with 600,000 non-meditators, insurance statistics showed that the use of medical care was 30 to 87 percent less for meditators in all but one of the 18 categories (childbirth) (McSherry, 1990; Orme-Johnson, 1987). Clients at the Harvard Community Health Plan who attended a six-week group that included meditation, had significantly fewer physician visits during the following six months at an average savings of $171 per client (*Alternative Medicine,* 1994). Despite the abundance of research indicating that meditation is a beneficial, low-cost intervention, it continues to be regarded as unconventional and is still ignored by many mainstream physicians (*Alternative Medicine,* 1994).

The Institute for the Scientific Study of Meditation has four current areas of investigation. Area 1 concerns meditative practices and their theoretical implications and developing theoretical models utilizing existing data related to meditative practices. Area 2 involves research on the neurophysiology of meditative practices exploring which parts of the brain function to generate the experience of meditation. The third area explores the effects of meditative practices on various physical and psychological conditions to determine its usefulness as adjunctive treatment in various diseases. The fourth area focuses on the training and education of meditative practices as well as the development of research fellowship training programs.

INTEGRATED NURSING PRACTICE

Progressive relaxation and meditation are used in a wide variety of clinical settings such as rehabilitation facilities, cardiac care units, postoperative units, stress management centers, behavioral counseling settings, and centers dedicated to health and wellness promotion. Thousands of hospitals, clinics, private practitioners, and universities offer training in meditation. In addition, audio tapes and books are available that make meditation more accessible to people with busy schedules. Many people practice meditation to reduce stress, anxiety, anger, and other negative emotions. But increasingly, health care practitioners prescribe meditation as part of the treatment for a large and growing number of medical conditions.

Progressive relaxation is a way of decreasing muscular tension. The relaxation response can be elicited by teaching clients two common techniques: progressive relaxation and body scan. Both focus on reducing muscle tone in the major muscle groups and take about 7–10 minutes. If possible, help the client find a quiet place with a comfortable temperature to do the exercise. It can be done in any comfortable position, although typically it is done with people lying on their back and begins with a focus of the breath, breathing gently, slowly, and deeply. The awareness is then shifted to different parts of the body in turn, by instructing the client to tense a muscle groups as tight as possible, hold the tension for several seconds, and then consciously relax it. This sequence is repeated for each of the major muscle groups in the body, usually beginning at the toes and slowly working up the body. Progressive relaxation is designed to help people with chronic tension experience the difference between a muscle that is tense and one that is relaxed. In the body scan exercise, clients are instructed to focus their attention on body parts, one at a time, often beginning at the feet and moving toward the head, and consciously relax each part. See Box 16.1 for directions of the body scan.

Box 16.1: Body Scan Meditation

- Lie on your back with your legs uncrossed, your arms at your sides, palms up, and your eyes closed.
- Focus on your breathing, breathing in peace and breathing out tension.
- As you begin to feel relaxed, direct your attention to your feet, paying attention to any sensations. Let your feet relax and feel the warmth spread throughout your feet.
- Then move your focus to your ankles. Follow the same procedure as you move up your lower legs, knees, thighs, hips, and so on all around the body.
- Pay particular attention to any areas that are painful or are the focus of any medical condition such as the lungs or heart.
- Finish the body scan by paying particular attention to the neck and head. Experience the warmth of the relaxation.

You can also teach clients to anchor the relaxation response with a sensory stimulus such as an aroma like lavender or rose or a touch such as pressing two fingers together. The sensory anchor should be done within 30 seconds of the relaxation exercise. After doing the sensory anchor for two weeks, the individual should be able to instantaneously relax by reexperiencing the particular sensory trigger, be it an aroma or a physical sensation.

Meditation is the next step following the mastery of progressive relaxation and body scan. Explain the two basic steps to clients: the repetition of a word, sound, prayer, phrase, or muscular activity and the disregard of everyday thoughts that interfere with the process. Box 16.2 lists focus words or prayers that you may suggest to clients. The word or phrase is silently repeated with each in-breath and out-breath. Some people choose to use one word for the in-breath and another for the out-breath. Some meditators choose an object of personal significance on which to focus. Every detail of the object is studied, including gradations of shape, color, texture, and so on. Flowers, candle flames, or religious statues are common choices.

Before sitting down to meditate, it is helpful to make sure that the area is clean and uncluttered, which helps keep the mind clear and fresh. No props are required for meditation, although some people may choose to include incense, candles, or religious symbols in their meditative practice. Beginners often start with 5–10 minutes of meditation and increase the time gradually. It is most important that time is scheduled each day, and many people find that meditating first thing in the morning, before the busy day begins, works well. Other people prefer to meditate in the evening. The key is to find a time when one is unlikely to be disturbed. It is best to wait about two hours after a big meal, during which time the blood flow is diverted from the brain to the gut, which makes falling asleep during meditation more likely.

All sitting meditative practices begin with finding a comfortable but erect position. The posture itself is a meditation. Slumping reflects low energy and passivity, while a ramrod-straight posture reflects tension and effort. It is easiest to meditate if the spine is straight and the body posture is symmetrical. Some people sit on the floor cross-legged using a firm cushion under their backside to support the spine. Others sit in a chair with a straight back, with both feet on the ground. The face relaxes, shoulders drop, and head, neck, and back move into easy alignment. The eyes may be either open or closed. Hands may be resting in the lap or may to held with palms together. It is believed that having the palms together with the fingertips touching completes a circuit of energy extending from the heart down the arms and through the chakras in the center of the palm of each hand as well as the chakras in the fingertips. People often experiment with various ways of positioning their hands during meditation until they find what is best for them (Collinge, 1998; Kabat-Zinn, 1994).

Box 16.2: Focus Words or Prayers

Secular Focus Words
  One
  Ocean
  Love
  Peace
  Well-being
  Let it be
  Relax
Religious Focus Words or Prayers
  Christian
    "Our Father who art in heaven"
    "The Lord is my shepherd"
    "Hail, Mary, full of grace"
    "Lord Jesus Christ have mercy on me"
  Jewish
    "Sh'ma Yisroel"
    "Shalom"
    "Echod"
    "The Lord is my shepherd"
  Islamic
    "Insha'allah"
  Hindu
    "Om"

Source: Benson, *Timeless Healing* (New York: Fireside Books, 1997).

Benson (1997, p. 136) describes the process he teaches his patients and the one he uses himself:

Step 1. Pick a focus word or short phrase that is firmly rooted in your belief system.

Step 2. Sit quietly in a comfortable position.

Step 3. Close your eyes.

Step 4. Relax your muscles.

Step 5. Breathe slowly and naturally, and as you do, repeat your focus word, phrase, or prayer silently to yourself as you exhale.

Step 6. Assume a passive attitude. Don't worry about how well you're doing. When other thoughts come to mind, simply say to yourself, "Oh, well," and gently return to the repetition.

Step 7. Continue for 10–20 minutes.

Step 8. Do not stand immediately. Continue sitting quietly for a minute or so, allowing other thoughts to return. Then open your eyes and sit for another minute before rising.

Step 9. Practice this technique once or twice daily.

Once people are adept at meditation, they can be taught to use "minis." Minis are small versions of meditation. Instruct the client to breathe deeply, releasing tension, while saying the chosen focus word, sound, phrase, or prayer. Minis are very helpful in the midst of busy, stressful times (Benson, 1997).

One type of meditation is an awareness of breathing meditation. In this form, the person concentrates on the sensation of the breath as it enters the nose and fills the chest and abdomen, and again as it passes out of the body. Alternatively, one can imagine the breath coming in from the toes, up the legs, through the belly, and into the chest and out the same pathway. It is helpful to imagine healing and relaxation flowing into the body with each in-breath, and stress or pain leaving the body with each out-breath. When thoughts arise, they are noticed, and then let go as attention is brought back to the breathing.

Another awareness of breathing practice you can teach clients is a simple technique used in Zen meditation. Instruct the clients to sit in a comfortable position with the spine straight. Ask them to gently close their eyes while breathing naturally and easily. To begin the exercise, have them count "one" to themselves as they exhale. On the next exhale, count "two," and so on up to "five." Then a new cycle is begun, counting "one" on the next exhale. Tell clients never to count higher than "five" and count only on the exhale. They will know their attention has wandered when they find themselves up to "eight" or "ten." When this occurs, have them gently refocus and restart on the count of "one." This form of meditation should be done for about ten minutes (Weil, 1995).

Any repetitive behavior can be used as a meditative focus. One of the most universally used practices is walking meditation. In walking meditation, one is not walking to get anyplace. Having no place to go makes it easier to be where one is. It is often done some place in nature, on a track, on a walking mandala, or even pushing a shopping cart through a supermarket. It can be practiced at any pace, from very slow to very brisk. The practice is to take each step as it comes and to be fully present with it. One notices the movements of

TRY THIS: *Loving-kindness Meditation*

Begin by focusing on your breathing and take a few slow, easy breaths. Feel your-self relax. Imagine a white light above you and slightly in front of you, pouring a waterfall of love and light over you. Let the light enter the top of your head and wash through you. See yourself totally enclosed in a cocoon of white light and repeat these loving-kindness blessings for yourself, with all the respect and love that you would have for your only child:

> May I be at peace
> May my heart remain open
> May I awaken to the light of my own true nature
> May I be healed
> May I be a source of healing for all beings.

Next, bring one or more loved ones to mind. See them in as much detail as pos-sible. Imagine the white light shining down on them and surrounding them. Then bless them:

> May you be at peace
> May your heart remain open
> May you awaken to the light of your own true nature
> May you be healed
> May you be a source of healing for all beings.

Next, think of a person or persons whom you hold in judgment or with whom you are angry and to whom you are ready to begin extending forgiveness. Place them in the white light and see the light washing away all their negativity, just as it did for you and your loved ones. Bless them:

> May you be at peace
> May your heart remain open
> May you awaken to the light of your own true nature
> May you be healed
> May you be a source of healing for all beings.

See our beautiful planet as it appears from outer space, a delicate jewel spinning in space. Imagine the green earth, the blue seas, the birds, the animals, the fish. Earth is a realm of opposites. Of day and night, good and evil, sickness and health, riches and poverty, female and male. Hold the earth as you offer these blessings:

> May there be peace on earth
> May the hearts of all people be open to themselves and to each other
> May all people awaken to the light of their own true nature
> May all creation be blessed and be a blessing to all that is.

Source: Borysenko and Borysenko, *The Power of the Mind to Heal* (Carlsbad, CA: Hay House, 1994); Collinge, *Subtle Energy* (New York: Warner Books, 1998); Kabat-Zinn, *Wher-ever You Go There You Are* (New York: Hyperion, 1994).

each foot, how it lifts, moves forward in space, and then descends again. Just as in other forms of meditation, when one begins to think, the thoughts are let go and awareness is returned to the physical sensations of walking (Borysenko and Borysenko, 1994).

An excellent book for nurses is Sherry Kahn's text, *The Nurse's Meditative Journal.* This book provides you, the nurse, with step-by-step instruction in meditation and journal writing as an aid in self-exploration and growth. Your ability to focus in the midst of chaos and understand in the midst of confusion can bring comfort to your clients and inspire your professional peers to find these same qualities within themselves.

There are as many ways to meditate as there are people. When people say they have tried meditation and cannot do it, they just have not found the right practice for them. One may want to sit, one do repetitive prayers, one swim or run, one walk, and one do yoga or T'ai Chi. Encourage clients to explore a variety of techniques and develop the habit of meditation on a daily basis.

REFERENCES

Alternative Medicine: Expanding Medical Horizons. 1994. A report to the National Institutes of Health on Alternative Medical Systems and Practices in the United States. U.S. Government Printing Office. Washington, DC.

BENSON, H. 1997. *Timeless Healing.* New York: Fireside Books.

BENSON, H. et al. 1994. Increases in positive psychological characteristics with a new relaxation-response curriculum in high school students. *J for Research and Development in Education.* 27: 226–231.

BENSON, H. 1975. *The Relaxation Response.* New York: Morrow.

BROOKS J. S. and T. SCARANO. 1985. Transcendental meditation in the treatment of post-Vietnam adjustment. *J Counseling and Development.* 65: 212–215.

BORYSENKO, J. and M. BORYSENKO. 1994. *The Power of the Mind to Heal.* Carlsbad, CA: Hay House.

CAUDILL, M. R. et al. 1991. Decreased clinic utilization by chronic pain patients: Response to behavioral medicine intervention. *Clinical J of Pain.* 7: 305–310.

COLLINGE, W. 1998. *Subtle Energy.* New York: Warner Books.

CRANSON, R. W. et al. 1991. Transcendental meditation and improved performance on intelligence-related measures: A longitudinal study. *Personality and Individual Differences.* 12: 1105–1116.

DAHLKE, R. 1992. *Mandalas of the World.* New York: Sterling Pub. Co.

DOMAR, A. D. et al. 1992. Psychological improvement in infertile women after behavioral treatment: A replication. *Fertility and Sterility.* 58: 144–147.

DRUBWANG, K. January–February 1998. Equalizing self and others. *YOGAChicago.* 5.

EVERLY, G. S., JR. and H. BENSON. 1989. Disorders of arousal and the relaxation response: Speculations on the nature and treatment of stress-related diseases. *Int J Psychosom.* 36: 15–21.

GOODALE, I. L., A. D. DOMAR, and H. BENSON. 1990. Alleviation of premenstrual syndrome symptoms with the relaxation response. *Obstetrics and Gynecology.* 75: 649–655.

JAHNKE, R. 1997. *The Healer Within.* San Francisco: Harper.

JACOBS, G. D., H. BENSON, and R. FRIEDMAN. 1993. Home-based central nervous system assessment of a multifactor behavioral intervention for chronic sleep-onset insomnia. *Behavior Therapy.* 24: 159–174.

JEVNING, R. et al. 1996. Effects on regional cerebral blood flow of transcendental meditation. *Physiol Behav.* 59(3): 399–402.

KABAT-ZINN, J. 1994. *Wherever You Go There You Are: Mindfulness Meditation in Everyday Life.* New York: Hyperion.

KABAT-ZINN, J. et al. 1986. Four-year follow-up of a meditation-based program for the self-regulation of chronic pain. *Clinical J Pain.* 2: 150–173.

KAHN, S. 1996. *The Nurse's Meditative Journal.* Albany: Delmar.

MacLEAN, C. R. K. et al. October 30, 1992. Altered cortisol response to stress after four month's practice of the transcendental meditation program. Presented at the 18th Annual Meeting of the Society for Neuroscience, Anaheim, CA.

MANDLE, C. L. et al. 1990. Relaxation response in femoral angiography. *Radiology.* 174: 737–739.

McSHERRY, E. 1990. Medical economics. In D. WEDDING, ed. *Medicine and Behavior.* St. Louis: Mosby, 463–484.

ORME-JOHNSON, D. W. 1987. Medical care utilization and the transcendental meditation program. *Psychosom Med.* 49: 493–507.

ROTH, B. and T. CREASER. 1997. Mindfulness meditation-based stress reduction: Experience with a bilingual inner-city program. *Nurse Practitioner.* 22(3): 150–176.

SCHNEIDER, R. H. et al. 1992. In search of an optimal behavioral treatment for hypertension. In E. H. JOHNSON, W. D. GENTRY, and S. JULIUS, eds. *Personality, Elevated Blood Pressure, and Essential Hypertension.* Washington, DC: Hemisphere.

SHARMA, H. M. et al. 1991. Maharishi Ayur-Veda: modern insights into ancient medicine. *JAMA.* 265: 2633–2634, 2637.

STUART, E. M. ET AL. 1987. Nonpharmacologic treatment of hypertension: A multiple-risk-factor approach. *J Cardiovascular Nursing.* 1: 1–14.

TELLES, S., R. NAGARATHNA, and H. R. NAGENDRA. 1995. Autonomic changes during "OM" meditation. *Indiana J Physiol Pharmacol.* 39(4): 418–420.

WEIL, A. 1995. *Natural Health, Natural Medicine.* Boston: Houghton Mifflin.

RESOURCES

American Chronic Pain Association
P.O. Box 850
Rocklin, CA 95677
916-632-0922

American Meditation Institute
P.O. Box 430
Averill Park, NY 12018
518-674-8714
email: postmaster@americanmeditation.org
www.americanmeditation.org

Mind-Body Medical Institute
Mercy Hospital and Medical Center
Stevenson Expressway at King Drive
Chicago, IL 60616-2477
312-567-6700

The Center for Mind-Body Studies
5225 Connecticut Ave. NW, Suite 414
Washington, DC 20015
202-966-7338

The Stress Reduction Clinic
Department of Medicine
University of Massachusetts Medical Center
Worcester, MA 01655
508-856-1616

World Research Foundation
15300 Ventura Blvd., Suite 405
Sherman Oaks, CA 91403
818-907-5483

Maharishi Medical Centers in the United States
www.maharishi-medical.com

www.mindtools.com

17 Hypnotherapy and Guided Imagery

Only the person who is relaxed can create,
and to that mind ideas flow like lightning.

Cicero

Tension is who you think you should be.
Relaxation is who you are.

Ancient Chinese proverb

Hypnotherapy is the application of hypnosis in a wide variety of medical and psychological disorders. Hypnosis is a state of attentive and focused concentration during which people are highly responsive to suggestion. Guided imagery, in a state of focused concentration, is a similar process that encourages changes in attitudes, behavior, and physiological reactions. Many people consider guided imagery to be a form of hypnosis.

Hypnotherapists and guided imagery therapists help people learn methods to take advantage of the mind/body/spirit connection through the medium of relaxation and imagination. The basic difference between meditation and hypnosis or guided imagery is that in meditation, one empties one's mind of images, while in hypnosis or guided imagery, one creates vivid mental images (Borysenko and Borysenko, 1994; Weil, 1995).

BACKGROUND

Around the world, shamans and traditional healers have used the power of suggested mental images for thousands of years. Hypnotic trances were used in a variety of healing practices and religious rituals such as holding sweat lodge ceremonies, drumming, and chanting. Inducing trance states and using therapeutic suggestion were central practices of the early Greek healing temples. People in the fourteenth century thought illness was related to evil spirits, and evil spirits were often treated with imagery and hypnotic techniques. During the Renaissance (fourteenth to sixteenth centuries), it was believed that dysfunctional imagination was the root of all pathology. It was even believed that the mother's imaginings during pregnancy could alter the growth and development of her fetus (Shames, 1996).

Hypnotherapy began in the late eighteenth century in Europe with an Austrian physician, Franz Anton Mesmer, who is considered the father of hypnosis. He is remembered for the term *mesmerize,* which described a process of inducing trance through a series of passes he made with his hands and/or magnets over people. He worked with psychic and electromagnetic energies that he called animal magnetism. The medical community eventually discredited him despite his considerable success treating a variety of ailments. In the mid-nineteenth century, James Braid, an English physician, successfully used hypnosis in pain control and as an anesthetic in surgery. Even after witnessing live demonstrations of a patient undergoing painless surgery, his colleagues dismissed him as a fake. Not long afterward, the discovery of chloroform led to the near abandonment of hypnotic anesthesia.

In the late nineteenth and early twentieth centuries, Emile Coue, a French physician, formulated the Laws of Suggestion, discussed later in this chapter and used to this day by hypnotherapists. He also discovered that giving positive suggestions when prescribing medication proved to be a more effective cure than prescribing medication alone. Sigmund Freud at first found hypnosis extremely effective in treating hysteria, and then, troubled by the sudden emergence of powerful emotions in his patients, he abandoned it in favor of psychoanalysis. Carl Jung did not actively use hypnosis, but he encouraged his patients to use active imagination to change old memories. He often used the concept of the inner guide in his healing work. Milton Erickson, an American psychologist and psychiatrist, is considered the father of modern hypnotherapy. He demonstrated how traumatic amnesia and psychosomatic symptoms can be resolved with hypnotherapy and was influential in the official acceptance of hypnotherapy by the American Medical Association in 1958 (Margolis, 1997; Rossi, 1993)

Since the 1970s, many books have been written on the use of guided imagery for healing. *Visualization* (Bry, 1972) and *Healing with Mind Power* (Shames and Sterin, 1978) were two of the first books that introduced imagery to the general public. *Creative Visualization* (Gawain, 1983) taught people how to improve their health, expand their mind, and achieve their life goals. Since then, hundreds of books and tapes have been published as people have become more interested in guided imagery.

PREPARATION

At present, no laws limit the use of hypnosis to clinical practitioners. While anyone can hypnotize other people, hypnotherapy is best practiced by a health care professional. Nurses, physicians, dentists, psychologists, social workers,

Box 17.1: Program Content for Nurses' Certificate Program in Interactive Imagery^{SM}

- Core concepts in mind/body medicine, psychoneuroimmunology, and holism
- Principles and theory of the imagery
- Self-care as an integral aspect of nursing practice
- A variety of relaxation and breathing techniques
- A multitude of guided imagery exercises
- The fundamentals of Interactive Imagery^{SM}
- Eight specific Interactive Imagery^{SM} techniques
- Opportunity for practice and case presentations

This program is approved for 110 C.E. hours by the American Holistic Nurses Association.

and counselors are eligible to take approved professional training in hypnotherapy. The American Society of Clinical Hypnosis (ASCH) and The Society for Clinical and Experimental Hypnosis (SCEH) share in the education and accrediting of people who meet professional requirements. Most practitioners do not identify themselves as hypnotists but as nurses, doctors, dentists, and others who use hypnosis as one of several modes of intervention.

The American Holistic Nurses Association and the Academy for Guided Imagery offer a Nurses Certificate Program in Interactive Imagery^{SM}. The program consists of 110 hours of in-depth, hands-on training to provide nurses with experience in relaxation and Interactive Imagery skills. An overview of the program content is found in Box 17.1.

CONCEPTS

Trance

To understand hypnotic trance, one must understand the functional difference between the conscious and subconscious mind. The conscious mind contains the short-term memory and the intellect. It functions like a computer, always analyzing, criticizing, and discriminating one's thoughts and perceptions. The language of the intellect is logic and reason. The subconscious mind contains emotions, creativity, imagination, intuition, long-term memory, and control of bodily functions. It also contains the habit center where persistent habits such as nail biting or test anxiety are located. The subconscious does not respond to reason and facts as does the intellect. The language of the subconscious is imagery and metaphor. During times of emotional turmoil or sudden trauma, people often become aware of the subconscious mind's power over bodily functions and intellect when they are unable to eat, sleep, or talk, and cannot think clearly. After years of ignoring feelings or "stuffing" them into the subconscious, in a hypnotic trance, people can access their subconscious mind, which allows them to tap into their creativity, access buried memories, change habits, unmask erroneous beliefs, repair self-esteem, and restore health.

A trance state is a form of heightened concentration. People in trance are aware of what is going on around them but choose not to focus on it and can return to normal awareness whenever they choose. The majority of people will tend to remember most of what happens in a controlled hypnotherapy or guided imagery session. Trance is not a form of sleep or stupor as is easily determined by observing the range of activities possible by people in a hypnotic trance.

People naturally flow in and out of hypnotic trances. When driving a familiar route, people may slip into a trance. They arrive at their destination, not sure exactly how they got there. During the trance they drive appropriately, stop at stop signs, obey traffic laws, and so on, but have no conscious awareness of doing these things. Another example of hypnotic trance occurs during movies. People enter the theater having set aside a specific period of time wherein they can enjoy themselves. The process of settling into theater seats relaxes moviegoers and puts them in a receptive frame of mind. The lights go down to reduce the distractions from the outside world and the big screen becomes the most noticeable aspect of one's perceptual world. Within moments, the audience is transported to another place and time. If the movie is frightening, many people experience a racing heart, rapid breathing, and muscle tension—yet they are well aware that no physical danger exists. They are responding to images and sounds alone. Movies work by similar mental mechanisms as hypnosis. First participants decide to let go of normal concerns and open the mind to a new experience. Then certain procedures relax the beta level of brain activity. Then, through the thoughtful use of metaphor and imagery, deeper levels of consciousness are reached. Finally, new images and perceptions can be introjected (Hamilton, 1998).

A trance is characterized by muscle relaxation, predominating alpha brain waves, feelings of well-being, diminished ability to vocalize, and an ability to accept new ideas if not in conflict with personal values. The perception of time is often distorted; thirty minutes may seem like five minutes. Feelings are more accessible while entranced, as well as memories from long ago. As one's awareness phases in and out, parts of the session may not be consciously remembered but are retained in the subconscious. People in trance describe their arms and legs feeling heavy like lead or light and tingly, almost numb. Some experience slight twitches as the nervous system relaxes, and respiration shifts to abdominal breathing. Coming out of the trance, people awaken with very pleasant, almost euphoric feelings of well-being.

Laws and Principles of Suggestion

The first law of suggestion, as formulated by Coue, is that of *concentrated attention*. When people focus their attention repeatedly on a goal or idea, that event tends to be realized. Based on this belief, practitioners repeat hypnotic suggestions three or four times during a session. The law of *dominant effect* states that stronger emotions tend to take precedence over weaker ones. An effective hypnotherapist, after assessing the client's emotional state, connects the hypnotic suggestion to the dominant emotions. The *carrot principle* is applied when the practitioner interjects comments about the person's goals with the hypnotic suggestions, thus linking motivation to the suggestions. The principle of *positive suggestion* is applied to help people override existing attitudes. Dr. Coue was known for encouraging his patients to say to themselves 20–30 times each night before going to sleep, "Everyday in every way, I am getting better and better." If someone is seeking hypnosis in an effort to lose weight, the positive suggestion is not, "You will not be hungry," which is unlikely and a negative rather than positive statement. Rather the positive suggestion might be, "You will be surprised to find how comfortable you will be. You treat your body with kindness and respect."

Memories

It is true that under hypnosis people often recall past forgotten events. It is also true that people under hypnosis often "remember" things quite vividly that never actually happened, but which have great personal significance nonetheless. These might be called fantasized life events. In a deep trance state, memories and fantasies may be intense, and the two may be indistinguishable. People are able to remember great detail of actual events and are also uniquely capable of making up details and experiencing them as if they were remembered. Recognizing the potential difficulties arising from what some call "false memory syndrome," several states in the United States now limit legal testimony to that obtained prior to any systematic hypnotic treatment. In 1985, the American Medical Association cautioned against the systematic use of hypnosis for memory recall for both its unreliability and its potential to create vivid false memories.

TREATMENT

Hypnotherapists do not "put" people into trances. They arrange circumstances to increase the likelihood that people will shift themselves into a trance state. About 20 percent of the population has a high capacity for trance; these people may go under hypnosis deeply. Another 20 percent has a slight capacity for trance, are easily distracted, and may not respond to hypnotherapy at all. People who cannot be hypnotized include those with organic brain disease, those with low IQ and those who do not want to be hypnotized. The remaining 60 percent of the population fall somewhere in between these extremes (Weil, 1995).

For people seeking hypnotherapy or guided imagery, the question arises as to whether the use of audio tapes would offer equal benefit. The answer to that question depends on several factors, including the nature and depth of the problem one wants to resolve. General self-hypnosis tapes will give one only general results. Personalized audio tapes, created by a therapist using the person's own images, are more effective. Working with an experienced practitioner is most effective because the procedure is individualized according to the client's expectations and preferences.

The first and most important step in hypnotherapy is establishing a relationship with the client. It is a cooperative venture, and if the suggestions are to be effective, the therapist and client must work together. The relationship is one in which clients permit themselves to be as receptive as possible and the therapist commits to working for the clients' well-being. The therapist gets to know clients, develops treatment plans, explains the hypnotic process, dispels myths and fears, answers questions, encourages positive attitudes about hypnosis, and with people's permission, trains them in self-inductive procedures. This process is as applicable for a short-term case of test anxiety as it is for a lengthy terminal illness. A measure of trust is needed to start the process and develop the relationship.

The induction phase is generally a period of relaxation or focus on the breathing that disengages people from other concerns and helps them focus their attention. In other words, the induction phase is similar to meditation and elicits the same physiological response. The induction starts with "easy" suggestions, such as focusing on breathing and closing the eyes. Directions are given to relax physically and mentally and to focus on the therapist's voice and words.

Training in induction may take one or two sessions. When the client is comfortable with entering the trance experience, the hypnotic suggestion begins. Based on the assessment process, the practitioner suggests an image known to be pleasurable to the client and related to the desired outcome. Hypnotic communications contain cues and explicit instructions for focusing attention and imagining in line with the aims of suggestions. The imagery is intensified by incorporating the five senses: the person is asked not only to visualize the scene but to smell the scents, touch things in the environment, hear the surrounding sounds, and even taste anything appropriate. The client is asked to focus attention on as many details about the situation as possible and is walked through the session focusing on the desired events. The suggestions of the hypnotherapist are translated by the client into ideas. These ideas then lead to corresponding behaviors in the nontrance state (Hammond, 1990; Keegan, 1994).

Trance removal is that time when clients are given suggestions which will return them to a nontrance state. The hypnotherapist, for example, may count to 10, asking clients to open their eyes at the count of 5, and to be fully alert at 10. Clients most commonly report that they feel relaxed during the session but may not be certain that they were hypnotized, since they could hear every word the therapist said. Many hypnotherapists provide guided audio tapes for their clients so they can practice the therapy at home.

Hypnosis cannot make people do anything against their will. If they really do not want to change, hypnosis will be a waste of time and money. If, for example, a person seeks hypnotherapy to stop smoking at a spouse's insistence but is poorly motivated, hypnotherapy will not be effective. Occasionally clients may demand that the hypnotherapist perform some magical incantation and remove thirty pounds or make the person never smoke again. This demand is the equivalent of insisting that their primary care provider cure them of hypertension while refusing to change their diet or follow a recommended medication schedule.

In some medical facilities, hypnosis and imagery are now routinely used with a variety of conditions, usually in conjunction with other forms of medical, surgical, psychiatric, or psychological treatment. They can be used with nonmedical clients as well, working through problems of living, situations of performance anxiety, and in changing bad habits. Depending on the complexity and seriousness of the complaint, treatment typically runs from two to ten sessions.

Much of the literature regarding the use of imagery for cancer is anecdotal but many people believe the reports must be respected. Jeanne Achterberg (1978, 1985) well known for her use of imagery in the treatment of cancer, believes that imagery is as essential as radiation and chemotherapy and must not be thought of as a "last alternative." She believes that imagery plays an important role in the biochemical healing process. She hypothesizes that images produced in the mind are converted to biochemical messages which somehow initiate a path of cancer-cell destruction or organ-cell reconstruction. Possibly this healing process inhibits the nervous and endocrine systems from secreting stress hormones. Of course, it is difficult to prove definitively that imagery is a direct cause of healing when it occurs, because imagery is never the sole treatment used.

Hypnotherapy and guided imagery can be used to help people gain self-control, improve self-esteem, and become more autonomous. People who are imprisoned by negative beliefs see themselves as hopeless, helpless victims. With guided imagery, they can learn how to substitute positive, empowering messages. Hypnosis and imagery can also be used as a mental rehearsal for procedures, treatments, or surgery. Clients are shown how to use their own images about the healing process or, alternatively, they are guided through a series of images that are intended to distract them from painful procedures or anxiety-producing situations. The practitioner may have them imagine themselves in a state of good health, well-being, or successfully achieved goals (*Alternative Medicine*, 1994).

People, especially children, are often able to rid themselves of warts by visualizing their disappearance in one way or another. Hypnosis and imagery are often used as a clinical treatment for Reynaud's disease, a condition in which the capillaries of the extremities constrict, with the result that hands and feet are cold and painful. When they learn to "think warm," people may find that the circulation to their hands and feet improves, resulting in less pain. Similarly, hand-warming frequently cuts down on both the incidence and severity of migraine headaches. The use of hypnosis in promoting feelings of comfort, distraction, and dissociation through imagery in those with chronic pain has been well established. Clients are often able to change their perceptual experience of pain by substituting numbness, a sense of pressure, or other sensation for an unwanted pain (Borysenko and Borysenko, 1994; Margolis, 1997).

Contraindications for hypnosis and imagery include poor motivation, such as "My husband sent me so I would lose weight," or an unwillingness even to try the treatment because of extreme fear or compelling religious objections. The procedure is unsuitable for people with active psychosis or somatic delusions. It is generally considered that these individuals are often bombarded with too many images already, and are unable to differentiate between voluntary and involuntary images (Dossey, 1995; Shames, 1996).

RESEARCH

Numerous studies indicate that mental imagery can bring about significant physiological and biochemical changes. Some of these findings are from well-controlled studies, while others are reports of single cases or small studies that have not been replicated. Nevertheless, the overriding conclusion points to a relationship between imagery of bodily change and actual bodily change (*Alternative Medicine*, 1994). These findings revealed that imagery could affect the following:

- Oxygen supply in tissues (Olness and Conroy, 1985)
- Vascular or thermal change (Green and Green, 1997)
- Heart rate and galvanic skin response (Jordan and Lenington, 1979)
- Gastrointestinal activity (Barber, 1978)
- Alleviation of nausea and vomiting associated with chemotherapy (Scott et al., 1986)
- More rapid healing of injuries in subjects diagnosed with knee and ankle injuries who used imagery, positive self-talk, and goal setting than in control subjects (Ievleva and Orlick, 1991)
- Mobilization of the immune system in people with cancer (Borysenko, 1987; Siegel, 1986; Simonton et al., 1978)
- Less post-operative anxiety (Holden-Lund, 1988), less post-operative pain (Daake and Gueldner, 1989; Manyande et al., 1995), and shorter hospital stays (Fazio, 1996; Rapkin et al., 1991) in surgical patients receiving relaxation and imagery instruction

The Academy for Guided Imagery in Mill Valley, California, is currently conducting research on imagery for people undergoing chemotherapy and as a part of preoperative instruction (Miller, 1998).

Modern research in hypnotherapy was initiated in 1933, and by 1977, Erickson and Hilgard had developed methodologies for objective studies. As of yet, no empirical tests assess whether a hypnotic state even exists. Studies have shown, however, that hypnosis can effect a wide variety of physical responses:

- Reduction in severity of episodes of hay fever and asthma (Mason and Black, 1958)
- Cure of warts (Surman et al., 1973; Ullman and Dudek, 1960)
- Raise immunoglobulin levels of healthy children (Olness et al., 1989)
- Shorter labors and more comfortable deliveries with predelivery hypnosis (Rossi, 1993)
- Reduction in migraine attacks in children and teenagers as shown in 12 controlled studies (*Alternative Medicine,* 1994)
- Changes in lymphocyte reactivity in adult cancer patients with metastatic disease (Hall, 1982–1983)

One of the difficulties in conducting research on hypnotherapy is that it is not simply one form of treatment. Hypnosis does not represent one standard set of suggestions which may account for the large number of studies that favor anecdotal, rather than controlled, evidence. For hypnosis to be most effective in a clinical setting, hypnotic suggestions are best formulated on the basis of the individual person's interests, style, motivation, and receptivity to hypnosis. It is not like administering a drug, where doses are standardized. In hypnosis, the personal and subjective matter a great deal. For those who are interested in basic research, Fromm and Nash's (1992) text on contemporary research provides information on theories, methodologies, research design, and the broad areas of actual research (Margolis, 1997).

INTEGRATED NURSING PRACTICE

As a nurse, you can employ guided imagery for personal and professional development. On a regular basis, take time to envision what kind of nurse you would like to be. Envision yourself as healthy, alert, balanced, compassionate, and competent in the clinical arena. You can also use imagery to learn new procedures or techniques. After learning the goals, steps, and processes of a new activity, you can envision yourself doing the procedure safely and skillfully several times as you integrate knowledge with psycho-motor skills. This "rehearsal" is a powerful tool to improve your technical nursing practice.

Some people fear that hypnosis and guided imagery may cause them to lose control of their minds to an outside force. The reality is quite the opposite because the individual is always under self-control. When clients learn a technique like imagery, it is entirely within their control, for use when, how, and where they want. It is a tool that can be used whenever a person feels particularly anxious, upset, or uncomfortable. That type of empowering, in itself, is healing, because people feel better and do better when they have a sense of mastery over what is happening to them.

Many kinds of imagery work well with clients. *Feeling-state imagery* is designed to simply help clients change their mood in a general way. You can suggest to people that they let their imagination take them to a favorite place, real or imagined. For example, some may imagine themselves at a beach and floating gently on the water, while feeling peaceful and relaxed. Others may imagine themselves as a young child sitting on the lap of a beloved grandparent. Clients can use this kind of imagery to move from a feeling state of tension and fear to one of peace and calm.

End-state imagery occurs when clients imagine themselves already in the situation or circumstances that they wish for. It may be seeing themselves as healthy, strong, and free from disease. Others may imagine themselves as successful, happy, and well loved.

Symptoms of disease are often thought to result from blocked energy. *Energetic imagery* involves imagining the life force energy, or qi, flowing smoothly and easily throughout the body. Clients can be taught to imagine that they are pulling up energy from the earth through the soles of their feet to replenish the body's energy.

Cellular imagery relates to imagining events at the cellular level. For example, you may teach clients to imagine their natural killer cells surrounding and attacking cancer cells. Cellular imagery is usually specific and focused on exactly what needs to be fixed. Remind clients that imagery does not have to be visual. Some people "hear" their imagery, others "feel" it, and some "taste" or "smell" it. Some people might choose to put a hand over the affected area and send healing images to the cells in that area.

Similar to cellular imagery, *physiological imagery,* involves the entire body. Thus, clients might be directed to imagine that their blood vessels are relaxed and wider in an effort to lower their blood pressure. People with back pain may imagine that all the muscles in their back are relaxing and softening. People with diabetes may put their hands over the abdomen and imagine insulin moving out of the pancreas to connect with hungry cells throughout the body.

Psychological imagery involves people's perception of themselves. For example, people who feel overly responsible may feel as though they have the weight of the world on their shoulders. Those who feel abandoned may feel the pain as a heartache. In guiding the imagery, you may direct them to focus on their sensation, put their hands on the hurting places, and breathe into the pain. Psychological imagery can also be interactive. When conflict is the issue, people can imagine a dialogue with the adversary that may bring a fresh perspective and new solutions to problems.

The goal of *spiritual imagery* is to make contact with God or the Divine or gain entrance into a larger world. Clients may use spiritual imagery to find guidance or inspiration. Some clients find it comforting to imagine that they are being held in the hands of God where they are perfectly safe (Naparstek, 1994).

Eight characteristics help to make imagery effective as a healing tool, especially with regard to cancer (Naparstek, 1994; Norris, 1992):

- Images must be personal. Images created by others appear to be less effective in the healing process.
- Images must feel right to the person and be congruent with who they are and their values. For example, for those people who see themselves as gentle and conciliatory, combative or warlike images are not appropriate.
- Imagery works best in a permissive, unforced atmosphere. What seems to be most effective is an attitude of allowing the imagery to happen.
- Images must be energetic and physical. People do best when they allow themselves to feel the sensations of their images.

- Images must be anatomically correct and accurate. The type of imagery is chosen on the basis of knowing the nature of the disease and understanding exactly what body part and/or system is affected.
- Skill at using imagery increases with practice. As people use imagery more, their response to it intensifies. Suggest to clients that they use imagery in 5–20 minute blocks of time, one or two times a day.
- Imagery should have an end-stage component. Encourage clients to see the imagery as a mission accomplished.
- If the person is receiving medical treatment concurrently, they should include it in the imagery. Clients who incorporate their chemotherapy or radiation treatment do better than those who ignore these medical procedures in their imagery.

Prior to beginning guided imagery, you should assess a client's belief system, desired outcome, and basic understanding of the pathophysiology involved, as well as the understanding of the effects of medications, treatments, or surgery. This information is necessary to formulate appropriate script content. Establish a quiet, safe environment free of unwanted distractions. Prior to the induction phase, take a few moments to center yourself. Let your mind and body release tension and tightness. Focus on letting your vocal cords relax to enhance a calming pitch, volume, and tone to your voice. Ask clients to assume a comfortable position, reclining if possible, and to close their eyes. Guide them through a progressive relaxation or body scan as described in chapter 16. Instruct them to go to a safe, comfortable place—an actual location or one conjured up in the imagination. Ask them to use all their senses to explore this place—what they see, hear, smell, taste, or feel. For example, you might ask them to identify the time of day or year, what flowers or trees they smell, the taste of any food that is around, and birds, train whistles, or any other sounds they hear.

Next, have clients focus on the problem at hand (e.g., the diagnosis of cancer, being HIV positive, wound or bone healing, or improved organ function). At this point you begin your script, directing them toward their previously discussed goals. You might say something like: "Imagine the broken edges of your bone. Now, bring lots of red blood cells to the area for extra nutrition and oxygen. Imagine new cells being formed and the bone edges growing together." After this type of individualized script, you should include an end-stage script, which might be something like: "Imagine that your broken leg is totally healed now. You have returned to your favorite ski hill. See yourself skiing down the slope. Your leg is strong and healthy and is pain free."

Following this phase of guided imagery, talk with clients about the meaning of what occurred during the session and reinforce the positive aspects of the experience. Some nurses make tapes of the individualized session to which clients may choose to listen as they practice on their own every day.

Gawain (1995) has developed an exercise from which most people can benefit. The pink bubble technique can be done as a one-time experience or regularly over a period of time. It is best to do the technique in the morning when you first wake up and/or in the evening right before sleep. This technique works as follows:

- Assume a comfortable position, breathe slowly, and go through a progressive relaxation or body scan procedure.
- Imagine something you would like to have or would like to have happen.
- Imagine that it has already happened. Picture the object or the situation as clearly as possible, with yourself in the picture.
- Surround this image with a pink bubble.
- Let go of the bubble and watch the bubble float off into the universe. See it becoming one with the higher power of the universe.

You can use guided imagery in many different clinical settings. In general, imagery can be used to move toward the following outcomes (Rossman and Bresler, 1982):

- Induce a state of physiologic relaxation
- Reduce stress
- Reduce pain
- Reduce anxiety
- Understand symptoms
- Stimulate healing responses
- Increase toleration of nursing and medical procedures
- Enhance motivation and self-care
- Find meaning in illness
- Resolve conflicts
- Enhance self-esteem
- Increase problem-solving ability
- Access positive inner resources

Shames (1996) describes numerous ways for nurses to incorporate the use of imagery with nursing procedures. She suggests that people receiving intravenous fluids envision the fluid flushing out cellular toxins while simultaneously nourishing the cells. You can teach people taking antibiotics to imagine

TRY THIS: *Renovating Your Day*

This exercise is designed to empower yourself with your thoughts by transforming negative thoughts and events through visualization. Do this every day for a week, prior to bedtime. Mentally go through your day and decide what you could have changed that would have brought better results. Then imagine that change occuring. For example, if someone said something to you that you did not like, imagine something more positive was said. If you did not like your test score, visualize the grade as a better one.

the medication attacking and destroying bacteria. Individuals experiencing illness or distress can be instructed to take a deep breath and send healing oxygen and a sense of peace to the lungs. On the out-breath, they can image all the toxins or tension leaving the body and disappearing into the air. When a specific organ or part of the body is disrupted, people can bring their awareness to that part and imagine healing resources migrating there to nourish and support the function. People experiencing pain can envision the pain flowing out of the body through the feet and fingertips. Some imagine the capillaries and veins expanding to become large pipes, carrying the pain out. Similarly, people can imagine the soothing effects of pain medication on the affected area and feel the softening and relaxing of the body as the pain lessens. Shames' book, *Creative Imagery in Nursing,* is a wonderful resource and provides many suggestions for clinical application of guided imagery. This technique allows you to use your creativity, intuition, and imagination as you support others on their healing journey.

TRY THIS: *Shrinking Antagonistic Forces*

If you are angry with or intimidated by another person, shrink that person and put him/her in the palm of your open hand. Dialog with that person but have that person talk in a different voice, such as a high, squeaky or cartoon voice. See that person getting smaller and smaller until the person disappears or you blow him/her off into space.

REFERENCES

ACHTERBERG, J. 1978. *Imagery and Cancer.* Champaign, IL: Institute for Personality and Ability Testing.

ACHTERBERG, J. 1985. *Imagery in Healing: Shamanism and Modern Medicine.* Boston: Shambhala Publications.

Alternative Medicine: Expanding Medical Horizons. 1994. A report to the National Institutes of Health on Alternative Medical Systems and Practices in the United States. U.S. Government Printing Office. Washington, DC.

BARBER, T. X. 1978. Hypnosis, suggestion, and psychosomatic phenomena. *Am J Clin Hypn.* 21: 12–27.

BORYSENKO, J. and M. BORYSENKO. 1994. *The Power of the Mind to Heal.* Carlsbad, CA: Hay House.

BORYSENKO, J. 1987. *Minding the Body, Mending the Mind.* New York: Bantam.

BRY, A. 1972. *Visualization: Directing the Movies of Your Mind.* New York: Barnes & Noble Books.

DAAKE, D. and S. GUELDNER. 1989. Imagery instruction and the control of postsurgical pain. *Appl Nurs Res.* 2: 114–120.

DOSSEY, B. 1995. Using imagery to help your patient heal. *Am J Nurs.* 95: 41–46.

FAZIO, V. 1996. Guided imagery proven a powerful adjunct to colorectal surgery. *Multispecialty News from the Cleveland Clinic 15.* XXX, Winter.

FROMM, E. and M. R. NASH, eds. 1992. *Contemporary Hypnosis Research.* New York: Guilford Press.

GAWAIN, S. 1995. *The Creative Visualization Workbook.* Novato, CA: New World Library.

GAWAIN, S. 1983. *Creative Visualization.* Berkeley, CA: Whatever Pub.

GREEN, E. and A. GREEN. 1997. *Beyond Biofeedback.* New York: Delta.

HALL, H. 1982–1983. Hypnosis and the immune system. *J Clin Hypn.* 25: 92–93.

HARDING, M. 1998. Hypnosis and Imagery. Personal communication.

HAMILTON, N. 1998. Understanding Hypnosis. Personal communication.

HAMMOND, D. C. 1990. *Handbook of Hypnotic Suggestions and Metaphors.* New York: W. W. Norton.

HOLDEN-LUND, C. 1988. Effects of relaxation with guided imagery on surgical stress and wound healing. *Res Nurs Health.* 11: 235–244.

IEVLEVA, L., and T. ORLICK. 1991. Mental links to enhanced healing: An exploratory study. *Sport Psychologist.* 5(1): 25–40.

JORDAN, C. S. and K. T. LENINGTON. 1979. Psychological correlates of eidetic imagery and induced anxiety. *J Mental Imagery.* 3: 31–42.

KEEGAN, L. 1994. *The Nurse as Healer.* Albany: Delmar Publishing.

MANYANDE, A. et al. 1995. Preoperative rehearsal of active coping imagery influences subjective and hormonal responses to abdominal surgery. *Psychosom Med.* 57: 177–182.

MARGOLIS, C. G. 1997. Hypnotic trance. Complementary and Alternative Therapies in Primary Care. *Primary Care: Clinics in Office Practice.* 24 (4): 809–823.

MASON, A. A. and S. BLACK. 1958. Allergic skin responses abolished under treatment of asthma and hay fever by hypnosis. *Lancet.* 1: 877–880.

MILLER, T. 1998. The value of imagery in perioperative nursing. *Seminars in Perioperative Nurs.* 7(2): 108–113.

NAPARSTEK, B. 1994. *Staying Well with Guided Imagery.* New York: Warner Books.

NORRIS, P. March 19, 1992. Psychoneuroimmunology: Visualization and imagery. Paper presented to the Association for Applied Psychophysiology and Biofeedback. Colorado Springs, CO.

OLNESS, K. and M. CONROY. 1985. A pilot study of voluntary control of transcutaneous PO by children. *Int J Clin Exp Hypn.* 33: 1.

OLNESS, K. et al. 1989. Self-regulation of salivary immunoglobulin A by children. *Pediatrics.* 83: 66–71.

ORNISH, D. 1990. Can lifestyle changes reverse coronary artery disease? *Lancet.* 336: 129.

RAPKIN, D. et al. 1991. Guided imagery, hypnosis and recovery from head and neck cancer surgery: An exploratory study. *Int J Clin Exp Hypn.* 39: 215–226.

ROSSI, E. L. 1993. *The Psychobiology of Mind-Body Healing,* 2d ed. New York: W. W. Norton.

ROSSMAN, M. and D. BRESLER. 1982. *Introductory Literature: Academy of Guided Imagery.* Mill Valley, CA: Academy of Guided Imagery.

SCOTT, D. W. et al. 1986. Comparative trial of clinical relaxation and an antiemetic drug regimen in reducing chemotherapy-related nausea and vomiting. *Cancer Nursing.* 9: 178–188.

SHAMES, K. H. 1996. *Creative Imagery in Nursing.* Albany: Delmar Publishing.

SHAMES, R. and C. STERIN. 1978. *Healing with Mind Power.* Emmaus, PA: Rodale Press.

SIEGEL, B. 1986. *Love, Medicine, and Miracles.* New York: Harper and Row.

SIMONTON, O. C., S. SIMONTON, and J. CREIGHTON. 1978. *Getting Well Again.* Los Angeles: JP Tarcher.

SURMAN, O. S. et al. 1973. Hypnosis in the treatment of warts. *Arch Gen Psychiatry.* 28: 439–441.

ULLMAN, M. and S. DUDEK. 1960. On the psyche and warts. *Psychosom Med.* 22: 68–76.

WEIL, A. 1995. *Natural Health, Natural Medicine.* Boston: Houghton Mifflin.

RESOURCES

Nursing

Beyond Ordinary Nursing
P.O. Box 8177
Foster City, CA 94404
650-570-6157
email: NCPII@aol.com
Administers the Nurses Certificate Program in Interactive Imagery[SM]

Academy for Guided Imagery
P.O. Box 2070
Mill Valley, CA 94942
800-726-2070

Simonton Cancer Center
P.O. Box 890
Pacific Palisades, CA 90272
310-459-4434

American Holistic Nurses Association
P.O. Box 2130
Flagstaff, AZ 86003
520-526-2196

General

American Institute of Hypnotherapy
16842 Von Karman, # 475
Irvine, CA 92714
800-USA-9996
email: aih@hypnosis.com
sysadmin@hypnosis.com

American Society of Clinical Hypnosis
2200 East Devon Ave., Suite 291
Des Plaines, IL 60018
847-297-3317

Society for Clinical and Experimental Hypnosis
128-A Kings Park Drive
Liverpool, NY 13090
315-652-7299

18 Dreamwork

> For God speaketh once, yea twice, yet a
> man perceiveth it not. In a dream, in a
> vision of the night, when sleep falleth
> upon men in slumberings upon the bed;
> then He openeth the ears of men, and
> speaketh their instructions, that he may
> withdraw man from his purpose and hide
> pride from man.
>
> *Job 33:14–16*

> Dreams must be heeded and accepted,
> for a great many of them come true.
>
> *Paracelsus, 1493–1541,*
> *Swiss physician*

In some ways, a great deal is known about dreaming, because it has been important to people for all time and across all cultures. In the twentieth century, the biology of the brain has been explored and increasingly understood. While this basic knowledge provides some facts underlying dreaming, it does not tell us what dreaming is. Thus, in a sense, little is known about dreaming, and scientists cannot yet agree on the basic nature of dreaming. Some believe dreams are nothing more than random firing of neurons during sleep. Others believe dreams are symbolic stories or metaphors people tell themselves that represent personal and social mythology. Others believe that dreaming is one of the ways that people reflect on and make sense out of their waking life events (Dombeck, 1995).

BACKGROUND

Virtually every culture has believed dreams carry important messages. To the ancient Greeks, dreams were great healers. People who were sick slept in special healing temples in hopes of receiving therapeutic dreams from the gods. The Talmud, the Hebrew sacred book of practical wisdom, states clearly that the Jews gave great importance both to the dream and to the dream interpreter. Mohammed began writing the Koran after an angel visited him in a dream. Tibetan Buddhists saw no distinction between dreaming and waking and considered all of life a dream.

Plato saw dreams as a release for fervent inner forces. Hippocrates thought dreams were windows on illness and that normal dream content indicated a state of wellness and bizarre content a state of illness. Aristotle believed that the beginning of illness could be felt in dreams before actual symptoms appeared. Likewise, Artemidorus, a physician in the Middle Ages, believed that dreams were like magnifying glasses that detected the small beginnings of physical illness.

The most famous dream book was written by Artemidorus of Daldi in the second century and the dreams recorded are remarkably similar to contemporary ones. Ghengis Khan is reported to have received his battle plans from his dreams, while Hannibal attributed the battle plan to attack Rome over the Alps with elephants as something that came to him in a dream.

During the late Middle Ages, dreams began to fall into disfavor by Christians in spite of the fact that throughout the Bible, God spoke directly to people through dreams and visions. St. Frances of Assisi founded the Franciscan Order as a dream directive from Jesus Christ (Steiger and Steiger, 1990).

In the United States, the traditional Iroquois were (and are) a people of dreams. Children were taught that dreams were the most important source of practical and spiritual guidance. The people of an Iroquois village began each day with dream-sharing. The entire village became involved in dreamwork, especially if a dream seemed to contain a warning of death or disease. "Big" dreams were thought to come about in one of two ways. During sleep, the dreamer would have an out-of-body experience and travel to many places, past, present, and future. Alternatively, the dreamer could receive a visit from a spiritual being. Dreams were considered to be central to healing by providing insight into the causes of illness, often before physical symptoms appeared. Dreams continue to be important tools for many traditional healers in the Native American population (Moss, 1996).

In 1900, Sigmund Freud wrote The *Interpretation of Dreams* and proposed that dreaming might represent a unique avenue by which unconscious motivation could be explored. Freud's theory was that dreams were disguised wish fulfillments of infantile sexual needs, which were repressed by censors in the waking mind. Freud's protege, Carl Jung, believed that humans were spiritual rather than instinctual and saw dreams as a compensatory mechanism whose function was to restore psychological balance. Jung said that the conscious and unconscious minds speak entirely different languages. The conscious mind is analytical, critical, and rational while the unconscious mind thinks in metaphor, simile, symbols, and intuition (Seaward, 1997).

Dr. Nathaniel Kleitman is considered to be the father of modern scientific dream research. In 1957, he and Eugene Aserinsky identified rapid eye movement (REM), demonstrating the activity of the brain during sleep. This active sleep stage has consequently been called REM sleep. Today hundreds of sleep clinics operate in the United States, and sleep disorders constitute the second most common health complaint after the common cold (Kelly, 1991).

PREPARATION

In a society that discounted dreams, Sigmund Freud introduced the concept of therapeutic dreamwork. He and his followers, however, began to associate dreams with illness rather than wellness and reserved dream interpretation for professionals who were deemed the only people competent to understand the latent content of dreams. This approach said, in effect, that individuals were not the experts on their own dreams. In contrast, Carl Jung (1965, pp. 170–171) stated that he "avoided all theoretical points of view and simply helped the patients to understand the dream-images by themselves, without application of rules and theories. . . . That is how dreams are intended." Many contemporary therapists believe that dreams belong to individuals and they are the final authority on the meaning of their own dreams. This viewpoint is not to minimize the fact that the meaning of many dreams is obscure and that other people may be able to help unlock hidden meaning (Moss, 1996).

Among indigenous peoples, shamans are recognized as dream counselors but not as "experts" in the Western sense. They are often called to their vocation by dreams. Shamans have a special relationship with the dreamworld, and through dreams are able to look into the future, communicate with spirits, and clarify the meaning of other's dreams (Moss, 1996).

CONCEPTS

Biology of Dreaming

Sleep can be divided into two distinct kinds: a quiet phase and an active phase. Changes in brain waves, eye movements, muscle tone, and the presence of dreams are used to define the two states. The quiet phase is divided into three substages. Stage one is the transitional state between drowsy wakefulness and light sleep. It is characterized by slow drifting eye movements and vivid, brief dream images. Stage two is genuine sleep and is characterized by unique patterns called "sleep spindles," which are waxing and waning brain waves. After 20–30 minutes, people sink into delta sleep, named after the regular, slow brain waves that are characteristic of this stage of quiet sleep. Delta sleep lasts about 30–40 minutes, during which the muscles are relaxed, although most people make major postural adjustments every 5–20 minutes. The dreaming that occurs during delta sleep is more poorly recalled, less vivid and visual, less emotional, and more pleasant than REM sleep dreaming. The sleep pattern then retraces the same stages in reverse order.

About 90 minutes after the onset of sleep, several abrupt physiological changes occur as the sleeper enters REM sleep, or the active phase, for the first time of the night. It is the sleep phase of vivid, memorable dreaming. Brain waves become desynchronized in a fast activity pattern that is similar, but not identical, to that of the waking state. An accompanying profound loss of muscle tone throughout the body causes a general paralysis except for the muscles of the eyes, middle ear ossicles, and respiration. Sometimes people awaken partially from REM sleep before the paralysis fades away, so that their body is still paralyzed, though they are otherwise awake. Sleep paralysis, as this state is called, can occur as people are falling asleep (rarely) or waking up (more frequently). Although the sensation may be terrifying, especially at the first occurrence, sleep paralysis is harmless.

During REM sleep, breathing may accelerate to a panting pace, and the rhythm of the heart may speed up or slow down. Typically, men have erections and women experience vaginal lubrication during every REM cycle, regardless of dream content. It is not unusual for men to ejaculate and women to experience orgasm during this time. During REM sleep, the cells of the brain, which have fired steadily throughout the wake state, fire in a wild and erratic pattern. Some neuroscientists believe dreaming is the attempt of the brain to impose meaning on these signals from random firings (Castleman, 1996; Kelly, 1991; LaBerge and Rheingold, 1990).

During a typical night's sleep, the average adult alternates between periods of REM sleep and quiet sleep at regular intervals 4–6 times each night. After the first REM period, the intervals between REM periods decrease throughout the night, while the length of each REM period increases. REM sleep is both the deepest and lightest stage of sleep. It is the stage when people are least likely to be aroused by environmental stimuli and it is also the stage when people are most likely to awaken spontaneously.

REM sleep is a primary means of brain development and maturation. Infants born 10 weeks prematurely spend 80 percent of the total sleep time in REM sleep and those born 2–4 weeks prematurely spend 60–65 percent in REM sleep. Full-term newborns spend about half of their sleeping time in REM sleep, which decreases to 30–35 percent by the age of two. REM sleep stabilizes at about 25 percent by 10 years of age and shows little change until people are in their 70s or 80s when it decreases to about 18 percent. Thus, the dreaming that occurs during REM sleep is thought to be an important source of internal stimulation necessary for proper maturation of the brain much as physical exercise is important in the development of muscles. This theory does not explain why dreaming continues after the brain has fully developed (Kelly, 1991).

Deprivation of REM sleep does not lead to psychosis, bizarre behavior, or anxiety, as was once feared. The interference with REM sleep may come from alcohol, sedatives, caffeine, drugs, anxiety, or depression. People with major depression dream considerably less than average and have limited dream recall. A sign that the depression is lifting is an increase in REM sleep and the reporting of more dreams. The most important effect of REM deprivation is a dramatic shift in subsequent sleep patterns. Reduction of REM sleep for several nights is followed by earlier onset and longer and more frequent periods of REM sleep. The longer the deprivation of REM sleep the larger and longer the REM rebound. This compensatory mechanism suggests that REM sleep is physiologically necessary (Kelly, 1991).

Functions of Dreaming

Dreaming is a process of making broad connections. Dreams connect with recent experiences, old memories, and imagination. Dreaming makes connections not made during the waking state. The waking state tends to be guided by a specific task or goal, whereas dreaming tends to wander and form unique combinations. For example, people awake and thinking of a house may recall a specific house in which they lived in in the past. People dreaming and thinking of a house may see a generic house or a combination of several houses or even a hotel. During dreaming, consolidation of thoughts and memories occurs, and the bizarre twists and images of dreams often represent the processing and reclassifying of old information. Dream symbols bring together ordinary awareness and deeper levels of knowing. Images mean different things to different people. As Moss (1996, p. 79) states, "A dream of teeth falling out might evoke fears of death or job loss in one person, the memory of a boyhood fistfight in another, and the need for a routine dental checkup to a third. A snake might warn of a sneak attack, arouse sexual fears or energies, or signal potential for healing or transformation." The dominant emotion of the dreamer guides the dreaming process to choose images in the memory related to that emotional concern. Dreams can be viewed as explanatory metaphors for the emotional state of the dreamer. "I leave my children in a house somewhere, and then I can't find them" may be a metaphorical description for the emotional state of guilt. If no single dominant emotion is present at the time, dreams may seem confused and almost random (Benson, 1997).

Jung believed that dreams are a remarkable way to reveal insights and solutions to deal with everyday problems encountered during the wake state. By and large, the language of dreams is anything but obvious, and for this reason it is easy to ignore the messages. What is bizarre to the conscious, rational mind is not so to the unconscious, which is rich in symbols. People who work on remembering and understanding their dreams often report that dreams provide insights to overcome and resolve problems and move ahead (Seaward, 1997).

While some dreams seem to be sequences of disconnected images, ideas, feelings, and sensations, others are storylike sequences that are dramatic and intricately detailed. They may have plots as coherent, funny, and profound as the best stories and plays. Some dreams are not told in a single episode and the dream series is concluded the following night and some may run for as long as a TV soap opera (LaBerge and Rheingold, 1990).

Types of Dreams

Dreams offer nightly gauges on the dreamer's physical, emotional, and spiritual health. When disease begins to develop, dreams often provide warnings of specific problems before physical symptoms are apparent. The warning may be in the form of a broken heart, an exploding head, or limbs falling off. Such early diagnosis dreams are entirely natural and are reminders of how illness is related to one's entire being. Dreams give advice on preventive measures and ways to provide for one's well-being. Dreams frequently suggest specific courses of treatment for different problems. These suggestions may involve lifestyle changes, conventional medical treatments, alternative therapies, or counseling that address the hidden sources of disease. People may neglect the warnings but the unconscious is highly inventive in rescripting the message in ways that make it harder and harder to ignore (Moss, 1996).

Nightmares are terrifying dreams with complex imagery and story lines that are usually vividly recalled. The most common scripts of nightmares include: being chased by a monster, being naked in public, falling through space, losing something precious, and being unprepared for an important exam. Nightmares are especially terrifying because in dreams, anything is possible. Most typically, the dreamer is alone with no chance for escape.

Because REM sleep becomes more physiologically intense as sleep continues, most nightmares occur in the early morning hours. Some factors that seem to contribute to nightmare frequency are fever, stress, and troubled relationships. Traumatic events can trigger a long-lasting series of recurrent nightmares. Alcohol, drugs, and some medications that suppress REM sleep can cause an increase in nightmares. The person sleeps soundly for the first five or six hours with little dreaming. When the effect of the substance has worn off, the brain makes up for the lost REM time. As a result, dreams are more intense than usual for the last few hours of sleep. L-dopa, used in the treatment of Parkinson's disease, and beta blockers, used in the treatment of cardiovascular disorders, seem to increase nightmares by increasing the activity during REM sleep (LaBerge and Rheingold, 1990).

Conscious dreaming, sometimes referred to as lucid dreaming, is being aware that one is dreaming during the experience. People in this unusual state of consciousness are simultaneously aware of their bodies lying on a bed, aware of the content of their dreams, and aware of watching themselves dreaming. Conscious dreaming may be triggered by various things such as doing something impossible in the dream like flying or walking on water. Likewise, auditory signals such as a doorbell or a siren may startle people into becoming aware they are dreaming. Individuals who wish to explore and use dreams constructively in their lives can learn techniques to increase their conscious dreaming time.

Precognition is knowing about an event before it actually occurs. Precognitive dreaming involves seeing people and situations from the future and is an event where individuals are not bound by space-time. As people learn to recall their dreams and record them in a dream journal, they often begin to recognize and work with precognitive material in their dreams. Precognitive dreams may indicate what may happen if certain courses of action are pursued or they may show a precise event that cannot be altered (Dossey, 1989; Steiger and Steiger,1990).

TREATMENT

Until recently, Western societies have discouraged dreamwork and dream-sharing. When dreams are recalled, the significance is often minimized. People tend to remember only bits and pieces from dreams and often jumble together parts from several dreams into a single confused story. By the time individuals are fully awake they have forgotten 90 percent, if not more, of their nighttime adventures. Thus, the remembered dream is often different from the fuller dream experience.

By paying closer attention to dreams, people often gain greater access to their inner lives. Some of the world's most successful business executives never make a decision until they have a chance to let it pass through their minds during sleep, allowing solutions to come during dreams. The first step in making sense of a dream is to own it. It belongs solely to the dreamer and is a personal story. Although many books have been written about dream symbols, they are best understood by the dreamer. Dreaming about a horse may be a symbol of comfort and security because the person always had a horse when she was growing up. A horse for another person may be a symbol of terror because he was kicked by a horse as a young child. A horse for another person may be a symbol for a challenge since she has wanted to learn to ride for some time. Thus, dream dictionaries do not have the answers to people's dream symbols; they are personal images taken from one's life representing one's unique experiences.

Journaling helps to mobilize intuition as people begin to understand their personal symbols. Because the dream journal is intensely personal, it should be kept private unless the dreamer chooses to share it with others. The entries should be dated so they can be correlated to significant life events in the present or future and recurring themes, places, and situations should be noted. Giving dreams titles or headlines like a newspaper headline often reveals a dream message that may be otherwise overlooked. People are encouraged to go back over their journals at regular intervals to note connections between dreams and waking events.

In the midst of nightmares, people who realize they are dreaming frequently choose to wake up. Many therapists believe, however, that the essential issue is to discover what elements from the past, mixed with current events are creating the nightmare. Insight into the source of the nightmare can help people face and overcome the terror while remaining in the dream. Nightmares can be transformed into more pleasant experiences. People are encouraged to remember that nothing in their dreams can hurt them.

Conscious dreaming, as a form of mental imagery, has potential to aid in the promotion of health and in the healing process. Evidence supports the idea that the vividness of mental imagery determines how strongly it affects physiology (Richardson, 1984). Dreams are the most vivid form of mental imagery most people experience and therefore, they are also likely to be a source of highly effective healing imagery.

Dreams can be immensely useful in gaining self-knowledge. Psychologist Ernest Rossi has proposed that an important function of dreaming is integration of split off parts of one's personality. According to Rossi (1985, p.142):

> In dreams we witness something more than mere wishes; we experience dramas reflecting our psychological state and the process of change taking place in it. Dreams are a laboratory for experimenting with changes in our psychic life. . . . This constructive or synthetic approach to dreams can be clearly stated: Dreaming is an endogenous process of psychological growth, change, and transformation.

The Tibetan Buddhist Tarthang Tulku (1978, p.77) writes:

> Experiences we gain from practices we do during our dream time can then be brought into our daytime experience. For example, we can learn to change the frightening images we see in our dreams into peaceful forms. Using the same process, we can transmute the negative emotions we feel during the daytime into increased awareness. Thus we can use our dream experiences to develop a more flexible life.

RESEARCH

Dream research is often accused of working from biased or otherwise inadequate samples. Some question whether people who remember dreams are different from other people. Some fear people do not report their dreams honestly. Many studies of high and low dream recallers demonstrate only small differences between them on a variety of personality and cognitive tests. High recallers differ primarily in their interest in dreams and their motivation to recall them. In many studies, subjects provide dream reports anonymously, which reduces the tendency to misreport. For most people, dreams are something that happens to them, so they do not see the dreams as a reflection on their self-image and are thus quite willing to report whatever they experience (Schneider, 1998).

Hall and Van de Castle (1966) cataloged more than 10,000 dreams from normal people and found that approximately 64 percent were associated with sadness, apprehension, or anger. Only 18 percent were happy or exciting. Hostile acts by or against the dreamer, such as murder or attack outnumbered friendly acts by more than two to one. Only 1 percent of dreams involved sexual feelings or acts. Other studies have shown that:

- Girls and women report more dreams than boys and men (Cowen and Levin, 1995; Hartmann,1989; Tonay, 1993).
- People are more likely to recall dreams that correspond to their current mood (Blaney, 1986; Bradley and Mathews, 1988).
- Pregnant women's dreams reflect somewhat predictable emotional concerns. Concerns early in pregnancy are related to physical changes and attractiveness and later concerns of what the baby will actually be like emerge (Garfield, 1988; Maybruck, 1989; Van de Castle, 1994).
- Remembering dreams is an immediate response to current psychological distress that serves a long-term adaptive role in processing emotional information, solving problems, and integrating painful experiences (Breger et al., 1971; Hartmann, 1995).
- Repeated exposure to life-threatening events such as war experiences or imprisonment in a concentration camp have been associated with decreases in dream recall (Kaminer and Lavie, 1991; Rofe and Lewin, 1980), whereas exposure to occasional and less severe trauma, such as major life changes increase dream recall (Cartwright, 1986).

INTEGRATED NURSING PRACTICE

Dreams are the doorway into the unconscious, which is also a domain of healing. Just as guided imagery can be used to direct people's attention to specific areas or organs of the body, so can dreams become a healing tool. For clients who are interested in cultivating healing dreams, they can follow a series of steps that you can teach them (Keegan, 1994):

- One half hour before bedtime, find a quiet place.
- Pay attention to the sounds and sensations of the outside environment as nature begins to settle down to rest.
- Spend a few minutes journaling the experiences and feelings you had during the day.
- Review your accomplishments of the day.
- Dwell for a moment on loving yourself and others with whom you interacted today.
- If you had conflict with others, put those thoughts and feelings away for now.
- Imagine yourself as part of the universe and feel a connection with all living things.
- Allow one issue of present concern to surface to your conscious mind.
- Ask for answers, solutions, or healing as you sleep and dream.
- On awakening, remember your previous night's request and let the answers come to your conscious mind.

A similar process is called dream incubation, which is a somewhat more deliberate format. Examples of the type of requests to make of our dreams are: How can I heal myself? Which path shall I choose? How can I solve (state problem)? How can I improve my relationship with (name)? How can I make (state project) a success? Should I do (state proposed action)? What shall I do now? Teach clients the following steps for dream incubation:

- Choose an important matter that you wish to explore.
- Write down a short, simple question about which you want to know.
- Meditate on the question for a few minutes. Repeat the question several times, followed by, "I give thanks for the answer, which will be in a dream that I remember."
- Envision yourself awakening, remembering, and receiving an answer.
- Write the question again.
- Place the paper with the question on it beneath your pillow.
- Upon awakening, follow the guideline in the TRY THIS box on improving dream recall.
- Watch for extra information that may come later during the day.
- Do not give up if success is not immediate.

Help clients understand that they need not seek professional help for bad dreams unless they frequently disrupt one's sleep. Other distress signals include regular bouts of fatigue or depression when you wake up or consistently feeling worse than when you went to bed. Remind people that nothing in their dreams can hurt them. Suggestions for reframing nightmare themes are presented in Box 18.1. Alternatively, nightmares can be managed through a process called dream reentry, which is practiced in the waking state. People begin by selecting the nightmare to relive, then come up with alternative ways of acting in the nightmare to transform the events into a more enjoyable experience. They relive the nightmare in imagination, incorporating the new action, and continue on with the dream until they see the result of their new behavior (LaBerge and Rheingold, 1990).

Spiritual care, in many settings, includes listening to clients' dreams. During times of transition, growth, or suffering, spiritual issues or struggles often occur and may be found in dreams as people wrestle with what is most important in their lives. Nurses have a unique opportunity to listen attentively to clients and help them work through this process. Sharing dreams with another person or with a group can provide a variety of insights into the many levels of the dream. Dream-sharing also builds a sense of community as people discover they have a great deal in common. If you are a nurse who is sensitive and empathic and you have good listening, communication, and group skills, you can facilitate a dream-sharing group (Dombeck, 1995).

If you want each member of the group to have time to work on a dream at every session, you will have to limit your numbers to six or eight. Members should be asked to make a commitment to attend regular sessions over a set time, usually for no less than six weeks. A typical group session is two to three hours. Dream-sharing requires mutual trust and respect. If people are going to share their innermost thoughts, they must have the assurance that they are in a place where they are protected and supported. The dream is always honored as a topic worthy of attention and thought. The protocol of dream-sharing is as follows (Dombeck, 1995; Moss, 1966):

- All members are given an opportunity to share dreams if they choose to, but are never pressured to do so.
- Dreams shared within the group should not be told to outsiders without the dreamer's permission.
- Sharing dreams does not mean giving up the right to privacy. Dreamers are free to share as much or as little about their dream or personal life as they wish.
- You are the final authority on the meaning of your dream.
- You cannot tell anyone else what her or his dream is about. You can only tell them what it would mean to you if it were your dream.

Box 18.1: Reframing Nightmares

Being Chased

Response: Stop running and face the chaser, which may cause it to disappear. If not, try to dialogue and reconcile with the person or animal. Alternatively, ask the adversary itself, what you are running away from.

Being Attacked

Response: Demonstrate your readiness to defend yourself, rather than giving in or running away. Then try to dialogue with the attacker in a soothing manner. Alternatively, enlist friendly and cooperative dream characters to help overcome the threatening character.

Falling

Response: Rather than waking up, go with it, relax, and land gently. Think about landing in a pleasant and interesting place. Alternatively, transform falling into flying.

Trapped or Paralyzed

Response: Relax and tell yourself you are dreaming. Go along with images or things that happen to the body, because none of it can be harmful in reality. Adopt an attitude of interest and curiosity about what happens.

Being Unprepared for an Exam or Speech

Response: Leave the exam room or the lecture hall. Alternatively, answer the text questions creatively or give a spontaneous talk on any topic of interest. The key is in transforming the experience into one that is fun.

Being Naked in Public

Response: Remember, modesty is a public convention and dreams are private experiences. Have fun with the idea. Try having everyone else in the dream remove their clothing also.

Sources: LaBerge and Rheingold, *Exploring the World of Lucid Dreaming* (New York: Ballantine Books, 1990); Moss, *Conscious Dreaming* (New York: Crown Trade Paperbacks, 1996).

TRY THIS: *Improving Dream Recall*

1. Clearly declare to yourself the intention to remember your dreams when you lie down to sleep.

2. Have your tools, notebook and pen or tape recorder, at your bedside.

3. If you awaken during the night while dreaming, record your dream immediately. Use a penlight to see if you do not wish to disturb your partner. If you tell yourself that you can go back to sleep and catch the dreams later, you will probably find you are wrong.

4. When you awaken in the morning, at first lie quietly before jumping out of bed. Then write whatever you remember, even if only one word or scene.

5. If you wake with no dream memories, move your body back into the position you were in as you began to awaken and you will be more likely to recall your most recent dream.

6. Don't censor your dreaming and don't try to interpret right away. Bizarre, weird, or trivial dreams may become important later.

7. Pay attention to your feelings. They are often your best guide to the dream's meaning and urgency.

8. Keep a journal for a month of the dreams you do remember. Look for important ideas or themes running through the dreams.

9. The more you practice these skills, the more dreams you will remember.

Source: Moss, *Conscious Dreaming* (New York: Crown Trade Paperbacks, 1996); Steiger and Steiger, *The Teaching Power of Dreams* (West Chester, PA: Whitford Press, 1990).

Even without a full understanding of what dreams signify, we can use their stories to know ourselves better. For many people—and you can be one of them—dreams really do come true.

REFERENCES

BENSON, H. 1997. *Timeless Healing.* New York: Fireside Book.

BLANEY, P. H. 1986. Affect and memory: A review. *Psychological Bulletin.* 99: 229–246.

BRADLEY, B. P. and A. MATHEWS. 1988. Memory bias in recovered clinical depressives. *Cognition and Emotion.* 2: 235–245.

BREGER., L., I. HUNTER, and R. W. LANE. 1971. The effect of stress on dreams. *Psychological Issues.* VII (3), Monograph 27.

CARTWRIGHT, R. 1986. Affect and dream work from an information processing point of view. *J Mind and Behavior.* 7: 411–427.

CASTLEMAN, M. 1996. *Nature's Cures.* Emmaus, PA: Rodale Press.

COWEN, D. and R. LEVIN, 1995. The use of the Hartmann boundary questionnaire with an adolescent population. *Dreaming.* 5: 105–114.

DOMBECK, M. T. B. 1995. Dream telling: A means of spiritual awareness. *Holistic Nurs Pract.* 9(2): 37–47.

DOSSEY, L. 1989. *Recovering the Soul.* New York: Bantam Books.

GARFIELD, P. 1988. *Women's Bodies, Women's Dreams.* New York: Ballantine Books.

HALL, C. S. and R. L. VAN DE CASTLE. 1966. *The Content Anaylsis of Dreams.* New York: Appleton-Century-Crofts.

HARTMANN, E. 1989. Boundaries of dreams, boundaries of dreamers. *Psychiatric J of the Univ of Ottawa.* 14: 557–560.

HARTMANN, E. 1995. Making connections in a safe place: Is dreaming psychotherapy? *Dreaming.* 5: 213–228.

JUNG, C. G. 1965. *Memories, Dreams, Reflections.* A. JAFFE, ed., R. WINSTON and C. WINSTON, trans. New York: Vintage.

KAMINER, H. and P. LAVIE. 1991. Sleep and dreaming in Holocaust survivors. *J Nervous and Mental Disease.* 179: 664–669.

KEEGAN, L. 1994. *The Nurse as Healer.* Albany: Delmar Publishers.

KELLY, D. D. 1991. Sleep and dreaming. In E. R. KANDEL, J. H. SCHWARTZ, and T. M. JESSEL, eds. *Principles of Neural Science,* 3rd ed. New York: Elsevier, 792–840.

LABERGE, S. and H. RHEINGOLD. 1990. *Exploring the World of Lucid Dreaming.* New York: Ballantine Books.

MAYBRUCK, P. 1989. *Pregnancy and Dreams.* Los Angeles: Jeremy P. Tarcher.

MOSS, R. 1996. *Conscious Dreaming: A Spiritual Path for Everyday Life.* New York: Crown Trade Paperbacks.

RICHARDSON, A. 1984. Strengthening the theoretical links between imaged stimuli and physiological responses. *J Mental Imagery.* 8: 113–126.

ROFE, Y. and I. LEWIN. 1980. Daydreaming in a war environment. *J Mental Imagery.* 4: 59–75.

ROSSI, E. 1985. *Dreams and the Growth of Personality,* 2d ed. New York: Brunner/ Mazel.

SCHNEIDER, A. 1998. Representative samples and the quality of the data. dreams@ zzyx.ucsc.edu

SEAWARD, B. L. 1997. *Stand Like Mountain Flow Like Water.* Deerfield Beach, FL: Health Communications, Inc.

STEIGER, S. and B. STEIGER. 1990. *The Teaching Power of Dreams.* West Chester, PA: Whitford Press.

Tonay, V. K. 1993. Personality correlates of dream recall: Who remembers? *Dreaming.* 3: 1–8.

Van de Castle, R. L. 1994. *Our Dreaming Mind.* New York: Ballantine Books.

RESOURCES

Association for the Study of Dreams
P.O. Box 1600
Vienna, VA 22183
703-242-0062
www.asdreams.org

Dream Network
1337 Powerhouse Lane, Suite 22
P.O. Box 1026
Moab, UT 84532-3031

Dreamwheel
191 Sudbury Rd.
Concord, MA 01742-3423
978-369-2634
email: dreamwheel@compuserve.com

The Lucidity Institute
2555 Park Blvd., Suite 2
Palo Alto, CA 94306-1919
800-465-8243
www.lucidity.com
email: info@lucidity.com

European Association for the Study of Dreams
39 rue Henri Maus
BP 400-Liege 1 Belgique
32-41 53 03 57
perso.club-internet.fr/oniros/EASD

Novato Dream Library and Archive
P.O. Box 866
Novato, CA 94948
415-898-2559
members.aol.com/dreammzzz/ncdarch.htm

Way of the Dreamer
P.O. Box 215
Troy, NY 12181
518–274–0506

Dream Gate
www.dreamgate.com

Sleep Home Pages from Brain Information Service
bisleep.medsch.ucla.edu

www.dr-dream.com/indexed.html

19 Biofeedback

> The only solid piece of scientific truth
> about which I feel totally confident
> is that we are profoundly ignorant
> about nature.
>
> *Lewis Thomas*

Biofeedback is a method for learned control of physiological responses of the body. It is a relaxation technique using electronic equipment to amplify the electrochemical energy produced by body responses. Normally out of conscious awareness, biofeedback provides perceptible information that individuals can use to gain voluntary control over various physiological processes.

BACKGROUND

The experimental data to support the feasibility of learned control first appeared in the 1950s. In 1961, experimental psychologist Neal Miller proposed that the autonomic nervous system was trainable, contrary to beliefs about human physiology at the time. As psychologists and physiologists continued this research, it became clear that dramatic gains could be achieved by using biofeedback information to assist people suffering from specific conditions, including headaches, ulcers, hypertension, and many other stress-related illnesses. The result of this work was the creation of biofeedback therapy, now widely used by both conventional and alternative practitioners. With the advent of computers, the technology has become more powerful (*Alternative Medicine,* 1994).

PREPARATION

Biofeedback does not belong to any particular field of heath care but is used in many disciplines including nursing, psychology, social work, chiropractic, medicine, dentistry, physical therapy, rehabilitation, psychiatry, respiratory therapy, occupational therapy, physician assistant, exercise physiology, and sports medicine. Since 1980, all biofeedback therapists must have certification from the Biofeedback Certification Institute of America (BCIA). Licensed RN's are accepted with an AA degree, while all other applicants must hold a bachelors degree or higher in one of the approved health care fields. Certification requires 60 hours in didactic biofeedback education as well as 140 hours in clinical experience. When applicants meet the requirements, they are allowed to sit for a qualifying examination that consists of both written and practical assessment. The BCIA provides directories of certified practitioners throughout the United States.

CONCEPTS

The nervous system has two major components—voluntary and involuntary or autonomic. The voluntary component is totally under a person's control. If someone decides to stand, the brain sends a message to the appropriate muscle groups, and the person stands. In contrast, the autonomic nervous system functions without conscious thought. Although people may be able to change their rate of respiration, for example, they are not able to stop breathing indefinitely.

People receive biofeedback from their bodies all the time. When they do not eat, they feel hungry. When they run, they get winded. When they experience stress, their muscles tense. Other types of biofeedback are more difficult to discern. With the use of technology, however, people can learn to adjust their thought processes to control bodily processes such as blood pressure, temperature, muscle tension, bronchial dilation, gastrointestinal functioning, and brain wave activity. The concept is simple: if individuals can develop sensory awareness of an involuntary function, they can learn to sense it. For example, if skin temperature in the hands is converted into an audible signal, the beeps give one's ears and brain feedback. As people learn to dilate the arteries in their hands, thus raising skin temperature, the beeps speed up, providing instant feedback on what is occurring in the body. Biofeedback teaches people what it feels like to be relaxed internally so they can recreate the feeling whenever they choose (Weil, 1995).

TREATMENT

Biofeedback instruments are highly sensitive electronic devices that monitor physiological processes. Signals from the body are amplified by the instrument and converted into usable information. The instruments may have meters, tones, or a computer display that presents the information to the trainee.

Temperature or thermal feedback is a primary tool for general relaxation training and treatment of specific vascular diseases. Blood flow in the hands responds to stress and relaxation, and the client learns to relax by watching the rise and fall of finger temperature. Electrodermal response (EDR) or galvanic skin response (GSR) feedback devices measure sweat gland activity of the finger tips or palm. This response is highly sensitive to emotions and thoughts. It is used in general relaxation training, helping people reduce the impact of significant stressors, and in treating excessive sweating. Electromyography (EMG) feedback measures muscle tension with sensors placed on the skin over appropriate muscles. EMG feedback is used for general relaxation training and is the primary tool for the treatment of tension headache, pain reduction, and muscle spasm or paralysis due to injury or stroke. Sensors on the fingers provide pulse feedback, which is used for people experiencing anxiety, hypertension, and some cardiac arrhythmias. Respiratory resistance (R(os)) biofeedback measures the rate, volume, and rhythm of respiration and is useful in both asthma and the hyperventilation of anxiety and panic attacks. Electroencephalograph (EEG) records information about brainwave activity from sensors placed on the scalp. Changes in brain waves reflect changes in attention as well as in states of arousal from sleep to alert wakefulness. This type of feedback is used for mind quieting, attention control, insomnia, pain control, and substance abuse treatment. Cardiovascular (EKG) feedback is available through portable heart-rate monitors to augment a person's ability to control heart rate. In addition to being used by persons with cardiac disease, many professional athletes use this system to aid their training. Sensors can now measure and report the activity of the internal and external rectal sphincters for the treatment of fecal incontinence, the activity of the detrusor muscle of the urinary bladder for the treatment of urinary incontinence, as well as esophageal motility and stomach acidity (*Alternative Medicine,* 1994; Castleman, 1996).

After the desired mode of treatment is determined for the specific disorder, electrodes are attached to the person in the area to be monitored. These electrodes feed the information to a computer that registers the results either with a sound tone that varies in pitch or speed or on a visual monitor. EEG measurements produce a kind of video game of brainwaves. The human brain produces different brain waves during various states of consciousness. Beta waves are associated with normal or waking consciousness; alpha waves are produced in an altered or relaxed state of consciousness; and theta and delta waves are associated with unconscious and sleeping states. When the client produces waves associated with concentration, the game speeds up. The game slows down when brainwaves associated with daydreaming are produced. This type of computer system can make learning control of body processes more interactive and fun, especially for children (Seaward, 1997).

A biofeedback therapist leads the client in mental exercises to help the person reach the desired result such as muscle relaxation or contraction or more of the alpha brain waves. Through trial and error, trainees eventually learn how to control the inner mechanism involved. Training typically requires 8–10 sessions, although people with long-term or severe disorders may require more sessions. Clients are expected to practice the skill 15–20 minutes a day throughout the training period to incorporate what they have learned into their lives.

Like other forms of therapy, biofeedback is more useful for some clinical problems than for others. Biofeedback is the preferred treatment in Raynaud's syndrome and in certain types of fecal and urinary incontinence. It is one of several preferred treatments for tension headaches, migraine headaches, irritable bowel syndrome, muscle reeducation, bruxism, temporomandibular joint syndrome (TMJ), and attention deficit disorder. Biofeedback is effective intervention in asthma, substance abuse, anxiety, cardiac arrhythmias, essential hypertension, epilepsy, and chronic pain syndromes (*Alternative Medicine,* 1994).

RESEARCH

Substantial research exists demonstrating the effectiveness of biofeedback in a number of conditions:

- People with essential hypertension were able to decrease their systolic pressure 17mm and their diastolic pressure by 7mm after four biofeedback sessions (Nakao, 1997).
- With one biofeedback session, individuals with advanced heart failure were able to increase their peripheral skin temperature in their feet and hands, increase cardiac output, decrease respiratory rate, and decrease vascular resistance (Moser, 1997).
- Children and adults experiencing migraine headaches were able to reduce the frequency of headaches (Allen and Shiver, 1997; Kropp et al., 1997).
- Individuals with drug-resistant epilepsy were able to significantly decrease the frequency of their seizures after 20 biofeedback sessions (Kotchoubey et al., 1977).
- Four weeks of biofeedback training had a positive effect on balance training for people experiencing hemiplegia following a stroke or traumatic brain injury (Wong et al., 1997).
- Asthma victims were able to decrease the frequency of attacks (Mass et al., 1996).

- People with diabetes were able to improve on average their daily blood glucose levels (McGrandy et al., 1996).
- EEG biofeedback is an effective alternative to stimulants in treating attention deficit hyperactivity disorder (Rossiter and LaVaque, 1995; Tan and Schneider, 1997).
- Biofeedback reduced the frequency of urinary incontinence (Kaplan et al., 1997; Tries and Brubaker, 1996).
- Biofeedback was effective in helping people with idiopathic constipation learn to coordinate defecating muscles during straining (Storrie, 1997).
- Women with ovarian cancer were able to boost their immune system (Lekander et al., 1997).
- Nine sessions of biofeedback significantly reduced the general intensity of pain in people with fibromyalgia (Sarnoch et al., 1997).
- School children identified by teachers as being anxious demonstrated a significant decrease in both state and trait anxiety following six sessions of EMG biofeedback and six sessions of thermal biofeedback training (Wenck et al., 1996).

Thousands of articles and more than 100 texts demonstrate the effectiveness of biofeedback. Further research questions include determining the full range of bodily responses that can be modified, the effects of motivation and expectations on success, situations in which biofeedback should be an adjunct versus a primary intervention, situations in which group instruction may be effective, and computer innovations that might advance biofeedback training.

INTEGRATED NURSING PRACTICE

Certified biofeedback therapists, many of whom are nurses, help interpret signals from monitoring devices while leading the client through physical and mental exercises to achieve the desired change in the body function being measured. As a nurse without specific training, your primary intervention is to provide information about biofeedback to appropriate clients. You can explain the types of monitoring devices and the conditions for which it is typically effective. In addition, you can help individuals find certified therapists. Explain that biofeedback creates a greater awareness of specific body parts and their functions. With training, clients can regulate these functions. Biofeedback helps people to relieve or eliminate symptoms, provides an internal locus of control, and helps them reduce their own health care costs.

TRY THIS: *Mind Control of Muscular Strength*

- Face your partner. Put your right hand on your partner's shoulder, palm up.
- Clench your fist, hold your arm straight.
- Have your partner grasp your elbow with both hands and pull down while you resist. The pull needs to be gradual until you both get a sense of how much force is needed to bend your arm.
- Then imagine you are a fire engine or pump. You are rooted to the earth and are drawing water up and it is pushing through your arm and out of your fingers at high speed with tremendous force. Such force that nothing can bend your arm.
- Then place your arm again on your partner's shoulder, this time with the fingers outstretched, holding onto the feeling and the image of the pump pushing water through your arm with great force.
- Ask your partner once more to apply gradual force to bend your arm. You will need to apply a little muscle power, but will find you can relax and hold steady with much less effort than before.

Source: Rutherford, *Principles of Shamanism* (San Francisco: Thorsons, 1996).

REFERENCES

ALLEN, K. D. and M. D. SHIVER. 1997. Enhanced performance feedback to strengthen biofeedback treatment outcome with childhood migraine. *Headache.* 37(3): 169–173.

Alternative Medicine: Expanding Medical Horizons. 1994. A report to the National Institutes of Health on Alternative Medical Systems and Practices in the United States. U.S. Government Printing Office. Washington, DC.

CASTLEMAN, M. 1996. *Nature's Cures.* Emmaus, PA: Rodale Press.

KAPLAN, S. A. et al. 1997. Pseudodyssynergia misdiagnosed as chronic nonbacterial prostatitis and the role of biofeedback as a therapeutic option. *J Urology.* 157(6): 2234–2237.

KOTCHOUBEY, B. et al. 1977. Self-regulation of slow cortical potentials in epilepsy. *Epilepsy Research.* 25(3): 269–276.

KROPP, P. et al. 1997. Behavioral treatment in migraine. *Functional Neurology.* 12(1): 17–24.

LEKANDER, M. et al. 1997. Immune effects of relaxation during chemotherapy for ovarian cancer. *Psychotherapy and Psychosomatics.* 66(4): 185–191.

MASS, R., R. RICHTER, and B. DAHME. 1996. Biofeedback-induced voluntary reduction of respiratory resistance in severe bronchial asthma. *Behavior Research and Therapy.* 34(10): 815–819.

MCGRANDY, A., G. GRAHAM, and A. BAILEY. 1996. Biofeedback-assisted relaxation in insulin-dependent diabetes—A replication and extension study. *Annals of Behavioral Med.* 18(3): 185–189.

MOSER, D. K. 1997. Voluntary control of vascular tone by using skin-temperature biofeedback-relaxation in patients with advanced heart failure. *Alternative Therapies in Health and Med.* 3(1): 51–59.

NAKAO, M. 1997. Clinical effects of blood pressure biofeedback on hypertension by autoshaping. *Psychosomatic Med.* 59(3): 331–338.

ROSSITER, T. R. and T. J. LAVAQUE. 1995. A comparison of EEG biofeedback and psychostimulants in treating attention deficit hyperactivity disorders. *J Neurotherapy.* 20: 48–59.

SARNOCH, H., F. ADLER, and O. B. SCHOLZ. 1997. Relevance of muscular sensitivity, muscular activity, and cognitive variables for pain reduction associated with EMG biofeedback in fibromyalgia. *Perceptual and Motor Skills.* 84(3, part 1): 1043–1050.

SEAWARD, B. L. 1997. *Managing Stress,* 2d ed. Boston: Jones and Bartlett Publishers.

STORRIE, J. B. 1997. Biofeedback: A first-line treatment for idiopathic constipation. *British J Nursing.* 6(3): 152–158.

TAN, G. and S. C. SCHNEIDER. 1997. Attention-deficit hyperactivity disorder. *Postgraduate Med.* 105(5): 201–204, 213–214, 216.

TRIES, J. and L. BRUBAKER. 1996. Application of biofeedback in the treatment of urinary incontinence. *Professional Psychology-Research and Practice.* 37(6): 548–553.

WEIL, A. 1995. *Natural Health, Natural Medicine.* Boston: Houghton Mifflin.

WENCK, L. S., P. W. LEU, and R. C. DAMATO. 1996. Evaluating the efficacy of a biofeedback intervention to reduce children's anxiety. *J Clinical Psychology.* 52(4): 469–473.

WONG, A. M. K. et al. 1997. The development and clinical evaluation of a standing biofeedback trainer. *J Rehabilitation Research and Development.* 34(3): 322–327.

RESOURCES

Association for Applied Psychophysiology and Biofeedback
Biofeedback Certification Institute
10200 West 44th Ave., Suite 304
Wheat Ridge, CO 80033-2840
800-477-8892
www.aapb.org/
email: AAPB@resourcenter.com

Association for Integrative Medicine
801 Beam Rd.
West Chester, PA 19380
610-738-8843
www.integrativemedicine.org/

Biofeedback Certification Institute of America
10200 West 44th Ave., Suite 304
Wheat Ridge, CO 80033-2840
303-420-2902
www.bcia.org/

Biofeedback Foundation of Europe
P.O. Box 21
3440 AA Woerden
The Netherlands
41-31 348 420 420
www.bfe.org/

EEG Spectrum
Dept. P
16100 Ventura Blvd., Suite 10
Encino, CA 91436
www.eegspectrum.com

Society for the Study of Neuronal Regulation
www.ssnr.com/

20 Movement-Oriented Therapies

> If you believe you can or if you believe you can't, you're right!
>
> *Henry Ford*

> To know who one is, an individual must be aware of what he feels.
>
> *Alexander Lowen*

A number of therapies focus on movement, body awareness, and breathing, and their purpose is to maintain health as well as to correct specific problems. This chapter presents two Eastern movement-oriented therapies: Qigong and T'ai Chi; and three Western movement-oriented therapies: the Alexander Technique, the Feldenkrais Method, and the Trager Approach. Common to these various approaches is the retraining of one's body to improve coordination and balance, to release and change postural faults, and to relieve structural and functional stress. A major principle is that awareness has to be experienced rather than taught verbally, which may then lead to more effective use of one's whole self (*Alternative Medicine*, 1994).

Qigong, also spelled as Chi Kung, Chi Gong, and Chi Gung, is pronounced "chee goong." Qigong is a Chinese discipline consisting of breathing and mental exercises that may be combined with modest arm movements. Qi is the term for vital energy and life force and gong means work or discipline. Qigong can be translated as "mastery of qi," "cultivation of energy," "air energy," "breath work," and "energy work." People discover how to generate more energy and conserve what they have in order to maintain health or treat illness (McGee et al., 1996).

T'ai Chi, sometimes spelled as taiji, is pronounced as "teye chee." T'ai Chi arose out of Qigong and is a discipline that combines physical fitness, meditation, and self-defense. Literally translated, it means "great ultimate fist" and is sometimes translated as "supreme boxing" or "root of all motion." Although it is considered a martial art, T'ai Chi is mainly practiced today as a health discipline (Castleman, 1996).

317

The Alexander Technique is a method to improve postural and movement dysfunction that can lead to pain and disease. It is designed to reduce and eliminate body misuse in daily activities especially in respect to the head, neck, and shoulders (Reiser, 1994). The Feldenkrais Method uses gentle movement and directed attention to improve movement and enhance functioning. The physics of body movement are combined with an awareness of the way people learn to move, behave, and interact. The Trager Approach uses light, rhythmic rocking, and shaking movements that loosen joints, ease movement, and release chronic patterns of tension (*Alternative Medicine,* 1994). All three of these Western approaches are considered to be educational in nature as opposed to medical interventions.

BACKGROUND

Written records on Qigong go back 4,000 years. For almost all of that time, this practice remained a closely guarded family secret, available only to the elite classes in China. This discipline was handed down covertly and was not revealed until the beginning of the twentieth century. In the late 1970s, the Chinese government funded several scientific studies of Qigong, which had been banned during the Cultural Revolution as superstitious practice. When a scientific basis was established, the government added Qigong to the list of treatment methods offered in Traditional Chinese Medicine Hospitals. T'ai Chi, a modern offshoot of Qigong, began in the fourteenth century, only 600 years ago, created by a Taoist priest. T'ai Chi gained popularity in the United States in the 1960s as people explored alternatives to conventional medicine. Some experts estimate that more than 800 million people practice Qigong or T'ai Chi internationally—nearly 20 percent of the world's population (McGee et al., 1996).

The Alexander Technique was developed more than a century ago by F. M. Alexander, an Australian actor who had lost his voice while performing. He carefully watched himself while speaking and observed that undue muscular tension accounted for his vocal problem. He sought a way to eliminate that restriction, and the technique he developed focused on correcting the misuse of the neuromuscular activity of the head, neck, and spine. The Alexander Technique is taught in the curriculum of music conservatories, theater schools, and universities throughout the world, as a foundation for improved health and creative exploration. It is also a useful tool to help people, able-bodied and disabled, maximize their movement potential (*Alexander Technique Resource Guide,* 1998).

The Feldenkrais Method was developed by Moshe Feldenkrais (1904–1984), a Russian-born Israeli physicist, mechanical engineer, and judo expert.

After suffering crippling knee injuries, Feldenkrais used his own body as his laboratory and taught himself to walk again. In the process, he developed a system for accessing the power of the central nervous system to improve human functioning (Rosenfeld, 1981).

The Trager Approach was developed by Milton Trager, in the early 1930s, on the basis of his experience as a boxing trainer. He spent the next 50 years, first as a lay practitioner and later as a physician, expanding and refining his discovery. It is a method of movement reeducation designed to produce positive, pleasurable feelings and tissue changes by means of sensory-motor feedback loops between the mind and the muscles (Juhan, 1995).

PREPARATION

For most people, Qigong and T'ai Chi are personal disciplines. Most practitioners spend 30–60 minutes a day doing the exercises. With more intensive practice over many years, some become masters. A T'ai Chi master is generally one who has exceptional skill in doing the form or in using the principles in boxing and in life. A Qigong master is one who has developed the ability to emit healing energy and has achieved proven success in healing with qi. Masters may also have qualities that are generally considered supernatural in the areas of special insight and spiritual transcendence. Rarely, if ever, will a true master call herself or himself a master. Rather, they say that "the practice is the teacher" and that "the qi is the teacher."

It is difficult to learn Qigong or T'ai Chi from a book, audio tape, or video. While simple forms may be grasped this way, the more complex forms are nearly impossible to learn without a teacher's guidance. In the Chinese tradition, one chooses and remains devoted to a teacher. The teacher-disciple relationship is revered as the only path to advanced skill. The honor and reverence that is bestowed on the teacher is part of the belief system that empowers the disciple (McGee et al., 1996).

The North American Society of Teachers of the Alexander Technique (NASTAT) is the certifying body for practitioners. A NASTAT-certified teacher must complete a 1,600-hour training program over a minimum of three years. The emphasis of the training is on observation and modification of human movement patterns to identify and eliminate sources of movement dysfunction.

All Feldenkrais practitioners must complete 800–1000 hours of training over a period of three to four years. The main purpose of the training is for practitioners to develop a deep understanding of movement, to become aware of their own movement, to become skillful observers of movement in others, and to be able to teach other people to increase their awareness and improve their skills of movement.

The Trager Institute provides training and certifies Trager practitioners. It takes an average of two years to complete the program's 269 hours of training and field work. Students learn the relationship between various groups of muscles and organs that produce patterns of posture and movement. The focus is on the mechanics of movement, the kinesthetic interaction, and principles of neuropatterning underlying movement. The Trager Institute is also approved to provide continuing education credits by the California Board of Registered Nursing.

CONCEPTS

Wide Applicability

Almost anyone can participate in movement-oriented therapies. These therapies can be learned by the young and old, by people physically challenged or physically fit, and by those in good health and those recovering from long-term injury or illness. In China, 80-, 90-, and 100-year-old people get up every morning before dawn and go out to the parks to practice Qigong or T'ai Chi, even in the middle of winter. These Eastern practices can be done alone, in pairs, or in large groups.

Qi

Qi is the invisible flow of energy that maintains physiologic function and the health and well-being of individuals. Imbalance of the flow of energy can be treated in a variety of ways including practicing Qigong and T'ai Chi. The principles underlying these movement-oriented therapies are the same as those in acupuncture (see chapter 12). The "forms," or sequences of movements, are specifically designed to stimulate pressure points all along the body, and to encourage deep, rhythmic breathing, which fills the body with life-giving qi. The ultimate goal is to strengthen the flow of qi through the body to promote health and well-being. When qi is flowing in balance, the body stays healthy, resistant to disease, and can activate its own healing efforts. Qigong and T'ai Chi consist of soft, slow, continuous movements that are circular in nature. When practiced by a master, the movements are so slow and fluid that they look like swimming in air. The softness of movements develops energy without nervousness. The slowness of movements requires attentive control that quiets the mind and develops one's powers of awareness and concentration. The continuous circular nature of the movements develops strength and endurance. Yin and yang refer to the balance of forces in the universe. T'ai Chi movements are designed to express these forces in balanced form by pairs of opposites. For example, a motion that ultimately involves turning to the right often begins with a small movement to the left. In Qigong, students learn to sense their qi and follow it as it moves around the body. As they become more skillful, they learn to strengthen their qi and direct it to specific areas of the body that are weak or ailing (Cassileth, 1998; Castleman, 1996).

Movement Patterns

The human body is viewed as a remarkable instrument, capable of responding with flexibility and resilience. But as the years pass, people often develop habitual reactions, beliefs, and movement patterns that cause physical and mental strain. These habits are typically expressed by tight muscles, collapsed posture, or lack of mobility. When muscles are working overtime, people eventually feel tight, tense, heavy, or tired. The sources of these problems are many—injury, illness, or stress. Lifelong misuse of muscles arises from sitting, standing, or walking incorrectly or too much sitting and too little walking. For example, after years of walking incorrectly, back or knee problems can occur. A knee replacement is a temporary solution only, because the real problem lies not in the knee, but in the way the person moves from the hip. Movement-oriented practitioners believe the only lasting remedy is in re-educating the body to walk correctly to avoid injuring the knee. Likewise, back problems can be eliminated by learning appropriate ways of moving (Juhan, 1995).

Sensory-movement activities are used to increase people's sense of postural awareness, free them from habitual patterns, and restore the proper use of muscles. Practitioners lead students though movements to enable them to discover a more fluid range of motion. As people develop new, alternative ways of moving, they experience positive sensory feelings and learn what it is like to be freer and lighter. The goal is to teach people how to move with minimum effort and maximum efficiency through increased consciousness of how their bodies work.

TREATMENT

Qigong is an easy and nontiring exercise that contains sets of moves designed to gather qi. Most people spend 30 minutes a day doing the exercises and another 30 minutes in meditation. Some forms are quite complex. For example, Wild Goose Qigong has two sections with 64 movements in each section. While it is difficult to learn, Wild Goose Qigong is exceptionally beautiful. In China, the goose is considered to be a marvelous creature who flies high into the clouds to gather cosmic energy and information and bring it to earth. Guo Lin Gong, a walking form of Qigong, is practiced in China particularly by people with cancer. Improvements have been documented in a wide range of conditions such as stroke, hypertension, spinal cord injuries, multiple sclerosis, joint disease, cerebral palsy, headaches, and many forms of cancer (McGee et al., 1996).

Yang is the most popular form of T'ai Chi and was developed in the early twentieth century by Yang Cheng Fu. It is composed of 108 separate motions which can take 6–12 months to learn. When they are strung together, the result is a cross between slow-motion shadow boxing and dancing. Each movement has a name, like "repulse the monkey," "the snake creeps down," "the white crane spreads its wings," or "parting the wild horse's mane," that describes what it looks like or what purpose it serves. For example, when one is trying to concentrate, monkey thoughts are distractions. As the monkey is pushed away, the person is not allowing distractions to take attention away from the process of the moment. T'ai Chi also has breathing exercises for the purpose of improving and strengthening the flow of qi. One form involves reversed breathing, which is contracting the stomach with the in-breath and expanding the stomach with the out-breath. The benefits of T'ai Chi are seen in conditions such as hypertension, osteoporosis, and arthritis. T'ai Chi can decrease stress and fatigue, improve mood, and increase energy. It is especially helpful in improving balance in older adults, which decreases the risk of falls (Castleman, 1996).

The Alexander Technique includes simple movements that improve balance, posture, and coordination and relieve pain. During a session, the client goes through a series of standing and seated exercises while the practitioner applies light pressure to points of contraction in the body. The techniques help people learn how to use their bodies with less tension and more awareness. The recommended course is 30 lessons, depending on the client's participation and initial level of functioning (*Alternative Medicine,* 1994).

The Feldenkrais Method consists of two parts—awareness through movement and functional integration. They are convenient labels for doing essentially the same thing in different ways. Awareness though movement is more like conventional exercises in format, with the teacher guiding a group class with words rather than by personal manipulation. The lessons consist of comfortable, easy movements that gradually increase in range and complexity designed for all levels of movement ability. Functional integration is a hands-on lesson which usually lasts 45 minutes to an hour and is performed with the client fully clothed and standing, sitting, or lying on a table. The practitioner touches and moves the client in gentle, noninvasive ways. The intent of this touch is to explore the person's responses to touch and movement and then suggest alternative ways of moving. Feldenkrais exercises are small, gentle movements, such as pelvic tilts—slowly and deliberately lifting the spine from the coccyx to the waist, one vertebra at a time. To be effective, the movements must be effortless. If exercise becomes painful, no learning takes place, because the brain is too focused on how to stop doing the painful activity. Feldenkrais exercises are said to improve flexibility, posture, range of motion, relaxation, ease of movement, physical performance, vitality, and well-being. They are also said to relieve joint pain, stress, muscle tension, low back pain, neck and shoulder pain, jaw pain, and headaches (Steffensen, 1998).

The Trager Approach is a process of using motion in muscles and joints to produce particular sensory feelings. These feelings are relayed to the central nervous system and then, through the process of feedback loops, they trigger changes in the tissues. A Trager session takes 60–90 minutes with the client wearing a swimming suit and lying on a well-padded table. The practitioner touches in such a gentle rhythmic way that the person actually experiences the possibility of being able to move each part of the body freely and effortlessly. Because active participation of the client is discouraged, the passive body can freely learn new movements. Trager practitioners work in a meditative state they call "hook-up." This state allows the practitioner to connect deeply with the client in an unforced way, to remain continually aware of the slightest responses, and to work efficiently without fatigue (Juhan, 1995).

Following this session, the student is given instruction in the use of *mentastics,* a system of simple, effortless movement sequences designed to maintain and even enhance the sense of lightness, freedom, and flexibility that was instilled during the treatment session. Mentastics, Dr. Trager's coined term for "mental gymnastics" is a powerful means of reinforcing positive changes. The Trager Approach is said to decrease various types of chronic pain, headaches, temporomandibular joint pain, improve muscle spasms, and aid in recovery from stroke and spinal cord injuries.

RESEARCH

Research in the medical effects of Qigong has been a subject of interest in China in recent years and has been the topic of nine international conferences since 1986. More than 800 abstracts have been translated into English and copies are available from the Qigong Institute, East-West Academy of Healing Arts. The practice of Qigong has been found to have the following benefits:

- Improve treatment for hypertension and coronary artery disease (*Alternative Medicine,* 1994)
- Elevate blood levels of superoxide dismutase (SOD), which scavenges harmful superoxide radicals and promotes immunologic function (Hefen et al., 1993)

- Demonstrate significant improvement in people with advanced cancer who were treated simultaneously with drugs and Qigong (Quizhi and Li, 1988)
- Improve the functional ability of 93 percent of clients in a group with paralysis (Huang, 1988)
- Improve the functional ability of nursing home residents with medical conditions considered to be untreatable (Chow, 1985)

T'ai Chi has been found to provide the following benefits:

- Improve the balance of older adults and reduce the risk of falls. 200 people over the age of 70 developed better stability using T'ai Chi than other balance-training techniques (Cassileth, 1998); a study of women aged 65–85 found that those in the experimental group of T'ai Chi had significantly better postural control thus decreasing the risk of falls and the risk of hip fractures that are a major contributor to dysfunction and death in elderly women (Castleman, 1996).
- Significantly lower the heart rate and blood pressure in people in cardiac rehabilitation programs compared to control groups participating in aerobic exercise or a nonexercise support group (Cassileth, 1998).
- In people with rheumatoid arthritis, T'ai Chi does not trigger joint inflammation the way most exercise does (Castleman, 1996).

A number of research studies have been conducted on the Alexander Technique. Success has been cited in relief of chronic pain (Fisher, 1988), postural management of scoliosis (Caplan, 1980), and improvement of respiratory muscular function (Austin and Ausubel, 1992). Among professional musicians, the Alexander Technique was found to be as effective as beta-blocker medications in controlling the stress response during performance (Nielsen, 1994).

Only limited clinical research studies have been conducted to document the Feldenkrais Method. Effectiveness has been cited in several review articles and clinical guidelines for physical therapy and pain management (DeRosa and Porterfield, 1992; Jackson, 1991; Lake, 1985; Shenkman and Butler, 1989). Ginsberg (1986) reported on Feldenkrais exercises for people recovering from spinal injury. Narula (1993) found increased walking performance and decreased pain in people with rheumatoid arthritis.

Several case histories describe long-term improvement for people using the Trager Approach in chest mobility with lung disease (Witt and MacKinnon, 1986) and in trunk mobility with childhood cerebral palsy (Witt and Paar, 1986). Other reports suggest success in treating chronic pain, multiple sclerosis, and recovery from stroke, spinal cord injuries, and polio (*Alternative Medicine,* 1994).

INTEGRATED NURSING PRACTICE

Like most moderate physical activities practiced on a daily basis, T'ai Chi and Qigong can improve stability, agility, flexibility, stamina, and muscle tone. They are good exercise for people who are already in shape. But they can also be adapted for older adults, children, or people with injury or illness. The movements are gentle and put less stress on the body than do other exercises. The breathing exercises are a form of meditation that quiets the mind and reduces the negative effects of stress.

If you or others you know are healthy and wish to maintain your health, learning T'ai Chi or Qigong is highly recommended. Experienced practitioners spend at least 20 and up to 60 minutes in daily practice. As a nurse, you can encourage your clients to consider practicing one of these forms. To increase health it is important that clients build up stamina over a period of time. Clients who are seriously ill may only be able to do the simple breath practice as they focus on absorbing healing qi from the environment. When they can manage it, they add simple hand gestures to the breathing. As they continue to improve, they sit in a chair and do the hand motions, moving to a standing position when they feel able. Finally, they do the walking form.

When starting T'ai Chi and Qigong, it is best to begin with simple exercises. You can teach people a few basic principles of standing and moving so they can begin to feel what it is like to inhabit their body with awareness. Getting the body into alignment is a most important part of these movement therapies. Instruct people to stand with their feet at shoulder-width apart, buttocks tucked in, spine straight, shoulder relaxed, knees unlocked, and the head straight and resting lightly on top of the spine as if a string from the top of the head were gently suspending the body from above. Standing in this position, have them pay attention to their own breathing, inhaling deeply and exhaling all the way out. Standing in this position, have people locate their tan t'ien (pronounced don-tee-en). It is the body's center of gravity and stability, located about one-and-a-half inches below the navel and into the center of the body. T'ai Chi and Qigong teach people to find and maintain their center through movement, whereas in meditation and yoga, centering is found in stillness. The tan t'ien is considered to be the source of energy and, as they practice, people will find that all the movements begin to flow more easily as they learn to move from the tan t'ien.

Two common movements in T'ai Chi that are part of various sequences are the T'ai Chi fist and the T'ai Chi ball. The fist is formed by imagining a robin's egg in the center of each palm and then slowly curling one finger at a time around the egg, beginning with the little finger and ending with the thumb resting lightly on top. Throughout all the forms, frequent references are made to "picking up the ball." Have people visualize forming a ball out of the air and picking it up and moving with it. The ball is designed to help movements flow more easily.

Standing like a tree or the horse riding stance contributes to a sense of rootedness and stability in the body. For this posture, instruct people to separate their legs wider than the shoulders and bend their knees, thus lowering the center of gravity closer to the earth. The top part of the body feels light while the lower half feels heavy. At first, the position may feel strenuous because the muscles in the legs have not been used in this way. With practice, people enjoy the feeling of stability it gives them. Next, direct people to bring their arms up as if embracing an invisible person, joining their fingertips in front of them. Direct them to slowly turn from side to side, letting their waist inititate the movement. Their legs should feel "soft," so that they follow the movement led by the waist. Their gaze should travel slowly across an imagined horizon.

T'ai Chi and Qigong are popular and available in most towns and cities. They are taught in health clubs, schools, YMCAs, community centers, hospi-

TRY THIS: *Feel Your Qi*

- Stand with your feet shoulder-width apart, your knees slightly bent, your spine upright, and your shoulders relaxed. Breathe easily.
- Start to flex or bounce gently at the knees.
- Still bouncing, shift your weight back and forth from your right to left leg.
- Keep your breathing relaxed and deep.
- Begin to snap all of your fingers, flipping each one past your thumb.
- Then, still bouncing and finger-snapping, twist at your waist, to the right, then to the left.
- While you are doing all this, make your exhale a sigh of relief. Do five of these sighs in a slow, relaxed manner.
- Now stop and close your eyes and turn your attention inward. Feel the buzzing, humming, or tingling sensation that is in your hands, legs, and body. This is qi. You are literally feeling the activity of the profound medicine you have produced within yourself.

Source: Roger Jahnke, Health Action, 243 Pebble Beach, Santa Barbara, CA 93117.

tals, clinics, and other facilities. Explain to your clients that it is useful, in most cases, to begin with a teacher. They can ask around to find a teacher whom others like, or they can observe a class or participate in a trial class. Some people try several teachers or forms before they find the one that meets their personal preferences. Encourage people to find general forms that they like and will do regularly. If possible, they should try to find a place to learn that is convenient. If it is too far, it may become difficult for people to continue in the practice. As T'ai Chi and Qigong have become more popular, people can be found practicing in parks. In some cases, individuals prefer to have time alone in nature. Often, however, people are happy to have others join them, and frequently informal groups form. These groups may develop socially as people get to know one another and socialize after the practice.

The claims for the Alexander Technique, the Feldenkrais Method, and the Trager Approach focus more on enhancing well-being that on healing illness. They are designed to relieve muscle tension, increase relaxation, reduce stress, and alter poor habits of posture and movement in those who are healthy. You can refer clients to the appropriate associations to locate certified teachers of these techniques.

REFERENCES

Alexander Technique Resource Guide. 1998. Minneapolis, MN: North American Society of Teachers of the Alexander Technique.

Alternative Medicine: Expanding Medical Horizons. 1994. A report to the National Institutes of Health on Alternative Medical Systems and Practices in the United States. U.S. Government Printing Office. Washington, DC.

AUSTIN, J. H. M. and P. AUSUBEL. 1992. Enhanced respiratory muscular function in normal adults after lessons in proprioceptive musculoskeletal education without exercises.*CHEST.* 102: 486–490.

CAPLAN, D. 1980. Postural management of scoliosis in the adolescent and adult based on the Alexander Technique. American Center for the Alexander Technique.

CASSILETH, B. R. 1998. *The Alternative Medicine Handbook.* New York: W. W. Norton.

CASTLEMAN, M. 1996. *Nature's Cures.* Emmaus, PA: Rodale Press.

CHOW, E. P. Y. 1985. *Integrated Healing System, Its Effects in Rehabilitation at the Lutheran Home for Aging.* San Francisco: The East-West Academy of Healing Arts.

DEROSA, C. and J. PORTERFIELD. 1992. A physical therapy model for the treatment of low back pain. *Phys Ther.* 72: 261–272.

FISHER, K. 1988. Early experiences of a multidisciplinary pain management programme. *Holistic Medicine.* 3(1): 47–56.

GINSBERG, C. Spring–Summer 1986. The shake-a-leg body awareness training program: Dealing with spinal injury and recovery in a new setting. *Somatics.* 31–42.

HEFEN, X. et al. 1993. Conical study of the anti-aging effect of Qigong. Jiangsu Provincial Institute of TCM, Nanjing, China. Presented at the Second World Conference on Academic Exchange of Medical Qigong, Beijing. (Abstract).

HUANG, M. 1988. A study of the effect of the emitted qi combined with self-practice of Qigong in treating paralysis. The General Hospital of PLA, Beijing, China. Presented at the First World Conference for the Academic Exchange of Medical Qigong. Beijing. (Abstract).

JACKSON, O. 1991. The Feldenkrais Method: A personalized learning model. In M. LISTER, ed. *Contemporary Management of Motor Control Problems.* Proceedings of the II-Step Conference. Foundation for Physical Therapy, 131–135.

JUHAN, D. 1995. *The Trager Approach: A Comprehensive Introduction.* Mill Valley, CA: The Trager Institute.

LAKE, B. 1985. Acute back pain: Treatment by the application of Feldenkrais principles. *Aust Fam Physician.* 14(11): 1175–1178.

MCGEE, C. T., K. SANCIER, and E. P. Y. CHOW. 1996. In M. S. MICOZZI, ed. *Fundamentals of Complementary and Alternative Medicine.* New York: Churchill Livingstone, 225–230.

NARULA, M. 1993. Effect of the six-week Awareness through Movement lessons—The Feldenkrais Method on selected functional movement parameters in individuals with rheumatoid arthritis. Unpublished Master's thesis, Oakland University, Rochester, MI.

NEILSEN, M. 1994. A study of stress amongst professional musicians. In C. STEVENS, ed. *The Alexander Technique: Medical and Physiological Aspects.* London: STAT Books.

QUIZHI, S. and Z. LI. 1988. A clinical observation of qigong as a therapeutic aid for advanced cancer patients. Kuangan Men's Hospital, China Academy of Traditional Chinese Medicine, Beijing. Presented at the First World Conference for the Academic Exchange of Medical Qigong. Beijing. (Abstract).

REISER, S. 1994. Stress Reduction and Optimal Psychological Functioning. Sixth International Montreux Congress on Stress.

ROSENFELD, A. 1981. Teaching the body how to program the brain is Moshe's "miracle." *Smithsonian.* 11(10): 52–58.

SenseAbility. 1997. A quarterly newsletter of Application of the Feldenkrais Method. The Feldenkrais Guild.

SHENKMAN, M. and R. BUTLER. 1989. A model for multisystem evaluation, interpretation, and treatment of individuals with neurologic dysfunction. *Phys.Ther.* 69: 538–547.

STEFFENSEN, S. 1998. No pain=gain. *YOGAChicago.* 5(2): 8.

WITT, P. and J. MACKINNON. 1986. Trager psychosocial integration: A method to improve chest mobility of patients with chronic lung disease. *Phys. Ther.* 66: 214–217.

WITT, P. and C. PARR. 1986. Effectiveness of Trager psychosocial integration in promoting trunk mobility in a child with cerebral palsy: A case report. *Physical Occupational Therapy in Pediatrics.* 8: 75–93.

RESOURCES

East-West Academy of Healing Arts
450 Sutter St., Suite 2104
San Francisco, CA 94108

Feldenkrais Guild of North America
524 Ellsworth St. SW, P.O. Box 489
Albany, OR 97321
800-775-2118
541-926-0981
www.feldngld@peak.org

North American Society of Teachers of the Alexander Technique (NASTAT)
3010 Hennepin Ave. South, Suite 10
Minneapolis, MN 55408
800-473-0620
612-824-5066
www.Alexandertech.com
email: NASTAT@ix.netcom.com

The Trager Institute
21 Locust Ave.
Mill Valley, CA 94941-2806
415-388-2688
www.trageradmin@trager.com
email: TragerD@trager.com

UNIT VI

SPIRITUAL THERAPIES

The most beautiful and most profound emotion
we can experience is the sensation of the mystical. It is the power of all true science.

Albert Einstein

21 Shamans

Earth Mother, Star Mother
you who are called by a thousand names,
May all remember
we are cells in your body
and dance together.
You are the grain and the loaf
that sustain us each day,
And as you are patient
with our struggles to learn
So shall we be patient
with ourselves and each other . . .

Starhawk

. . . there is an important and potentially
very happy marriage between the spiritual, the mystical and scientific world
views, because they are all methods for
looking at the nature of reality.

Elizabeth Rauscher

Shaman (pronounced SHAH-min) is a word from the Tungus people of
Siberia. This term has been adopted widely by anthropologists to refer to
those known in the West as "medicine men," "witch doctors," "witches," "magicians," and "seers." Not every kind of medicine person or witch doctor,
however, is a shaman. A shaman is a woman or man who enters an altered
state of consciousness, at will, to contact and utilize another type of reality to
acquire knowledge and power and to help other people. Shamans use ancient
techniques to achieve and maintain well-being and healing for themselves
and members of their communities, serving as a link between the worlds of
matter and spirit. Shamanism is not a belief system. Rather, it is a broad umbrella covering ancient, indigenous, and holistic healing practices worldwide
(Harner, 1990). For further information on Native American healers, see
chapter 5.

BACKGROUND

The origins of shamanism go back at least 40,000–50,000 years to Stone Age times, making it the oldest of all healing therapies. All over the world evidence from ancient cave drawings and similar records supports the conclusions that indigenous peoples shared a similar understanding of how the universe works, how to maintain health and strength, how to cope with serious illness, and how to deal with the trauma of death. One of the most remarkable aspects of shamanism is that concepts and treatment methods are similar in widely separated and remote parts of the planet among peoples isolated from one another. Anthropologists have studied shamanism in North, Central, and South America, Africa, Australia, Indonesia, Malaysia, Bali, Tibet, Korea, Siberia, and across Europe and found that shamans functioned fundamentally in much the same way and with similar techniques worldwide. The basic uniformity suggests that, through trial and error, people arrived at the same conclusions (Harner, 1990; Rutherford, 1996; Vitebsky, 1995).

Today, shamanism survives in less "developed" regions of the world in spite of the advent of Western scientific medicine. The field of holistic medicine is reclaiming many techniques long practiced in shamanism, such as visualization, altered state of consciousness, hypnotherapy, meditation, positive attitude, and stress reduction. Shamanic healing is rapidly gaining popularity among urban Americans as people turn back to the old cultures for help and guidance in finding a better balance with nature and with themselves. Shamanic practice and biomedical treatment are not in conflict. Contemporary shamans are perfectly willing to have their patients see a conventional physician, because the primary goal is wellness. Any kind of technological treatment or medication that will contribute to the strength of the patient is welcomed (Harner, 1990).

PREPARATION

People discover in a wide variety of ways that their purpose in life is to become a shaman. Often potential healers have prophetic dreams about their future calling. The dream may even include details about locating a teacher and how long the training period will be. In some cases, people are led to shamanism through personal and private mystical experiences, while in others, they are drawn from the ranks of cured patients (Quinn, 1994).

The journey from apprentice to shaman is illustrated in the following example of Native American shamans. The first step is "embracing personal history." This process includes working through old traumas, fears, anger, hate, abandonment, betrayals, and wounds. The purpose is to heal the emotions so that one is no longer controlled by them but rather, consciously guided by feelings. The second step is "facing death and making death an ally." This step means examining one's attitudes and beliefs to "put to death" any that are inaccurate or outdated. It includes remembering that bodies are temporary and will one day be claimed by death. It is moving beyond personal history and recognizing that all people are part of a family, village, tribe, city, country, and ultimately all humanity. The third step is "stopping the world," which involves clearing the mind of its mental garbage. The fourth step is "controlling the dream and finding new vision and purpose." It is the time to quest for vision and seek direct connection with the dream world and its spiritual teachers. The Vision Quest is part of many old world cultures and is a time when one fasts and prays in a sacred place, often a mountaintop, for up to four days and nights. The person prays for a vision and thus a reconnection with the Creator and Creation. Following the Vision Quest, the person is expected to make life changes that were called for. The fifth and final step is taking full responsibility for all of one's actions without guilt or shame. Apprentice shamans go through this path of transformation as they become healers and helpers in service to other people (Rutherford, 1996).

Shamanic initiation is experiential and often gradual. Shamans must learn how to achieve the shamanic state of consciousness, must become familiar with their own guardian spirits, and must successfully help others as a shaman. After learning the basic principles and methods, new shamans extend their knowledge and power by shamanic journeying. Many years of shamanic experience are necessary for the few shamans who become true masters of knowledge, power, and healing.

CONCEPTS

Environment

For the shaman, everything exists as part of an infinite web of life. Plants, stones, the earth herself, are all perceptive beings; they are all consciously aware and have a story to tell. In the shamanistic tradition, people communicate intimately and lovingly with "all their relations," as the Lakota would say, talking not just with other people, but also with animals, plants, and all the elements of the environment, including rocks and water. From the shaman's viewpoint, one's surroundings are not "environment," but family. A deep respect for all forms of life is present, with a great awareness of one's dependence on the environment. Shamans believe their powers are the powers of the animals, of the plants, of the sun, of the basic energies of the universe. They are expected to live in harmony with nature and to provide strength in daily life and help save others from illness and death (Harner, 1990).

Power

In shamanism, the preservation of one's personal power is fundamental to well-being. Specific shamanic methods restore and maintain personal power and use it to help others who are weak, ill, or injured. In shamanism, the word *medicine* means vital force or energy. A person's medicine is their power, their knowledge, and their expression of their life energy.

Many shamans keep power objects, their medicine, in a medicine bundle. This bundle is normally kept wrapped up and is unrolled publicly only on ritual occasions. The objects inside are highly personal and, as with other matters of power, one does not boast of them because to do so might result in power loss. Almost any small object can be included, but the quartz crystal is highly prized among the shamans of North and South America, Australia, Southeast Asia, and elsewhere. Quartz crystals are six-sided stones that are usually transparent to milky white and in a sense, appear to be "solidified light." The quartz crystal is considered the strongest power object and is viewed as a spirit helper. For thousands of years, shamans have used their quartz crystals for power in seeing and divination. Interestingly, in modern physics, the quartz crystal is also involved in the manipulation of power. Its remarkable electronic properties made it a basic component in early radio transmitters and receivers. Later, quartz crystals became basic components for modern electronic hardware such as computers and timepieces (Harner, 1990).

State of Consciousness

The Ordinary State of Consciousness (OSC) is an agreed-upon consensus of what reality is. This OSC, also called ordinary reality or simply "reality," is determined by every society and learned by individuals from childhood. Reality, then, is predetermined expectations. For example, in Western societies, people are not surprised when they put a card in a machine and money comes out. Another characteristic of Western ordinary reality is that it can be measured and quantified. As Candace Pert (1997, p. 21) states, "Measurement! It is the very foundation of the modern scientific method, the means by which the material world is admitted into existence. Unless we can measure something, science won't concede it exists, which is why science refuses to deal with such 'nonthings' as the emotions, the mind, the soul, or the spirit."

Nonordinary realities are other levels of consciousness. They can be experienced during dreaming, or induced by drugs, fasting, sleep deprivation, or environmental factors. In Western society, this level of consciousness is often viewed as psychosis rather than another legitimate reality.

Shamans move, at will and with serious intention, between an Ordinary State of Consciousness and a Shamanic State of Consciousness (SSC). The SSC is an altered state of consciousness that may vary from a light to a deep trance. Shamans journey back and forth between these realities for the specific purpose of healing or in some manner aiding the community. Shamans operate in nonordinary reality or SSC only a small portion of the time and then only as needed to perform shamanic tasks. During this trance state, shamans' souls are believed to leave their bodies and ascend to either the upper world or lower world. Unlike the altered state of consciousness during dreaming, the SSC is a conscious waking state and at any time shamans can will themselves out of it, back into the OSC. The experience is like a waking dream in which shamans can control their actions and direct their adventures. Unlike a mind-altering drug experience, the SSC experience is not dependent on a chemically determined length of time, nor does it risk the possibility of being locked into a "bad trip" (Harner, 1990).

Shamanic Cosmology

Shamanic cultures throughout the world have a three-tiered cosmology or way of viewing the universe. The middle world is the world of OSC or ordinary reality. It is the world of matter and the world in which people live their daily lives. The lower world and the upper world are SSC worlds, nonordinary reality, or worlds of the spirit, not to be confused with heaven and hell. These worlds are just as real as the ordinary reality of the middle world.

The lower world is the world of power animals. These archetypical energies take the form of animal guides who have knowledge and wisdom to share and help people navigate through life. Power animals tend to provide practical help and guidance. The capability of power animals to speak to humans is taken as an indication of their power. The belief that shamans can shape-shift into the form of their power animal is common to many cultures. Sharing the identity of one's power animal varies among shamans. Some speak publicly about them while others fear that disclosing the animal's identity may cause it to leave the person. Many cultures believe that every person is born with a particular animal spirit that is to be their guide throughout life. A similar belief in Western cultures is that of guardian angels watching over people, especially children (Rutherford, 1996).

The upper world is the world of spirit guides. Spirit guides are beings that look more like people and are more familiar to most individuals. It is in the upper world that people meet their guardian angels. The help from spirit guides tends to be more general and philosophical in comparison to the practical help from the lower world. These worlds are complementary and equal, and neither is superior to the other.

Power animals and spirit guides teach people how to empower themselves, improve their lives, and even heal themselves. One does not have to be a shaman to make contact with one's personal power animal and spirit guide. The most traditional method of accessing this nonordinary reality is the shamanic journey.

Imagination

Most indigenous people make little distinction between what Westerners call imagination and reality. Imagination is just as real and just as concrete as ordinary reality. In fact, most of the material things of the "real" world were someone's imagination first. Automobiles, televisions, and computers have come from the imaginary realm. In fact, logic and reason have always been preceded by imagination. Western people often ask whether the power animals and guardian spirits are real or imagined. If the information that is received from power animals and guardian spirits empowers people, improves their lives, and helps them heal, the question does not apply. It is real because people's lives are changed (Sandore, 1997).

VIEW OF HEALTH AND ILLNESS

In the shamanic world view, the ability to maintain good health is a matter of power. If the body is power-full, it resists the intrusion of external, harmful forces. No room is available for disease and illness in a power-filled body. Being power-full is like having a protective force field surrounding the body. Possession of guardian spirit power is also fundamental to health. From a shamanic point of view, illnesses usually are intrusions that break the force field of power-fullness. In some ways this concept is not too different from the biomedical concept of infection. Serious illness and other misfortunes are usually only possible when people are dis-spirited, meaning they have lost their power and their guardian spirits. This loss results in an inability to fight off unwanted intrusions. Illness is viewed as a separation—from one's power, from one's guardians, from nature, from community, and from the Great Spirit. Even Western everyday language reflects this view when people say, "I'm having a low-energy day," or "I wasn't myself last night."

Severe trauma can result in soul loss, a natural survival mechanism. It is believed that a part of one's self or soul goes into hiding to ensure that the individual will survive the extreme stress. Western psychiatrists refer to this phenomenon as dissociation. Sometimes people's souls remain lost until they go through a process of soul retrieval. Symptoms of soul loss are an inability to focus and concentrate, a lack of connection to one's emotions, a feeling of being "spaced out" and not really present, a feeling of being an observer of life, or chronic depression. Soul retrieval brings buried memories and emotions back to the surface, much like the process of psychotherapy (Rutherford, 1996).

TREATMENT

Shamans may be called upon to help those who have become ill or those who have lost their power, their spirit guides, or even their souls. In such cases, shamans use the shamanic journey to recover that which was lost. Shamans also journey to gather information to help and guide individuals or groups, solve problems, and answer questions. Shamans, by offering their total commitment to a patient for as long as several days, develop intense relationships that underscore the importance of caring as well as curing in the shamanic healing tradition. In old cultures, shamans would do the journeying for patients, but in today's world, anyone can experience a shamanic journey. It is through this process that people meet and talk with their power animals and spirit guides and restore their own power and self-healing (Harner, 1990; Rutherford, 1996).

Basic tools for entering the SSC prior to the shamanic journey are the drum, providing lower vibrations, and the rattle, providing higher vibrations. A drum beat at a steady 200 to 280 beats a minute serves as a focus for concentration and quiets the chattering mind. The pace of the drumbeat corresponds to theta brainwaves associated with the hypnotic state, facilitating the move into nonordinary reality. It is a remarkably safe practice for most people, because one can return to an ordinary state of consciousness at any time. Some people add dancing or chanting to the drum beat as another way to reach this altered state of consciousness (Rutherford, 1996).

Some shamans use teacher plants as a catalyst to the shamanic journey. Throughout the world are many teacher plants: peyote, San Pedro cactus, ayahuasca, psilocybin, and red and white mushrooms are some examples. Shamans consider these plants to be gifts to be used with care and awareness. The use is never intended to be recreational but rather as a part of a sacred ceremony (Rutherford, 1996).

Sometimes communities share in a group healing ceremony. An example is found among the indigenous people of Hawaii, who come together as a group and experience a forgiveness ritual before the shaman begins the healing work. Family and community members convey concern for the patient by their participation in the ritual. This process underscores the belief that no one lives in isolation but is connected to and affected by other people. When people join together in a show of community support, new levels of healing are possible (Collinge, 1998).

RESEARCH

Clinical evidence of results from shamanic healing is anecdotal, and most published studies have been done by social scientists, folklorists, and historians.
In another sense, the ancient methods of shamanism have been tested immea-
surably longer than biomedicine. The similarities between shamans and scientists include an awareness of the complexity of the universe and the vast array
of knowledge still to be uncovered and understood. As Harner (1990, p. 45)
describes the similarity:

> Both shamans and scientists personally pursue research into the mysteries of the
> universe, and both believe that the underlying causal processes of that universe
> are hidden from ordinary view. And neither master shamans nor master scien-
> tists allow the dogma of ecclesiastical and political authorities to interfere with
> their explorations. It was no accident that Galileo was accused of witchcraft
> [shamanism].

Research has demonstrated that drumming produces changes in the
brain. The beat of the drum contains many sound frequencies that transmit impulses along the nerve pathways in the central nervous system. Shamanic
drumming produces frequencies in the theta wave range of 4–7 cycles per second. Studies have found that the rhythmic auditory stimulation of drumming
increases the production of theta waves, the brain waves of the trance state
(Neher, 1961, 1962; Wright, 1995).

INTEGRATED NURSING PRACTICE

Albert Schweitzer reportedly once observed, "The witch doctor succeeds for
the same reason all the rest of us [doctors] succeed. Each patient carries his
own doctor inside him. They come to us not knowing this truth. We are at our
best when we give the doctor who resides within each patient a chance to go
to work" (Harner, 1990). This belief is almost identical to Florence Nightingale's basic premise that healing is a function of nature that comes from within
the individual.

A current example of a combination of the techniques of shamanism
with biomedicine is the well-known work of Dr. O. Carl Simonton and
Stephanie Matthews-Simonton in treating people with cancer. As part of their
treatment, clients are taught to relax and visualize themselves on a walking
journey until they meet an "inner guide," which is a person or animal. The
client then asks the guide for help in getting well. The process is similar to a
shamanic journey and the meeting of a power animal (Harner, 1990).

Contemporary shamans work among today's Native American and other indigenous cultures. Their repertoire of curative powers now includes some modern and biomedical practices, and they may collaborate with conventional health care practitioners. Today, many shamans share their knowledge about healing with others, which has contributed to a recent renewal of interest in this oldest of healing therapies. Lectures, retreats, and weekend meetings, where shamans teach the principles of living in balance with nature, are now available to the general public (Cassileth, 1998).

In sharing information with clients, you can explain that shamanism offers a chance for contemplation. Guides offer more in the way of introspection and insight than physical cure. A shamanic journey may increase self-understanding, guidance for living, and a spiritual rejuvenation, all of which are important for the healing process.

In the old cultures, shamans would do the journeying while an apprentice or helper drummed. In today's world, it is more appropriate for each of us to learn to journey for ourselves and restore our own power. Personal power is believed to be basic to health and well-being. Some of your clients may wish to meet in drumming circles every one or two weeks while others prefer to work alone. Drumming tapes have been designed and produced for shamanic journeying. As in any other field of learning, it may be more effective to work firsthand with a professional during a workshop or retreat.

The shamanic journey begins with the drum. Among all the instruments used in healing, the drum produces some of the most powerful effects. Drumming has been used in organizations ranging from therapy groups and twelve-step programs to rehabilitation centers. Human bodies are multidimensional rhythm machines with everything pulsing in synchrony. Drumming can influence how strongly and harmoniously life moves within and around us (Campbell, 1997). The TRY THIS exercise presents an overview of the shamanic journey that you may want to experience for yourself.

In the shamanic tradition, healing is not just for the individual but also for the community. In shamanism, ultimately no distinction is made between helping others and helping yourself. By helping others, one becomes more powerful, self-fulfilled, and joyful. The broader purpose is the helping of humankind. The desire to help others is what draws many people into the profession of nursing.

The North American Nursing Diagnosis Association identifies the diagnoses of potential for enhanced community coping and ineffective community coping. It is expected that nurses apply the nursing process with individual clients, families, groups, and communities. Perhaps someday we will see a modern version of the shaman working side by side with us. This cooperation is already starting to take place where native shamans live, as on some North American Indian reservations and in some places in

TRY THIS: *Shamanic Journey*

- Find a private, secure place where you will not be disturbed.

- Assume a comfortable position, either sitting or lying down. You may want to cover your eyes to block out room light.

- Set the intent of your journey—if you want to go to the upper world or lower and the intent to meet your guardian spirit or your power animal.

- Turn on a drumming tape. Let your body relax, let it sink down into Mother Earth. Take a few deep, slow breaths. Let the drum beat become part of you; feel it resonate through your body.

- In your mind, bring yourself to a place in nature that is special for you, one that holds personal meaning. It might be a tree you climbed as a child, the lake you swam in on summer vacations, the place you now walk your dog. Imagine that place and go there in your mind. Feel the energy of that place.

- If you are going to the lower world, find a place you can enter the earth such as a hollowed out tree stump, an animal den, a cave, or whatever you want to imagine. When you enter the earth, you will be in a long cave. Take your time and follow it. Eventually it will open up into the lower world. Walk around and enjoy the beauty of the lower world. Explore. Soon you will come in contact with power animals. Introduce yourself. Dialogue with the animal, and ask what information the animal has for you.

- If you are going to the upper world, find a way to get up into the sky. You may climb a mountain or a tall bean stalk, use a hot air balloon, or even shape-shift into the form of an eagle and fly up. Eventually, you will come to the interface between the middle world and the upper world. Find a way through this interface, which is something like a membrane. The upper world is an ethereal, light, crystalline place. Explore. Soon you will meet your guardian spirit. Introduce yourself. Dialogue with the spirit, and ask what information the spirit has for you.

- Eventually, the journey has to end. It can end when you decide to end it, when no more information remains to be gained, or when the drum beat changes, signaling an end. Return home by the same path you took to get there.

- Allow the information to sink into your consciousness. It is best if you write the information down in a notebook, in a concrete form you will remember. The shamanic journey is much like a dream—it will leave you quickly. Writing it down is a method to keep the information you gained during the journey.

Richard Sandore, M.D., personal communication, 1998.

Australia. Equally exciting is the idea of nurses being trained in shamanic techniques and health maintenance so they can combine both approaches in their practice.

REFERENCES

Alternative Medicine: Expanding Medical Horizons. 1994. A report to the National Institutes of Health on Alternative Medical Systems and Practices in the United States. U.S. Government Printing Office. Washington, DC.

CAMPBELL, D. 1997. *The Mozart Effect.* New York: Avon Books.

CASSILETH, B. R. 1998. *The Alternative Medicine Handbook.* New York: W. W. Norton.

COLLINGE. W. 1998. *Subtle Energy.* New York: Warner Books.

HARNER, M. 1990. *The Way of the Shaman.* San Francisco: Harper.

NEHER, A. 1962. A physiological explanation of unusual behavior in ceremonies involving drums. *Human Biology.* 34(2): 151–160.

NEHER, A. 1961. Auditory driving observed with scalp electrodes in normal subjects. *Electroencephalography and Clinical Neurophysiology.* 13(3): 449–451.

PERT, C. 1997. *Molecules of Emotion.* New York: Scribner.

QUINN, J. F. 1994. Caring for the caregiver. In J. WATSON, ed. *Applying the Art and Science of Human Caring.* New York: National League for Nursing Press.

RUTHERFORD, L. 1996. *Principles of Shamanism.* San Francisco: Thorsons.

SANDORE, R. 1997. *Introduction to the Shamanic Journey.* Prone Stone Recording. Soaring Spirit.

VITEBSKY, P. 1995. *The Shaman.* Boston: Little, Brown & Co.

WRIGHT, P. A. 1995. The interconnectivity of mind, brain, and behavior in altered states of consciousness: Focus on shamanism. *Alternative Therapies in Health and Medicine.* 1(3): 50–56.

RESOURCES

The Foundation for Shamanic Studies
P.O. Box 1939
Mill Valley, CA 94942
415-380-8282

Upaya Foundation
1404 Cerro Gordo
Santa Fe, NM 87501

Eagle's Wing Centre for Contemporary Shamanism
BCM Box 7475
London, England WC1N 3XX

www.deoxy.org/shaman.htm

22   Faith and Prayer

In the end, Mother Teresa is bound to be canonized. The requisite miracle? Not that she helped the blind to see. Her life was devoted to the belief that no one should die untouched and unloved.

USA Today *editorial, September 8, 1997*

Man has no body distinct from his soul.

William Blake

Health care sciences have begun to demonstrate that faith and religious commitment may play a role in promoting health and reducing illness. Nurse clinicians and researchers, as well as others, are becoming more interested in the connection between religious faith and survival. Increasingly, people are beginning to recognize that faith is good medicine.

Religion can be described in a number of ways. The definition chosen for this text is one developed by Mickley, Carson, and Soeken (1995), three nursing researchers. They believe that religion develops and changes over time and is comprised of people's beliefs, attitudes, and patterns of behavior that relate to the supernatural—God, the Divine One, the Great Spirit, Creator, etc. Religion usually includes a group of people who hold similar beliefs and participate in shared traditions. A community of religious people may or may not have a formal organizational structure.

The U.S. population would seem to be religious, with 95 percent of the general public expressing a belief in God (Gallup, 1985) and more than two-thirds claiming that they base their entire approach to life on their religious beliefs (Bergin and Jensen, 1990). For decades, surveys have found that more than 90 percent of the U.S. population reportedly pray (Gallup, 1985; Levin and Taylor, 1997). Recently both *Time* (June 22, 1996, pp. 26, 58–62) and *Newsweek* (March 31, 1997, pp. 56–65) devoted cover stories to the popular and sometimes controversial topic of prayer and religious healing. The *Newsweek* poll found that 54 percent of Americans pray daily, with 29 percent reporting that they pray more than once a day (Woodward, 1997).

Prayer is most often defined simply as a form of communication and fellowship with the Deity or Creator. The universality of prayer is evidenced in all cultures having some form of prayer. Prayer has been and continues to be used in times of difficulty and illness even in the most secular societies. A common image of prayer in the United States is something like this: "Prayer is talking aloud to yourself, to a white, male, cosmic parent figure, who prefers to be addressed in English" (Dossey, 1997, p. 10). This cultural view of prayer fails to encompass how prayer is regarded by many people throughout the world. For some, prayer is more a state of being than of doing; for others, prayer is silence rather than words; for some, prayer is a thought or a desire of the heart; others pray to a female Goddess or a Divine Being who looks like they do. Buddhists do not believe in a personal God as creator and ruler of the world. Yet prayers, offered to the universe, are central to the Buddhist tradition. Prayer may be simply being still and knowing that God is God. Prayer is part of many religious traditions and rituals and may be individual or communal, public or private (Burkhardt and Nagai-Jacobson, 1997; Dossey, 1997). Larry Dossey (1997, p. 11) provides a broad definition of prayer: "Prayer is communication with the Absolute. This definition is inclusive, not exclusive; it affirms religious tolerance; and it invites people to define for themselves what 'communication' is, and who or what 'the Absolute' may be." According to a Sufi saying, prayer is when you talk to God and meditation is when God talks to you. In this definition, meditation is thought of as passive and receptive and prayer as active and engaging. The boundaries between meditation and prayer, however, are often blurred.

BACKGROUND

Until the last 200 years, medicine and religion were so thoroughly united that healers and priests were often the same individuals. The first hospitals were founded in monasteries by physicians who were usually monks. Today, many cultures throughout the world continue to regard their healers as a source for guidance in matters of faith and wellness. In the West, religion and medicine were fused until the end of the Middle Ages in the mid-1400s. Philosophers such as Descartes (1596–1650), Locke (1632–1704), and Hume (1711–1766) promoted the scientific basis of knowledge, believing that truth could only be realized through the examination of empirical data and the rational, scientific method. Centuries later, Western societies continue to experience the consequences of this split between religion and medicine. Western physicians are educated to think primarily in terms of what can be empirically proven in the laboratory. Discussions of spirituality and religion are considered by many physicians to be "off limits" with such discussion belonging to spiritual or religious leaders. In the past, when arguments arose between religion and medicine, religion usually did not fare well. Thus, many religious leaders today are cautious about what science is beginning to say about their faith. As nurses such as Dossey, Burkhardt, and Nagai-Jacobson and physicians such as Dossey, Matthews, and Benson research and write more about the blending of religion and health care, the practice of these professions will evolve to once again, include the forgotten "faith factor" in health care.

Research has shown that religious practices such as worship attendance and prayer have significant health and survival implications. People's religiousness not only influences healthy behaviors but also influences how individuals view and define illness. A study of elderly inpatients found that one-third of those surveyed believed that sickness was a punishment from God, and nearly four-fifths felt that good health was a blessing from God (Bearon and Koenig, 1990). A study of hospitalized psychiatric patients found that nearly half of those surveyed believed that leading a moral life could protect against illness, and almost three-quarters attributed their illness to a sin against God (Sheehan and Kroll, 1990). Some religions stress prayer as the way to mobilize self-healing and believe that biomedical interventions, such as surgery or blood transfusions, are harmful or sinful.

In some situations, religion may have a negative impact on people's lives. Religious participation can lead to more, not fewer, problems when unscrupulous leaders coerce or manipulate others to give up all personal autonomy. Problems also occur when religion fosters excessive guilt or shame or encourages people to avoid dealing with life's problems. Some religious groups urge their members to avoid all conventional medical care, which can lead to life-threatening situations (Matthews and Clark, 1998; Mickley et al., 1995).

CONCEPTS

Universality of Faith

Throughout history and around the world, people have called upon a Divine Being to sustain them. People are nourished by life-affirming beliefs and philosophies. They meditate and say prayers that elicit physiological calm and a sense of peacefulness, both of which contribute to longer survival. Benson (1997) believes that a genetic blueprint makes believing in the Great Mystery part of people's nature. Through the process of natural selection, mutating genes retain the impulses of faith, hope, and love, and faith is a natural physiologic reaction to the threats to mortality everyone faces. Benson (1997, p. 212) goes on to say that "according to my investigations, it does not matter which God you worship, nor which theology you adopt as your own. Spiritual life, in general, is very healthy."

Crises

Serious illness presents a spiritual crisis. As long as people are well, they maintain their autonomy and their ability to function at home, work, or school. Their feelings of self-worth are supported as they find meaning and purpose in their many activities. Once serious illness occurs, some of these things change. Ill people may have to depend on others for personal care and experience other radical lifestyle changes. Body concept changes may threaten self-esteem. In these situations, most people are forced to reevaluate life's meaning and purpose. Religious people draw heavily on their resources of faith to see them through difficult situations like serious illness. According to a number of studies, religiously involved individuals suffer less death anxiety than do nonreligious people. Highly religious people have the least fear of death and the strongest belief in an afterlife. Even people with terminal illness may experience a profound sense of psychological and spiritual well-being and wholeness as they grapple with imminent death (Matthews and Clark, 1998; Richardson et al., 1983; Waldfogel, 1997).

Twelve Remedies

Numerous studies demonstrate that religious involvement promotes health. It appears at this time that a number of religious "ingredients" promote health and well-being. Although some may be found in nonreligious settings, they are more commonly found operating together in religious organizations. Matthews and Clark (1998) have termed these religious remedies, a listing of which appears in Box 22.1.

The first remedy is the relaxation response, which can be evoked with meditation and prayer (Matthews and Clark, 1998). The relaxation response buffers stress by clearing the mind and freeing the body from everyday tension. Practiced regularly, the relaxation response decreases heart rate, lowers metabolic rate, decreases respirations, and slows brain waves. In addition, it enhances measures of immunity. Benson (1997) found that when religious beliefs were added to relaxation response activities, worries and fears improved significantly when compared to the relaxation response alone. Most worship services provide time for silent prayer or meditation as well as help people take time out from busy schedules. With regular practice of the relaxation response, people report experiencing an increase in spirituality. They often describe the presence of an energy, a power, or God, that is beyond themselves. Those who feel this presence often experience the greatest medical benefits (Benson, 1997).

The second remedy is one of healthful living (Matthews and Clark, 1998). Some religious groups actively promote a healthy lifestyle as part of

Box 22.1: Religious Remedies

1. Relaxation response
2. Healthful living
3. Aesthetics of worship
4. Whole-being worship
5. Confession and absolution
6. Support network
7. Shared beliefs
8. Ritual
9. Purpose in life
10. Turning over to a Higher Power
11. Positive expectations
12. Love for self and others

Source: Matthews and Clark, *The Faith Factor* (New York: Viking, 1998).

their doctrine. Religious proscriptions may include dietary moderation, rules about sexual behavior, and regulations regarding hygiene as well as avoidance of tobacco, alcohol, and drugs. In one survey of college students, researchers found that the more religious students avoided health-compromising behaviors and engaged in more frequent health-enhancing behaviors than those students who were less religiously involved (Oleckno and Blacconiere, 1991).

Remedy number three is the aesthetics of worship, which taps into a universal appreciation for beauty. Visual symbols of faith are reassuring and calming images. Stained-glass windows, beautiful architecture, and floral arrangements all provide an experience of harmony and balance. Sacred music uses audible beauty to communicate the splendor of God. The smell of incense may evoke a deep sense of peace and quietude (Matthews and Clark, 1998).

The fourth remedy is whole-being worship. Christians who sing familiar hymns, Jews who sing "Torah Ora" when the Torah scroll is presented, and Buddhists who chant their prayers all participate in whole-being worship through music. This combination of physical activity (singing), cognitive activity (reading the words), and spiritual activity (prayer through song) evokes a sense of peace. Movements such as kneeling, standing, bowing heads, folding hands, or even dancing engage people on all levels of being. As people worship with body, mind, and spirit, they go through a unifying experience that is as good for them as it feels (Matthews and Clark, 1998).

Remedy number five is confession and absolution. Harboring guilty feelings can literally make people sick. In many religions, people are encouraged to confess their sins, repent, and are given assurance of forgiveness and absolution. This process allows individuals to review their mistakes, share their personal pain, and learn from and move on rather than becoming preoccupied with personal shortcomings (Matthews and Clark, 1998).

The sixth remedy is one's support network—those family members and friends who offer practical help, emotional support, and spiritual encouragement in the time of need. People are social beings whose health often deteriorates when they become isolated and lonely. Lack of human companionship has been linked to depression of the immune system and a lowered production of endorphins, the neurotransmitter that produces the feeling of well-being. A 10-year study of 2,754 people found that men who volunteered regularly and had social contact with others were less likely to die than those who volunteered less and had less social contact (House et al., 1982). Spiegel and colleagues (1989) found that women with metastatic breast cancer who participated in support groups lived 18 months longer on average than women who did not. Oxman, Freeman, and Manheimer (1995) studied elderly patients undergoing heart surgery and found that those who participated in community and social groups, like those who received comfort from their religious beliefs were three times more likely to survive. But those who participated in both social activities and received comfort from their religious faith were 10 times more likely to survive. Interaction with others can help people transform their attitudes and emotions, which magnifies the effect of self-healing and health enhancement efforts. Religious organizations often provide many opportunities for social interaction from religious services to sacred study groups, to youth, women's, and men's groups, and to community outreach groups (Benson, 1997; Matthews and Clark, 1998). Jahnke (1997) describes some of the benefits from group interaction, which offers a sense of partnership, helps with coping, creates a sense of community and safety, encourages a cooperative approach to problem solving, helps to change behaviors and thoughts, supports taking control, and encourages personal action.

Remedy number seven is shared beliefs. Most people prefer to associate with individuals who share similar beliefs and points of view. Great things can be achieved when groups are unified around common values. Religious traditions are opportunities for people to share common beliefs. Individuals who feel they are part of a group find they are not alone and gain strength from the power of shared beliefs. Participation in regular worship not only helps people feel connected and helps them rise above their differences, but it also is an antidote to the alienation often prevalent in Western society (Matthews and Clark, 1998).

The eighth remedy is ritual. Ceremony and ritual are ways of creating sacred space and time, when normal ways of relating are put aside and people can listen and pray with an open heart to their Divine Being. Religious ritual is a powerful healing mechanism that has soothing and calming effects. As Benson (1997, p. 177) states:

> There is something very influential about invoking a ritual that you may first have practiced in childhood, about regenerating the neural pathways that were formed in your youthful experience of faith. . . . Even if you experience the ritual from an entirely different perspective of maturity and life history, the words you read, the songs you sing, and the prayers you invoke will soothe you in the same way they did in what was perhaps a simpler time in your life.

Rituals provide people a link with tradition and give them a sense of security (Matthews and Clark, 1998).

The ninth remedy is that of finding a purpose in life (Matthews and Clark, 1998). Victor Frankl (1984) describes people's search for meaning as being the primary motivation in their lives. This search for meaning becomes more intense during periods of illness as people struggle with age-old questions such as: Why me? Why now? Did I do something to deserve this? Religion and worship attendance provide a framework of meaning, a sense of purpose in life, and a meaningful interpretation for difficult times. People who are dying often seem to arrive at a sense of what life's purpose is. As they tell it, the purpose of life is to grow in wisdom and to learn to love better. They discover that health is not an end but rather a means. In other words, health enables people to serve a purpose in life, but health is not the purpose in life (Remen, 1988).

Remedy number ten is turning one's life over to the Great Mystery or God. It is an acknowledgment that no one has total control over her or his life. Religion provides an avenue for asking for guidance, intervention, and strength. Faith in a God who is loving and caring provides comfort for those going through difficult times. Worship services often leave people feeling less burdened and anxious, as well as more peaceful (Matthews and Clark, 1998).

The eleventh remedy is that of positive expectations. During a time of illness or distress, religion often provides a sense of hope and the strength to endure that which has happened. The expectancy of help from the Divine Source works in the same way as does the expectancy of help from a medication, procedure, or caregiver. Various holy writings promise health and healing to the faithful, and researchers are beginning to document the effect of this expectation on the outcome of disease (Benson, 1997; Matthews and Clark, 1998).

The twelfth, and last, remedy is love for self and others. All religions focus on loving God and other people. This love includes helping others, strangers as well as family and friends (Matthews and Clark, 1998). When people love and help others, they often experience better health than those who do not. Luks (1993) surveyed thousands of volunteers across the United States and found that people who help others consistently report better health than peers in their age group. They identified that helping others on a regular basis gave them a good physical sensation and greater calm and relaxation.

These 12 religious remedies can be found outside of religious organizations. Frequent religious participation however, provides many these remedies in one context. Research is demonstrating that religious participation is an important factor in the prevention of disease, achievement of well-being, healing from illness, and extension of life span. One mystery that remains, however, is why some people are cured and others are not. One can be very spiritual and still get sick and die. It must be remembered that religious participation and spirituality are no guarantee for physical health. Failure to recognize this basic reality can result in inappropriate self-blame (Matthews and Clark, 1998).

How Prayer Works

No one knows how praying for others works. Skeptics say it cannot happen, because no accepted scientific theory explains it. In the development of theories, however, empirical facts often lead to the development of an explanatory theory. For example, it was well known that penicillin worked before anyone discovered how it worked. The debate has now shifted from *whether* prayer works to *how* prayer works.

Larry Dossey (1993) has proposed that prayer is "nonlocal," an idea derived from the field of quantum physics. The word *local* means that something is present in the here and now; each of us exists here and not somewhere else and now and not at some other time. The word *nonlocal* means that something is not confined by place or time. All the major theistic (belief in a personal God as creator) religions agree on the nonlocal nature of God; that (S)He is everywhere, is not confined by space and location, and exists throughout time. According to the concept of nonlocality, consciousness cannot be localized or confined to one's brain or body, nor can it be confined to the present moment. Consciousness is basic to the universe, perhaps similar to matter and energy. According to this theory, neither energy nor information travels from one mind to another, because the two minds are not separate but rather interconnected and omniscient. Dossey has proposed that consciousness-mediated events such as prayer, telepathy, precognition, and clairvoyance may be explainable as developments continue in quantum physics. As in any new theory, the nonlocal theory raises more questions than it answers. Evidence exists that prayer works, even though the exact mechanism is unknown at this time.

TREATMENT

Some people seek out nurses, doctors, counselors, and therapists who focus on spiritual concerns as well as physical and emotional concerns. This focus is especially helpful for those who are dealing with issues related to meaning and purpose in life. Alternatively, people may seek the help of a religious leader who includes healing practices in her or his religious practice. Faith healing has not been scientifically proven but remains a popular option for many. Some people go to specific places for healing. The Catholic church has documented 36 "miracles" at Lourdes, for example. A variety of spiritually focused healing groups are also available. People with addictive disorders benefit from 12-step programs, which rely on both group support and the specific invocation of a Higher Power.

Two different types of prayer are directed and nondirected. In directed prayer, the praying person asks for a specific outcome, such as for the cancer to go away or for the baby to be born healthy. In contrast, in nondirected prayer, no specific outcome is asked. The praying person simply asks for the best thing to occur in a given situation. Studies show that both approaches are effective in promoting health (Dossey, 1993).

Prayer can also be described according to form. Colloquial prayer is an informal talk with God, as if one were talking to a good friend. Petitional prayer or intercessory prayer is asking God for things for oneself or others. The focus is on what God can provide. Intercessory prayer is often called "distant" prayer, because the person being prayed for is often remote from the person who is praying. This form of prayer is of current interest to researchers. Ritual prayer is the use of formal prayers or rituals such as prayers from a prayer book or in the Jewish *siddur,* or the Catholic practice of saying the rosary. Meditative prayer, also known as contemplative prayer, is similar to meditation and is a process of focusing the mind on an aspect of God for a period of time (Matthews and Clark, 1998).

RESEARCH

The research data support the premise that religion is good for people's health. Many studies meet the standards of scientific inquiry. In one review, over 75 percent of 325 studies of different types have produced findings indicating the benefit of religious involvement to health and well-being. Although the studies have not established cause-and-effect relationships, they strongly support the existence of an important connection between religious practice and good health (Matthews and Clark, 1998). More religiously strict groups appear to have greater health benefits, most likely related to their religious commitment and healthy lifestyle. Seventh Day Adventists have lower rates of cardiac and oncologic disease than other populations (Berkel and deWaard, 1993); active Mormons have lower occurrences of cancer and cardiovascular disease and lower mortality rates than other populations (Enstrom, 1989); and among immigrants to Israel, the most orthodox Jews had the lowest mortality rates and secular Jews the highest mortality in a 23-year follow-up study (Goldbount et al., 1993).

The most famous prayer study was conducted by Randolph Byrd and published in 1988. Patients were randomly assigned to two groups. One group of 192 patients was prayed for by religious strangers who made a commitment to pray regularly for each patient, knowing only the patients' names and clinical status. The control group of 201 patients did not receive the experimental prayer. The patients, the nurses, and the doctors all knew who was participating in the study but did not know to which group the patients had been assigned. Both groups received standard medical care. During the course of hospitalization, measurements were made of variables related to more severe illness and/or complications including episodes of congestive heart failure, use of diuretics, episodes of cardiopulmonary arrest, episodes of pneumonia, use of antibiotics, and the need for intubation. The findings were statistically significant: patients in the control group were nearly twice as likely to suffer complications than were patients in the prayer group—27 percent as opposed to 15 percent. A flaw in the study was the inability to control for intercessory prayer by people outside the experiment or of the control group for themselves. At the present time, researchers at the University of California, San Francisco, are studying the effects of distant prayer on the immune systems of AIDS patients and Harvard's Mind/Body Medical Institute is conducting a major study of healing through distant prayer.

Other studies related to religious practice and prayer have demonstrated the following:

- Elderly African Americans who attend church frequently are nearly twice as likely as other African Americans to be alive five years later, even when controlling for sociodemographic, health, and activity levels (Bryant and Rokowski, 1992).
- One study focused on 30 elderly women recovering from surgical correction of a broken hip. Those with strong religious beliefs were able to walk significantly farther and were less likely to be depressed (Pressman et al., 1990).
- A classic 1972 study of 91,909 people living in Maryland found that those who attended church at least once a week had significantly lower death rates from the following: 50 percent reduction in coronary artery disease; a 56 percent reduction in emphysema; a 74 percent reduction in cirrhosis of the liver; and a 53 percent reduction in suicide (Comstock and Partridge, 1972).
- Individuals who have a strong religious commitment are less likely to develop alcoholism (Koenig et al., 1994). Nearly 90 percent of people surveyed with narcotic addiction lost interest in religion during their

teenage years, compared with 20 percent of community controls who lost interest during the same age period (Cancellaro et al., 1982).

The benefits of religious involvement have been well documented since the 1970s. Findings have been summarized in Matthews, Larson, and Barry's four-volume bibliography, *The Faith Factor.*

INTEGRATED NURSING PRACTICE

Every serious illness is a spiritual crisis because it is a confrontation with one's own mortality. Every nurse, regardless of personal belief, must recognize that religion is often an essential part of the life of those entrusted to her or his care. To avoid these issues is to fail to truly be a nurse healer because our task is to address the physical, psychological, and spiritual needs of clients. Respecting people's beliefs and experiences also means that nurses do not force spiritual issues on clients, push religion on them, or attempt to convert them to a particular faith. Doing so violates the trust that is basic to the nurse-client relationship. Promoting the benefits of faith and prayer includes respecting client's choices about doctrine and denomination (Matthews and Clark, 1998).

Surveys by *USA Today Weekend* and *Time* (McNichol, 1996; Wallis, 1996) indicate that nearly two out of three Americans would like their physicians to address spiritual issues and to pray with them, if they so request. In a study of people who were hospitalized, more than 75 percent believed that their physician should address spiritual issues as a part of their medical care. Not only did they want them to discuss these issues, but nearly half wanted their physician to pray with them. Unfortunately, these same clients reported that spirituality and religion were hardly ever addressed, less than 1 percent of the time, as part of their medical care (King and Bushwick, 1994). One might make the assumption that clients have these same expectations from nurses.

Of course, some nurses and physicians do incorporate faith and prayer into their care. Dr. Alijani, a faculty member at Georgetown University Medical School and a well-known surgeon, believes that faith plays a significant role in his patient's well-being. He sees prayer as the literal lifeline between health and spirituality: "Just as my body needs water, carbohydrates, protein, and lipids, my mind needs Allah, and the only way to receive Allah is to pray" (Matthews and Clark, 1998, p. 73).

Why is it that some nurses do not incorporate faith and prayer into their professional practice? Some nurses are unaware of the research data regarding the faith factor. That situation is beginning to change as schools of nursing develop courses to teach students about the faith-health connection. Some nurses have been told specifically that they are not to mix nursing and faith. This recommendation was made out of a concern that we might blur the professional-personal boundaries and cause harm to our clients. As more research is being documented, nurses are reexamining the relationship between nursing and faith. Other nurses do not incorporate faith and prayer into their practice because they have not been educated to address spiritual beliefs, practices, and experiences. As curricula and continuing education programs address this issue, the discomfort of nurses should decrease (Matthews and Clark, 1998).

Health care practitioners are not meant to replace clergy. The roles are distinct. Although many clients may want their spiritual needs addressed by nurses and physicians, others do not, preferring to have these issues addressed by clergy. The practitioner needs to take into account, however, where and how the client's belief enters into the healing process. Nor should health care practitioners be forced against their wishes into participating in client's religious practices. In the best of worlds, health care professionals and clergy work closely together to provide meaningful holistic care.

You can, as a nurse, incorporate faith and prayer issues in your care of clients, regardless of your own personal religious beliefs or world views. When you remember that people are spiritual beings, you will be more alert to spiritual concerns. It is important that you promote an atmosphere that accepts and encourages many forms of spiritual expression (Burkhardt and Nagai-Jacobson, 1997).

Faith and prayer can be explored effectively with people of most age groups. The depth and focus of the conversation will vary based on the cognitive and developmental ability of the individual or family. Health maintenance visits provide an opportunity to explore spiritual beliefs and practices in the context of an overall assessment of lifestyle, risks, and resources. Doors can be opened in a nonthreatening, nonurgent fashion, and the topic can be validated for future discussion. In the face of major illness, terminal disease, or dying, the discussion of faith and prayer is even more relevant. Clearly though, discussion of this topic should not be restricted to these types of client encounters (Maugans, 1996). Box 22.2 provides an example of a nursing assessment regarding faith and prayer.

Although intercessory prayer is guided by beliefs, experiences, and faith traditions, you can provide some basic guidelines on how clients can incorporate the benefits of intercessory prayer into their lives (Matthews and Clark, 1998):

- If you are ill, ask specifically for people's prayers for healing. It may involve clergy, members of a congregation, adding your name to a prayer list, or asking family and friends to pray for you on a regular basis.
- Pray for your own healing.
- Seek out healing services. Many churches and synagogues offer opportunities to participate in a prayer service or healing service.
- Pray persistently. Keep praying regardless of apparent results. Continuing prayer is an expression of faith and hope.
- Pray for others who are suffering.

Box 22.2: Faith and Prayer Assessment

What does your faith mean to you? Has it changed during your illness?

What is the importance of this faith in your daily life?

Do your beliefs influence the way you think about your health or look at your illness?

How important is your religious identification? Do you belong to an organized group?

Tell me about your religious practices, such as worship, prayer, or meditation.

What is the role of prayer in your life?

How are your prayers answered?

What aspects of your faith would you like me to keep in mind as I care for you?

Would you like to discuss religious implications of your care?

Sources: Burkhardt and Nagai-Jacobson, "Spirituality in healing," *Core Curriculum for Holistic Nursing* ((City): Aspen Pub., 1997); Matthews and Clark, *The Faith Factor* (New York: Viking, 1998); Maugans, "The Spiritual History," *Arch Fam Med* 5, (1996), 11–16.

As a nurse, you can also teach people to take time out to count their blessings and say "thanks" for the good things in life. Paying attention to what they already have and what is going right helps alleviate stress, anxiety, and depression. An act of gratitude often restores a sense of balance and perspective. You can make the following suggestions:

- Remember to say "thank you." Make it a habit whenever someone helps you out, gives you a compliment, or gives you a gift.
- Create rituals of thanks; for example, saying grace before meals or daily prayers. Practice them until they become a habit.
- Every night before you go to bed, make a list of five things you are grateful for. It will help take the focus off the stresses in your life.
- Take the time to give back. Look for opportunities to help others and recycle the good fortune you have in your life.
- Once a day, strike a grateful pose. It could be kneeling in prayer or standing with your arms extended joyfully to the sky.

TRY THIS: *Projecting Love*

1. Visualize someone for whom you have loving feelings. Let the love you feel surround your whole body inside and out. Concentrate on these feelings and project them to this person.

2. Next, visualize someone toward whom you have warm feelings that are not as strong as for the first person. As you focus, send these feelings of love and appreciation to that person.

3. Next, visualize someone toward whom you have neutral feelings, nothing strong either way. As you focus on the person, bring the same intensity of love and appreciation you felt for the first two people to the third. Send these feelings to that person.

4. Now visualize someone you have some difficulty with, perhaps whom you dislike but not very intensely. Bring to this person the same feelings of love and appreciation.

5. Finally, visualize someone you have a strong dislike for, and again, as you focus on this person, bring the same degree of love and appreciation you felt for the others. It may be helpful to focus on the person's heart as you do this exercise. Send these feelings to that person.

Source: Collinge, *Subtle Energy* (New York: Warner Books, 1998).

- Take ten minutes each day to be grateful. Go outside into nature, meditate, or pray. Whatever you do, take the time to appreciate all that you have right now.

As nurses, we must educate ourselves about the clinical relevance of faith and prayer for our clients. The time has come to give more than lip service to the spiritual aspects of our nursing care. It is important that we let our clients know that we will do everything we can do scientifically but that science and technology have their limitations. Perhaps it is appropriate also to let them know that we may pray for guidance in providing competent and compassionate care.

REFERENCES

BEARON, L. B. and H. G. KOENIG. 1990. Religious cognitions and use of prayer in health and illness. *Gerontologist.* 30(2): 249–253.

BENSON, H. 1997. *Timeless Healing.* New York: Fireside Book.

BERGIN, A. E. and J. P. JENSEN. 1990. Religiosity of psychotherapists: a national study. *Psychotherapy.* 27(1): 3–7.

BERKEL, J. and F. DE WAARD. 1993. Mortality pattern and life expectancy of Seventh-Day Adventists in the Netherlands. *International J Epidemiology.* 12(4): 455–459.

BRYANT, S. and W. ROKOWSKI. 1992. Predictors of mortality among elderly African Americans. *Research on Aging.* 14(1): 50–67.

BURKHARDT, M. A. and M. G. NAGAI-JACOBSON. 1997. Spirituality and healing. In B. M. DOSSEY, ed. *Core Curriculum for Holistic Nursing.* Gaithersburg, MD: Aspen Pub.

BYRD, R. B. 1988. Positive therapeutic effects of intercessory prayer in a coronary care unit population. *Southern Med J.* 81: 826–829.

CANCELLARO, L. A., D. B. LARSON, and W. P. WILSON. 1982. Religious life of narcotics addicts. *South Med J.* 75(10): 1166–1168.

COLLINGE, W. 1998. *Subtle Energy.* New York: Warner Books.

COMSTOCK, G. W. and K. B. PARTRIDGE. 1972. Church attendance and health. *J Chronic Diseases.* 25: 665–672.

DOSSEY, L. 1997. The return of prayer. *Alternative Therapies.* 3(6): 10–17, 113–120.

DOSSEY, L. 1993. *Healing Words: The Power of Prayer and the Practice of Medicine.* San Francisco: Harper.

ENSTROM, J. E. 1989. Health practices and cancer mortality among active California Mormons. *J National Cancer Institute.* 81: 1807–1814.

FRANKL, V. 1984. *Man's Search for Meaning.* New York: Simon & Schuster.

Gallup Report No. 236. May 1985. *Religion in America.* Princeton, NJ: The Gallup Organization.

GOLDBOUNT, U., S. YAARIS, and J. H. MEDALIE. 1993. Factors predictive of long-term coronary heart disease mortality among 10,059 male Israeli civil servants and municipal employees. *Cardiology.* 82: 100–121.

HOUSE, J. S., C. ROBBINS, and H. L. METZNER. 1982. The association of social relationships and activities with mortality. *Am J Epidemiology.* 116: 123–140.

JAHNKE, R. 1997. *The Healer Within.* San Francisco: Harper.

KING, D. E. and B. BUSHWICK. 1994. Beliefs and attitudes of hospital inpatients about faith healing and prayer. *J Fam Pract.* 39: 349–352.

KOENIG, H. G. et al. 1994. Religious practices and alcoholism in a southern adult population. *Hosp Community Psychiatry.* 45(3): 225–231.

LEVIN, J. S. and R. J. TAYLOR. 1997. Age differences in patterns and correlates of the frequency of prayer. *Gerontologist.* 37(1): 75–88.

LUKS, A. 1993. *The Healing Power of Doing Good.* New York: Ballantine.

MATTHEWS, D. A. and C. CLARK. 1998. *The Faith Factor: Proof of the Healing Power of Prayer.* New York: Viking.

MATTHEWS, D. A., D. B. LARSON, and C. P. BARRY. 1993. *The Faith Factor: An Annotated Bibliography of Clinical Research on Spiritual Subjects.* Rockville, MD: National Institute for Healthcare Research.

MAUGANS, T. A. 1996. The spiritual history. *Arch Fam Med.* 5: 11–16.

McNichol, T. April 5–7, 1996. The new faith in medicine. *USA Today Weekend.* 4–5.

Mickley, J. R., V. Carson, and K. L. Soeken. 1995. Religion and adult mental health. *Issues Mental Health Nursing.* 16: 345–360.

Oleckno, W. A. and M. A. Blacconiere. 1991. Relationship of religiosity to wellness and other health-related behaviors and outcomes. *Psycholo Rep.* 68: 819–826.

Oxman, T. E., D. H. Freeman, and E. D. Manheimer. 1995. Lack of social participation or religious strength and comfort as risk factors for death after cardiac surgery in the elderly. *Psychosomatic Med.* 57: 5–15.

Pressman, P. J. et al. 1990. Religious belief, depression, and ambulation statues in elderly women with broken hips. *Am J Psychiatry.* 147: 758–760.

Remen, R. N. Autumn 1988. Spirit: Resource for healing. *Noetic Science Review.* 61–65.

Richardson, V., S. Berman, and M. Piwowarski. 1983. Projective assessment of the relationships between the salience of death, religion and age among adults in America. *J General Psychology.* 109: 149–156.

Sheehan, W. and J. Kroll 1990. Psychiatric patients belief in general health factors and sin as causes of illness. *Am J Psychiatry.* 147: 112–113.

Spiegel, D. et al. 1989. Effect of psychosocial treatment on survival of patients with metastatic breast cancer. *Lancet.* 2: 888–891.

Waldfogel, S. 1997. Spirituality in medicine. Complementary and Alternative Therapies in Primary Care. *Primary Care: Clinics in Office Practice.* 24(4): 963–976.

Wallis, C. June 24, 1996. Faith and healing. *Time.* 62.

Woodward, K. L. March 31, 1997. Is God listening? *Newsweek.* 129(13): 56–57.

RESOURCES

Common Boundary
4905 Del Ray Ave., Suite 210
Bethesda, MD 20814
301-652-9495
www.commonboundary.org
email: connect@commonboundary.org

Fellowship in Prayer, Inc.
291 Witherspoon St.
Princeton, NJ 08542-3227
609-924-6863
www.fip.org

The Interface Between Medicine and Religion
John Templeton Foundation
P.O. Box 8322
Radnor, PA 19087-8322
610-687-8942
www.templeton.org
email: info@templeton.org

National Center for Jewish Healing
9 East 69th Street
New York, NY 10021
212-772-6601

Shalem Institute for Spiritual Formation
5430 Grosvenor Rd.
Bethesda, MD 20814
301-897-7334
www.shalem.org

UNIT VII
OTHER THERAPIES

The old gods are dead or dying
and people everywhere are searching,
asking: What is the new mythology to be,
the mythology of this unified earth
as one harmonious being?

Joseph Campbell

23 Bioelectromagnetics

> Energy is not obtained from the gross
> molecular aspects of food and air, but
> rather from what can be called its "vibra-
> tional" essence or its electromagnetism.
>
> *Dr. Stephen T. Chang*

Bioelectromagnetics (BEM) is the emerging science that studies how living organisms interact with electromagnetic (EM) fields. What underlies all of biochemistry is electromagnetism, a form of energy. Quantum physics has demonstrated that what people see as solid matter, be that a person or an object, is actually 99.9999 percent empty space filled with energy. Everything is, in fact, energy vibrating at different rates (*Alternative Medicine,* 1994; Simpson, 1997).

The earth is 85 percent crystal. Its crust is largely silicon and oxygen, combined with aluminum, iron, calcium, sodium, potassium, and magnesium. From these chemicals comes a wide variety of crystal colors, shapes, sizes, and hardness. Different crystals are formed under varying conditions of temperature, pressure, space, and time. Diamonds, for example, are found only at a few locations in the world because the exact conditions for their formation are relatively rare (Simpson, 1997).

Crystals are solid minerals with a symmetrical internal atomic structure and can be classified according to their external appearance: cubic, tetragonal, hexagonal, trigonal, orthorhombic, monoclinic, and triclinic. The most desirable crystals are called precious or semiprecious gemstones such as diamonds, amethyst, aquamarine, rose quartz, opal, topaz, and turquoise. Crystal healing works on the principle that every animal, plant, and mineral has an electromagnetic field which enables organic beings and inorganic objects, such as crystals, to communicate and interact as part of a single, unified energy system. Imitation or synthetic gemstones are material made to look like a gem but have a different chemical structure and physical properties. An example would be blue glass cut to imitate sapphire.

BACKGROUND

In the eighteenth century, Guigi Galvani, an Italian physician conducted experiments on frog muscle to demonstrate that bioelectricity exists within living tissue. Shortly after that, Alessandro Volta, a physicist, found that animal
tissue was not needed to produce a current and went on to invent the electric
battery in 1800. Michael Faraday, a British chemist, became the greatest ex-
perimentalist in electricity and magnetism of the nineteenth century, produced
the first electric motor, and succeeded in showing that a magnet could induce
electricity. From this early work came many devices for the diagnosis and
treatment of disease, including many that are in use today (*Alternative Medicine*, 1994).

In the late 1950s in Japan, doctors began to see a new syndrome of
low energy, insomnia, and generalized aches and pains. After extensive research it was discovered that these complaints came from people who spent
large amounts of time in metal buildings and were thus shielded from
the earth's natural magnetic field. The disorder was labeled "magnetic field
deficiency syndrome," and symptoms were alleviated by the external application of magnetic fields to the patients' bodies. Today, magnetic healing continues to be a significant part of mainstream medicine in Japan.
Similarly, early Russian cosmonauts who spent more than a year in space
were amazed to find that they had lost nearly 80 percent of their bone
density. As a result, spacecrafts were designed to include strong artificial
magnetic fields on board to avoid this problem. Both of these examples illus-
trate how magnetic fields are essential to good health and well-being
(Collinge, 1998)

Throughout the ages, crystals have been a part of cultural development.
Early people used crystals to make tools and weapons and to generate a spark
with which to make fire. Crystals, or gemstones, were also portable forms of
wealth and status. The oldest examples of jewelry made of gold, silver, and
semi-precious stones were found in the tomb of Queen Pu-abi at Ur, which
dates back to 3000 B.C. Early Egyptians, the first to develop cosmetics, high-
lighted their eyes with powdered malachite (green) and lapis lazuli (blue).
Gemstones were worn as amulets, objects believed to bring good luck, protect
against evil, and ensure safe travel after death into the next life. The contemporary custom of wearing birthstones is a reflection of this history. Native
Americans believed quartz crystals to be the home of supernatural forces that
would bring good luck to their hunting trips.The first known reference to
the healing power of certain crystals comes from an Egyptian papyrus from
1600 B.C. It gave directions for curative use, such as placing crystals on various areas of the body and grinding them up and mixing with a liquid for internal consumption (Simpson, 1997).

CONCEPTS

Geomagnetic Field

Every atom and cell of the body is a small magnetic field that radiates out into space, decreasing in strength with distance and ultimately becoming lost in the jumble of other magnetic fields. Like the human body, the earth radiates an energy field outwardly, called the geomagnetic field. This energy originates in the earth's core and radiates out beyond the atmosphere, stimulating and protecting all of life on earth. Migrating birds or fish returning to their spawning grounds navigate over great distances with the help of magnetic field receptors in their brains. It is believed that they tune in to the magnetic field of the earth to determine location and direction. Animals are attuned to the geomagnetic field and can sense subtle changes in it. For example, dogs, horses, and cattle often become agitated just before an earthquake (*Alternative Medicine,* 1994; Collinge, 1998).

A magnetic field is like a generator, generating internal energy that can penetrate the body as if it were air. A strong magnet held on one side of the hand can easily deflect a compass needle on the other side of the same hand. As the magnetic field penetrates the body, it causes one's atomic particles to fly around faster and interact with more force.

Subtle changes occur in the strength of the geomagnetic field with the time of day. The day side of the planet, that side facing the sun, always has a slightly weaker field, because the energy coming out of the earth is being "pushed" back and compressed by the radiation from the sun. Thus, the magnetic field passing through the human body is stronger on the nighttime side, away from the sun. Chemical reactions, the healing process, and other cellular activities accelerate in the presence of a stronger field, and thus they are improved slightly at night because of the stronger field (Collinge, 1998).

Like a giant mirror, the moon reflects radiation from the sun toward the earth, thus affecting the earth's energy field. The full moon and the new moon are opposite in their effect on the geomagnetic field. The greatest amount of solar radiation is reflected toward the earth during a full moon, which pushes back and compresses the earth's energy, resulting in a weaker magnetic field than during a new moon. Study results have been mixed as to the effect on human behavior but a study done throughout the calendar year 1993 in Las Vegas found that the full moon was associated with a rise in psychotic behavior, an increase in suicide rates, and an abrupt increase in crisis calls to "911" (Collinge, 1998).

A stronger magnetic field is more conducive to sleep, which makes sleep at night more refreshing and healing than sleep in the daytime. In addition, the sun "agitates" the earth's field with sunspot activity. These intense magnetic

explosions on the sun spray additional radiation on the earth, in turn disturb-
ing the geomagnetic field. During these periods of geomagnetic disturbance,
higher admission rates to psychiatric facilities and higher rates of violence are
characteristic. On the other hand, when the earth's magnetic field is most quiet,
more paranormal experiences like mental telepathy, clairvoyance, and precognition take place (Collinge, 1998).

Endogenous Magnetic Fields

Endogenous magnetic fields are those produced within the body. This electrical activity demonstrates patterns that provide medically useful information.
EKGs and EEGs, for example, provide information about the endogenous
magnetic fields of the heart and brain and are diagnostic in any number of conditions. New technologies in developing instruments that are extremely sensitive have opened new lines of research. For example, a study using transcranial
magnetic stimulation (TMS) found that people who experience migraine
headaches with an aura, have a more excitable occipital cortex when compared
with normal controls (Aurora, 1998).

Like other kinds of magnetic fields, the human energy field is strongest
at its source and fades with distance. Another name for this energy field is
"aura" and is the field that surrounds the body as far as the outstretched arms
and from head to toe. The human energy field is both an information center
and a highly sensitive perceptual system that transmits and receives messages
as people interact with their surrounding environment. Patterns of circulation
of energy within the body include the meridian system and the chakras. Virtually every alternative healing therapy has a way of interpreting these subtle energy fields (Myss, 1996).

Recent research has uncovered a form of endogenous radiation, an extremely low-level light known as biophoton emission. It is believed that biophoton emission may be important in gene expression, membrane transport,
and bioregulation. Externally applied energy fields may alter biophoton emission to the benefit or detriment of the organism. This, as well as other endogenous fields of the body may prove to be involved in energetic therapies
such as Therapeutic Touch (*Alternative Medicine,* 1994).

Exogenous Magnetic Fields

Exogenous magnetic fields are those produced by sources outside the body
and can be classified as either artificial or natural. Artificial exogenous fields
are created by such things as power lines, transformers, appliances, radio transmitters, and medical devices. Some of these may be harmful, such as those
fields emitted by power lines, which are linked to an increased risk of child-

hood leukemia. Artificial electromagnetic fields are unpolarized. Their behavior is chaotic and disordered as they pass through the body's cells. This chaotic nature disturbs the endogenous magnetic fields, resulting in damage to the body's tissues (*Alternative Medicine,* 1994; Collinge, 1998).

The earth's geomagnetic field is one example of a natural exogenous field. Another example is moving water. When people are at beaches, on river banks, beside waterfalls, or even walking outside after a powerful rainstorm, they often experience feelings of relaxation and peace. While these feelings may be attributed to the psychological cues from these environments, they also have an energetic basis. When water moves or flows, it releases negative ions into the air. When people are surrounded by negative ions, they seem to balance their energy fields. As Collinge (1998, p. 93) states, "It is as if the metaphors of "cleansing" and "washing away" that we associate with moving waters have a real basis in their impact on the field of emotional energy that surrounds and penetrates our body."

Ionizing/Nonionizing Fields

Electromagnetic fields can also be classified as ionizing or nonionizing. A field is ionizing if its energy is high enough to dislodge electrons from an atom or molecule such as gamma rays or x-rays. Because these rays are strongly ionizing in biological matter, prolonged exposure is harmful. Nonionizing electromagnetic fields may have nonharmful and even beneficial effects on biological tissue. This effect is the basis for bioelectromagnetic (BEM) application and research (*Alternative Medicine,* 1994).

The actual mechanism by which BEM produces biological effects is under intense study. It is likely that BEM affects the cell membrane, perhaps at the receptors where neurotransmitters and neurohormones bind. Alteration in the binding process then alters the cell's internal processes. Interestingly, some specific frequencies of BEM affect specific target tissues, just as drugs affect specific tissues.

Resonance

Another principle, related to electromagnetics, is resonance, which is simply defined as sympathetic vibration. For example, when a tuning fork turned to note A is sounded near a piano or guitar, any string that is tuned to that same tone will pick up the vibration and begin to move, while the other strings will not. Crystals possess electromagnetic properties and are capable of resonating in harmony with another form. It is believed that when the body's natural frequencies become unbalanced, people experience dis-ease. The resonance of crystals is believed to harmonize and balance the body's frequencies back to optimum, healthy levels. The disrupted field (the ill person) receives energy from the stronger field (the crystal) until the two find their own balance and resonate in harmony. At the current time, however, no explanations for crystal healing fit within known scientific facts (Simpson, 1997).

TREATMENT

Magnetic and crystal healing work best in combination with other healing modalities and are considered to be adjunct treatments to conventional medicine. They should not be used by themselves for any major disease or medical condition (Null, 1998).

Nonionizing BEM medical applications are classified into two types, thermal or nonthermal. Thermal or heat applications include radio frequency (RF) hyperthermia, laser and RF surgery, and RF diathermy. The most important BEM modalities in alternative medicine are the nonthermal applications. The term *nonthermal* means that it causes no significant gross tissue heating. An example is microwave resonance therapy where the mechanism of action is thought to be in the modification of the cell membrane. The major alternative healing applications of nonthermal, nonionizing electromagnetic fields are: bone repair, nerve stimulation, wound healing, the treatment of osteoarthritis, electroacupuncture, tissue regeneration, immune system stimulation, and neuroendocrine modulations (*Alternative Medicine,* 1994). Box 23.1 describes these applications for stimulation and measurement of nerve activity.

Cell Specific Cancer Therapy (CSCT) is available only outside the United States, in Santo Domingo, at this time. The CSCT device identifies cancer cells by their excess of positively charged ions. As the cancer cells are identified, a physician marks the locations on the patient's skin. When the entire body has been scanned, the frequency of the electromagnetic field is changed to that appropriate for killing the cancer cells. Some researchers say not enough evidence shows that BEM has any value in treating cancer while others believe BEM can possibly reverse cancer. More research is needed before the efficacy of this technology is proven or disproven ("Medicine on the Holodeck," 1998).

Being immersed in a field of negative ions seems to balance people's energy and relieve pain. Physicians specializing in orthopedics and sports medicine have been recommending magnets since 1993. Athletic performance is enhanced and risk of serious injury is decreased when magnets are used to warm up muscles and joints. People wear magnets on their wrists, elbows, and knees for joint pain or on their heads for headaches. Magnets are used to speed

Box 23.1: Applications of Nonthermal, Nonionizing Electromagnetic Fields in Stimulation and Measurement of Nerve Activity

Transcultaneous electrical nerve stimulation (TENS)	Used for pain relief
Transcranial electrostimulation (TCES)	Used to reduce symptoms of depression, anxiety, and insomnia; may be effective in drug dependence
Neuromagnetic stimulation	Used in place of electro-convulsive therapy in certain types of mood disorders; used in diagnostic nerve conduction studies
Electromyography	Used to diagnose and treat carpal tunnel syndrome and other movement disorders
Electroencephalography	Along with EEG biofeedback, used to treat attention deficit disorder, learning disabilities, stroke, and alcoholism
Electroretinography	Noninvasive monitoring of rapid eye movement sleep
Low energy emission therapy	Used to treat insomnia and hypertension

Source: *Alternative Medicine,* (Washington, DC: U.S. Government Printing Office, 1994).

the healing of wounds. Though not recognized as medical devices by the Food and Drug Administration, magnets have been widely used in Asia for years. Blood cells, believed to have tiny positive charges at one end and negative charges at the other end, respond to the pull of magnets, thus increasing blood flow to the area. The increased blood flow brings in more healing nutrients and carries off toxins. Magnets appear to block pain by altering the electro-magnetic balance between negatively charged and positively charged ions in the nerve pathways that carry pain messages. The magnets used are about

5–10 times as strong as refrigerator door magnets and cost between $12 and $28 a pair depending on the size.

A few contraindications for magnetic therapy need to be observed. Until further research is conducted, pregnant women should not wear magnets over the abdominal area. Magnets should not be used by persons wearing pacemakers, defibrillators, or other implanted electrical devices. Magnets decrease the stickiness of platelets, which contributes to increased bleeding. For that reason, they should not be used with people on anticoagulants or who have an actively bleeding wound (Null, 1998).

Crystal healing is based on tuning in to the natural vibrations of a mineral from the earth, which has infused it with its energies. For this reason, neither imitation nor synthetic crystals are suitable for healing. In electrocrystal therapy, the body is initially scanned with a specially adapted video camera that relays a colored picture of the auric field on to a computer screen. The therapist marks those areas where the color of the aura is inappropriate, indicating stress or dysfunction. Electrocrystal therapy uses quartz crystals in saline solution that are enclosed in a sealed, glass electrode connected to a battery. Up to five electrodes are placed against the affected area or over a chakra point. The crystals are electrically stimulated, which amplifies their natural healing vibrations until they vibrate and resonate at a desired frequency. This treatment is thought to bring the endogenous fields back to a harmonious state (Simpson, 1997).

Crystal cards, meant to be worn on the body, were developed as a result of the NASA space program. Astronauts travel into space with a number of pyramid-shaped quartz crystals, electronically charged to vibrate at the frequency of the earth's geomagnetic field, to combat the negative effects of spending time outside the earth's magnetic field. The crystal cards sold in stores contain a number of tiny corundum crystals that are electrochemically etched with hydrochloric acid. The acid changes the form of the crystals, which produces beneficial negative ions and harmonizes cellular activity (Simpson, 1997).

Electronic gem therapy blends modern technology with traditional Ayurvedic medicine by combining gemstones or crystals, colored light, and electronic amplification. Depending on the condition, patients either require cooling gems such as emerald, topaz, or carnelian or warming gems such as ruby, chrysoberyl, or citrine. During treatment the gemstone is electronically vibrated at a frequency set for a specific condition. The energy from the gemstone is focused by special colored lamps called gem transducers on to the part of the body requiring treatment. It is believed the treatment provides additional energy needed to bring about self-healing. The seven chakras are assigned different gemstones corresponding to their vibratory rates. In crystal bodywork, people place crystals on the chakras as they meditate (Simpson, 1997). Box 23.2 lists the gemstones or crystals associated with each chakra.

> **Box 23.2: Crystals, Gemstones, and Chakras**
>
> **Root Chakra**
> Agate, bloodstone, tiger's eye, hematite
>
> **Sexual Chakra**
> Moonstone, tiger's eye, citrine, carnelian
>
> **Solar Plexus Chakra**
> Citrine, rose quartz, aventurine quartz, malachite
>
> **Heart Chakra**
> Jade, aventurine quartz, watermelon tourmaline, rose quartz
>
> **Throat Chakra**
> Aquamarine, lapis lazuli, turquoise, celestite
>
> **Third Eye Chakra**
> Amethyst, fluorite, lapis lazuli, sodalite
>
> **Crown Chakra**
> Amethyst, celestite, jade, rock crystal (clear quartz)

RESEARCH

No known published articles demonstrate the effectiveness of crystal healing via clinical trials. Little research has been conducted in the United States regarding the clinical effects of magnets. In Europe and Russia, however, where magnetism is well-regarded, hundreds of scientific studies have been documented. Extensive research in the United States regarding BEM applications is illustrated in the following few examples:

- Double-blind clinical trials have demonstrated the efficacy of BEM bone repair treatment in promoting healing in nonunion bone fractures (Barker et al., 1984; Sharrard, 1990).
- In cases of retarded or arrested wound healing, BEM applications may trigger healing to occur (Lee et al., 1993; Vodovnik and Karba, 1992).

- Pulsed fields promote cell activation and proliferation in the treatment of venous skin ulcers (Stiller et al., 1992).
- BEM applications act to suppress inflammatory responses at the cell membrane level in people with osteoarthritis (O'Connor et al., 1990).
- Electrostimulation with acupuncture is beneficial in the treatment of postoperative pain (Christensen and Noreng, 1989); in chemotherapy-induced sickness in cancer patients (Dundee and Ghaly, 1989); and in the treatment of renal colic (Lee et al., 1992).
- Daily left prefrontal repetitive transcranial magnetic stimulation has antidepressant effects in some severely depressed patients (George, 1997; Kirkcaldie et al., 1997).
- Low intensity, external magnetic field treatment significantly reduces seizures (Anninos et al., 1991; Sandyk and Anninos, 1992).
- People suffering from migraine, tension, and/or cervical headaches received good to excellent relief from pulsating electromagnetic fields. Those with posttraumatic or cluster headaches received no benefit (Prusinski et al., 1988).

For extensive lists of peer-reviewed scientific studies, refer to Null (1998) pages 101–215 and *Alternative Medicine* (1994) pages 54–56. These studies include subjects with Alzheimer's disease, arthritis, bone fractures, cancer, cardiovascular disease, depression, epilepsy, headache, kidney problems, multiple sclerosis, neurological disorders, osteoporosis, Parkinson's disease, sleep disorders, ulcers, and wound healing.

INTEGRATED NURSING PRACTICE

Many people use crystals in combination with other healing modalities. Some people choose crystals intuitively while others select crystals on the basis of therapeutic qualities. You can help individuals determine which crystal is "right" for them by asking them the following questions (Simpson, 1997):

- What do you want the crystal for—healing, meditation, energizing your environment, as a focus for visualization, or for decoration?
- Which crystals are most appealing—geometrically shaped, such as clear quartz, or "massive," such as rose quartz?
- Which colors are appealing to you—pale or deep shades? Do you prefer clear or opaque?
- What size crystal are you looking for?

- Do you prefer cut and polished crystals or ones that are completely natural?
- How much are you prepared to spend?

Members of the quartz family, such as clear quartz, amethyst, and rose quartz, are the crystals used most frequently in healing. Amethyst is the "stone of meditation," creating a state of enhanced spirituality and contentment. Clear quartz represents the clarity of mind that people hope to achieve through meditation. Chapter 16 provides general guidelines for meditation. Building on this process, you can encourage clients to try a crystal focus meditation. Maintaining a focus on a crystal helps quiet one's thoughts during meditation. Instruct clients to hold the crystal or place it in front of them on the floor or on a small table. Some people take three similar crystals and position them in an equilateral triangle, forming a charged energy field in which to sit. Explain that they are to half-close their eyes and gaze at the crystal, concentrating on its color, shape, and size during their meditation. As they come out of the meditative state, they should continue to focus on the crystal and open their eyes gradually.

People who are experiencing illness or disease may find that crystal imagery improves the healing process. Explain imagery to clients as described in chapter 17 and add the following steps (Simpson, 1997):

- Assume your meditative position and focus on the crystal in front of you.
- Close your eyes, while continuing to visualize the crystal.
- Allow this image of the crystal to become bigger and bigger until it completely surrounds you.
- Imagine that you are at the center of the crystal.
- Notice that you have become one with the crystal.
- Image the illness or disease leaving your body as you become one with the crystal.
- Consider how it feels to share the same perfection and clarity as the crystal. Be aware that you are whole and complete as you are one with the crystal.
- Contemplate how the crystal forms a protective shield around you so that you are totally safe and secure.
- When you sense that your inner journey is completed, begin to separate yourself from the crystal.
- Reduce the crystal to its normal size.
- Fade this picture from your mind, open your eyes, and take a few deep breaths to bring yourself back into the here and now.
- Be aware of any thoughts, feelings, or emotions that come to you.

Awareness of magnetic healing is gaining credibility in the United States and is being applied by increasing numbers of conventional as well as alternative health-care practitioners as an adjunctive therapy. Increasing numbers of people are sleeping on magnetic beds at night and wearing small magnets during the day for pain relief, greater energy, and healing.

Some controversy surrounds the issue of when to use the north, or negative pole, and when to use the south, or positive pole. Some people believe that the north pole of a magnet enhances healing and health while the south pole exacerbates disease. Practitioners in Japan and Russia believe no strong evidence supports the use of one pole over the other but rather that the entirety of the magnet is doing the healing.

Explain to clients that the effectiveness of magnetic treatment depends on the number of magnets used and their strength, thickness, and spacing. Magnets vary in strength and those used for healing purposes are generally between 1,000 and 5,000 gauss. In general, healing magnets are unipolar and are either circular or rectangular. Several can be stacked for increased gauss strength and, therefore, greater effectiveness. The thicker the magnet, the greater the depth of penetration. The problem with this is that, with increasing thickness, the magnet becomes more uncomfortable to wear. Most people wear magnets between 1/4 and 3/8 of an inch thick. In general, the magnet should be larger than the size of the area being treated. Clients who are treating finger joints for arthritis will use a small magnet, while those who are treating the lower back will apply a much larger magnet.

When teaching clients about magnetic therapy, you can explain that the most common use is in the treatment of pain, with reports of successful treatment in arthritis, rheumatism, fibromyalgia, back pain, headaches, muscle sprains and strains, joint pain, tendonitis, shoulder pain, carpal tunnel syndrome, and torn ligaments. A magnetic field can also function like an antibiotic by lowering acidity, which is a hostile environment for microorganisms. A magnetic field applied to the head has a sedating effect by stimulating the hormone melatonin. Biomagnetic therapy increases general well-being by enhancing energy through the repolarization of cells. Many professional athletes revitalize their bodies by sleeping on a magnetic mattress pad. Some even participate in their sport with dozens of magnets taped to their bodies (Null, 1998).

Magnetic therapy may be one of the most effective methods for achieving relief from arthritis, especially in the hands and feet. People with carpal tunnel syndrome can apply magnets to the front and back of the wrist to help control symptoms. Individuals diagnosed with fibromyalgia can sleep on a magnetic mattress pad and use a magnetic pillow, as well as using magnets over the painful areas during the day. Magnetic insoles increase circulation and help conditions such as numbness, burning, aches, restlessness, and leg cramps. If you have a client with phantom pain following an amputation, you may suggest the use of magnets which improve the flow of blood in the stump and

TRY THIS: *Absorbing Earth Energy*

Find a grassy, open area that is in its relatively natural state. You may choose to use a blanket or not. Lie face down with your arms and legs extended in a spreading out fashion. Notice that all your chakras are in direct contact with the earth. Visualize an exchange of energy as you release to the earth, with each out-breath, any stress or negativity you have been carrying. With each in-breath, imagine that your chakras are receiving fresh, balanced, healing energy from the earth. Do this relaxation breathing for at least 20 minutes. You should feel yourself in a pleasant and refreshed state.

cause the phantom pain to disappear. People with asthma and bronchitis may find that wearing a strong neodymium magnet over the chest and at an equal level on the back will help return breathing to a normal state. For minor burns, people can place a magnet over the site of injury to speed up the healing and reduce the pain (Null, 1998).

It is unclear at this time whether you should suggest that clients wear the magnets full time or intermittently. This recommendation will need to be determined through further research. At this time you can encourage clients to experiment with time periods that seem most effective. As our scientific and clinical understanding increases, we will be able to provide greater knowledge about how to manipulate magnets for the best effects.

TRY THIS: *Going to the Mountains*

If you live near hills or mountains, go to the highest natural point you can reach. High places are concentrations of energy and seem to lift us above our normal conflicting energies. Looking down below, get a sense of the differences in the two energetic environments. The higher point you are on may feel like clear, focused energy while the area below may feel like a mixture of many different energies. After a while you should experience clearer thinking and a sense of inspiration.

Source: Collinge, *Subtle Energy* (New York: Warner Books, 1998).

REFERENCES

Alternative Medicine: Expanding Medical Horizons. 1994. A report to the National Institutes of Health on Alternative Medical Systems and Practices in the United States. U.S. Government Printing Office. Washington, DC.

ANNINOS, P. A. et al. 1991. Magnetic stimulation in the treatment of partial seizures. *International J Neurosci.* 60(3–4): 141–171.

AURORA, S. K. 1998. Transcranial magnetic stimulation confirms hyperexcitability of occipital cortex in migraine. *Neurology.* 50: 1111–1114.

BARKER, A. T. et al. 1984. Pulsed magnetic field therapy for tibial nonunion. *Lancet.* 1(8384): 994–996.

CHRISTENSEN, P. A. and M. NORENG. 1989. Electroacupuncture and postoperative pain. *Br J Anaesth.* 62: 258–262.

COLLINGE, W. 1998. *Subtle Energy.* New York: Warner Books.

DUNDEE, J. W. and R. G. GHALY. 1989. Acupuncture prophylaxis of cancer chemotherapy-induced sickness. *J R Soc. Med.* 82: 268–271.

GEORGE, M. S. 1997. Mood improvement following daily left prefrontal repetitive transcranial magnetic stimulation in patients with depression. *Am J Psychiatry.* 154: 1752–1756.

KIRKCALDIE, M. T. et al. 1997. Transcranial magnetic stimulation as therapy for depression and other disorders. *Aust N Z J Psychiatry.* 31(2): 264–272.

LEE, R. C. et al. 1993. A review of the biophysical basis for the clinical application of electric fields in soft tissue repair. *J Burn Care Rehabil.* 14: 319–335.

LEE, Y. H. et al. 1992. Acupuncture in the treatment of renal colic. *J Urol.* 147: 16–18.

Medicine on the Holodeck. 1998. *New Age Journal.* 100–102.

MYSS, C. 1996. *Anatomy of the Spirit.* New York: Three Rivers Press.

NULL, G. 1998. *Healing with Magnets.* New York: Carroll & Graf Pub.

O'CONNOR, M. E. et al. 1990. *Emerging Electromagnetic Medicine* (conference proceedings). New York: Springer-Verlag.

PRUSINKSI, A. et al. 1988. Pulsating electromagnetic field in the therapy of headaches. *J Bioelectr.* 7(1): 127–128.

SANDYK, R. and P. A. ANNINOS. 1992. Magnetic fields alter the circadian periodicity of seizures. *International J Neurosci.* 63(3–4): 265–274.

SHARRARD, W. J. W. 1990. A double-blind trial of pulsed electromagnetic fields for delayed union of tibia fractures. *J Bone Joint Surg.* 72B: 347–355.

SIMPSON, L. 1997. *The Book of Crystal Healing.* New York: Sterling Pub. Co.

STILLER, M. J. et al. 1992. A portable pulsed electromagnetic field (PEMF) device to enhance healing of recalcitrant venous ulcers. *Br J Dermatol.* 127: 147–154.

VODOVNIK, L. and R. KARBA. May 1992. Treatment of chronic wounds by means of electric and electromagnetic fields. Part 1: literature review. *Med Biol Eng and Comput.* 257–266.

RESOURCES

Bio-Electro-Magnetics Institute
2490 West Moana Lane
Reno, NV 89509
702-827-9099

Center for Specific Cancer Therapy
Santo Domingo
809-534-2090
www.csct.com

International Society for the Study of Subtle
Energies and Energy Medicine (ISSSEEM)
356 Goldco Circle
Golden, CO 80403
303-425-4625
www.vitalenergy.com/issseem
email: 74040.1273@compuserve.com

BEMI
Dr. John Zimmerman
2490 W. Moana Lane
Reno, NV 89509
702-827-9099

24 Detoxifying Therapies

The most beautiful thing we can experience is the mysterious. Recognition of
the mystery of the universe is the course
of all true Science.

Albert Einstein

The greatest discovery of any generation
is that human beings can alter their lives
by altering the attitude of their minds.

Albert Schweitzer

Many cultures and religions, past and present, define what is "unclean" and also have rituals of purification. In Western cultures, some people are currently fascinated with the concept of detoxification, the belief that physical impurities and toxins must be cleared from the body to achieve better health. This chapter provides an overview of several ways people purge their bodies: hydrotherapy, colonics, and chelation therapy.

HYDROTHERAPY

Background

Water has been a part of healing practices from ancient times and great healing powers have been attributed to it as seen in phrases "healing waters" and the "fountain of youth." The Romans built bathhouses throughout their empire. Saunas have been popular in Scandinavian countries for many years and have risen in popularity in the United States in the latter half of the twentieth century. In Europe and the United States, people go for periods of rest and rejuvenation to spas that have been built around the mineral waters of natural hot springs. Today, hydrotherapy, or water-based therapy, is used to treat wounds, injuries, and burns, to promote physical rehabilitation, and to manage stress (Cassileth, 1998).

Preparation

The use of water as a healing treatment is known as hydrotherapy. Nurses, chiropractors, physical therapists, naturopaths, massage therapists, yoga masters, and conventional physicians incorporate various forms of hydrotherapy in their professional practice. Programs of study in each discipline cover the use of hydrotherapy techniques that are appropriate for one's professional practice.

Treatment

Hydrotherapy, the use of hot and cold moisture in the form of solid, liquid, or gas, makes use of the body's response to heat and cold. The primary effect of both heat and cold is stimulation. The secondary effects of heat are drowsiness, sedation, and relaxed muscles. Heat also dilates blood vessels, increasing the circulation to the area being heated. The secondary effects of cold are invigoration and restoration. Cold constricts blood vessels, reducing circulation to that area of the body. Hydrotherapy is used to decrease pain, decrease fever, reduce swelling, lessen cramps, induce sleep, and improve physical and mental tone. It must be used with great care in the young and the old who have poor heat regulation and also with people experiencing a prolonged illness or fatigue (Krohn et al., 1996).

Three basic types of hydrotherapy are compresses, bathing, and sweat baths. The general use of compresses involves towels wrung out in hot and cold water and alternately applied to the body. The intense fluctuations in temperature are believed to improve the circulation to the stomach, liver, kidneys, and intestines, thereby improving digestion and the elimination of metabolic wastes. Other examples of compresses include ice packs to reduce the swelling of sprained ankles and hot water packs for muscle pain.

Baths, as a form of hydrotherapy, involve local baths such as a foot, sitz, and full immersion baths. They may be hot or cold or alternating. Hot water, and the substances sometimes added to the water, increase blood flow to the skin, open pores, and increase sweating, all of which lead to a faster release of toxins. Warm water is often used to irrigate and cleanse wounds. Full immersion baths are used for physical rehabilitation. Exercising in water can be more effective and cause less strain to the skeleton and joints than exercise out of water.

Sweat baths are a method of detoxification that enables the body to eliminate salt, drugs, and a variety of toxins. They are typically done in a steam room or a sauna. Pregnant women should never use sweat bathing as the heat may cause neural tube defects in the first trimester. Sweat baths are also contraindicated for people with heart disease, kidney disease, or anemia (Cassileth, 1998; Collinge, 1996; Krohn et al., 1996).

A process in yoga called *neti* (pronounced NAY-tee) involves various methods for cleansing the nasal passages. One method is to sniff warm water into the nostrils and spit it out of the mouth. Neti bottles are also available and are designed to pour water into one nostril, which will then come out the other nostril.

COLONICS

Background

Written documents of ancient Egypt and Greece contain references to colon therapy. For hundreds of years, nurses and physicians have advocated enemas as internal body baths. Colon therapy was introduced to the United States at the end of the nineteenth century, and it rapidly became popular. Healthy people used enemas to cleanse and rejuvenate themselves. Others used enemas to treat heart disease, hypertension, arthritis, depression, and various infections. In the mid-twentieth century, as antibiotics and other medications became available, colon therapy began to fade from popular use. In the 1980s a resurgence of colonics took place in the United States among people who believe that their bodies are full of harmful chemicals, by-products, food residues, or accumulated intestinal waste. This desire for cleansing has created a growing market for products and treatments that claim to detoxify the body and restore it to a state of purity (Cassileth, 1998).

Preparation

The International Association for Colon Hydrotherapy (I-ACT) is the certifying body for colon hydrotherapy training. A list of schools teaching the I-ACT syllabus, as well as names of colon therapists, is available from the association. The foundation level of education includes a 100-hour course of colon hydrotherapy training from an approved school or certified instructor as well as a 100-hour internship. In addition, students must pass a written exam. The intermediate level requirements include 500 hours of course work, a demonstration of expertise, and an intermediate exam. The instructor level requirements include 1,000 hours of training or three years of practice. In addition, teaching skills must be demonstrated.

Treatment

Colonics, or colon therapy, is based on the idea that high-fat, Western diets lead to an accumulation of a thick, gluelike substance in the colon, which in turn produces toxins that lead to disease. Colonics, also called colonic irrigation or high colonics, is a procedure for washing the inner wall of the colon by filling it with water or herbal solutions and then draining it. Colonics is a technique for removing any material that may be present high in the colon and cleans the entire five feet of the colon compared to enemas, which clean only the lower 8–12 inches of the colon. Colonics are administered by a colon therapist using 2–6 liters of liquid at a time. The therapist then massages the colon through the abdomen, and the water is eliminated through a waste tube. The procedure is repeated over a period of 30–45 minutes and using more than 20 gallons of water per session.

Colon cleansing is a controversial method of detoxification, and there tends to be no middle ground in the beliefs about the usefulness of colonics. People tend to either strongly support or challenge the practice of colonics. Those who support colonics believe that toxicity can build up in the pockets of the colon through years of a diet heavy in fried foods, white flour, sugar, refined and processed foods, dairy products, carbonated beverages, and not enough fiber. The use of prescriptive drugs, smoking, and drinking alcoholic beverages are additional sources of toxicity. Substances generally used for colonics include water, coffee, herbal teas, a mild soap solution, meat broth, wheat grass juice, and barley juice. I-ACT recommends the use of colonics twice yearly as a maintenance regimen. Contraindications for colonics include people in a weakened state and those having ulcerative colitis, diverticulitis, Crohn's disease, severe hemorrhoids, or tumors of the large intestine or rectum (Berry, 1997; Krohn et al., 1996).

Those who oppose the use of colonics believe no medical reason supports them. It is believed that diet, water, and exercise should be enough to maintain the health of the colon. Andrew Weil (1995, p. 209) states, "I have reviewed many systems of colon cleansing, including colonic irrigation (colonics) and the use of natural laxatives and herbal mixtures. If you eat a high-fiber diet, drink plenty of water, exercise, and move your bowels regularly, you shouldn't need any of them. The best way to care for the colon is to let its own natural physiological action keep it clean and in good working order." Problems that may result from colonics include enzyme imbalance, perforation of the colon, and general weakening of the body.

CHELATION THERAPY

Background

Chelation comes from the Greek work *chele* or "claw." When chelation chemicals are introduced into the bloodstream, they bind, or claw, to heavy metals in the body. Ethylene diamine tetraacetic acid (EDTA) is a synthetic amino acid that readily binds to heavy metals. EDTA was synthesized in the 1940s and was originally used by the United States Navy to remove calcium from pipes and boilers. In the 1950s, EDTA was tried with success in curing people with lead poisoning who were working in battery plants, and the U.S. Navy used it on people who had acquired lead poisoning from repainting old ships. Not only did EDTA eliminate the poisoning but physicians noted that patients also showed considerable improvement in cardiovascular symptoms. The FDA has approved EDTA for the treatment of lead poisoning, hypercalcemia, and ventricular fibrillation secondary to digitalis toxicity. EDTA is legally available for a physician's use and it is quite legal for a licensed physician to utilize a drug for any purpose which, in that physician's judgment, is best for the patient. Thus, since the 1960s, EDTA has been used to treat cardiovascular disease coupled with dietary changes and nutritional supplements (Leviton, 1997).

Preparation

Only licensed physicians are able to provide chelation therapy in the United States. In some facilities the physicians oversee the procedure, which is actually implemented by registered nurses.

Treatment

In conventional medicine, EDTA is used as the preferred treatment for lead poisoning as well as for removing a number of other toxic metals. EDTA circulates through the blood vessels and "chelates" or binds to excess amounts of iron, copper, lead, mercury, cadmium, aluminum, and calcium. EDTA, with its load of metal, is then eliminated quickly through the urine.

It is the free radical-chelation connection that makes chelation therapy a form of alternative therapy for atherosclerosis and other degenerative diseases. As the body goes through its normal processes, and oxygen is used to provide cellular fuel, some of the oxygen molecules lose one of their pair of electrons. When this happens, the formerly stable oxygen molecules become dangerous free radicals that try to stabilize themselves by stealing another electron from stable molecules, thus damaging them and creating more free radicals. Free radicals are normally kept under control through the production of enzymes that act as free radical scavengers to search out and neutralize dangerous free radicals. Metals that are loose and free-floating inhibit this enzyme function and also increase free radical production. In addition, the production of prostaglandins is put into imbalance by free radicals, the two most important, in relation to blood vessels and atherosclerosis, being prostacyclin and thromboxane. The proper balance of these must be maintained to protect against injury and hemorrhage on the one hand, and to maintain normal circulation on the other. Free radicals block production of prostacyclin, which results in overactivity of thromboxane thus causing spasm and blood clots in arteries.

EDTA helps reestablish prostaglandin hormone balance by removing the metallic ions and blocking the free radical chain reactions. EDTA may also function as a kind of "calcium-blocking agent," a category of drugs known to have potent coronary vasodilating effects (Cranton, 1996).

The American Heart Association does not approve of chelation therapy. The conventional approach to treating severe atherosclerosis is angioplasty, a mechanical method of scrubbing the inside of clogged arteries with an inflated balloon catheter to flatten the deposits of plaque, or bypass surgery (*Alternative Medicine,* 1994; Leviton, 1997).

In early experiments, EDTA was often used in doses up to ten times the amount now recommended. This resulted in serious adverse effects including renal failure. With the lower doses and with the use of kidney function tests, and by following recommended protocols, the present-day procedure is considered to be safe.

Chelation therapy is performed in an outpatient or physician's office setting. EDTA is given as an intravenous infusion over a period of 3–4 hours. Usually 20–30 treatments, at an average cost of $80 to $100 each, are administered at the rate of 1–3 sessions per week. The average cost of a course of treatment is $3,000 to $5,000, compared to the average cost of balloon angioplasty at $12,000 and bypass surgery in excess of $30,000.

In late 1996, an oral chelation substance was introduced to the market. It is a three-month program designed to detoxify and balance the cardiovascular system. The oral route is advisable for people with potential heart problems but whose condition does not yet require rapid action. The advantages of oral chelation are that it does not require a physician's supervision or expensive blood tests to monitor and is much lower in cost. The primary disadvantage is the longer time to get the same benefits as intravenous chelation (Leviton, 1997).

RESEARCH

Ice packs, hot compresses, and warm baths are good examples of self-help techniques that work on a number of common problems. The data are primarily anecdotal rather than scientifically researched. No data support the claims or beliefs on which colonics is based. Conventional physicians often warn against the use of this procedure.

A large retrospective study of 2,870 patients in Brazil showed that 89 percent of the patients treated with EDTA had marked improvement (Olszewer and Carter, 1989). This study was followed by a double-blind clinical trial of EDTA for men with peripheral vascular disease. The group showing dramatic improvements was identified as those receiving EDTA (Olszewer et al., 1990).

Much of the long-term benefit derives from EDTA's ability to undo the under-lying cause of arterial blockage.

For obvious reasons, double-blind studies have never been done to prove or disprove the clinical benefits from balloon angioplasty or bypass surgery. Given this situation, the effectiveness of EDTA chelation therapy has been clinically proven to the same extent as those procedures.

Hundreds of conventional physicians are convinced that EDTA chelation therapy is of greater benefit to their patients than more dangerous and costly treatments such as bypass surgery. Chelation is available throughout the United States as well as many foreign countries. In the U.S., the four major organizations promoting acceptance of chelation therapy are the American Board of Chelation Therapy, the American College for Advancement in Medi-cine, the Great Lakes Association of Clinical Medicine, and the International Bioxidative Medicine Association.

INTEGRATED NURSING PRACTICE

Sweating, as a natural method of purification, can be recommended to many people, especially to people who smoke, drink, or use other drugs, suffer chemical exposures, or eat a lot of salt. Remember to warn pregnant women, or those who think they might be pregnant, to avoid saunas and steam baths because they may cause neural tube defects in the first trimester. The complete recommended program is to exercise for 20 minutes, sauna or steam bath for a maximum of 30 minutes, take a cleansing shower, and then have a massage. Caution people to be careful as they emerge from the sauna or steam bath as they may be weak, dizzy, or unstable on their feet. It is especially important that you teach people to drink plenty of water throughout the program to re-place the fluids that have been lost. Even after the sweat, fluid intake should be high to continue the flushing out of toxins and to prevent dehydration.

Steam inhalation is an excellent remedy for respiratory problems such as chest congestion, bronchitis, bronchial cough, laryngitis, and sinusitis. Adding sage and eucalyptus to the steam is both soothing and antibacterial, which de-creases the chance of secondary bacterial infection in viral respiratory diseases (Weil, 1995). Steam inhalation can be done with a commercial steam vapor-izer or through making one's own steam tent. A towel draped over one's head and over the top of a pot of boiling water is quite effective. Great care must be taken not to set the towel on fire if the source of heat is a gas burner.

Hot, wet compresses are good treatment for localized infections. Instruct people to wet a towel, wring it out, and if possible, heat it in the microwave. Care must be taken to avoid temperatures hot enough to burn. Place on the infected area for 15 minutes at least three or four times a day. Heat is also effective for sore muscles as well as menstrual and intestinal cramps. This therapy can be accomplished with heating pads or with gel packs designed to be heated in a microwave. Cold compresses are good for bruises, sprains, traumatized joints, burns, bites, and stings. Instruct people to make a cold compress using ice cubes or a package of frozen peas wrapped in a towel. A home first aid kit should include a gel ice pack which can be stored in the freezer until it is needed. For campers, instant ice packs are available and simply need to be squeezed, stretched, and applied. A cold compress will reduce leakage of fluid into injured tissues, reduce swelling and pain, and slow the spread of any toxins into the system. It should be kept in place for most of the first few hours and then used intermittently for 24 hours after the injury.

Intense sweating, at the very start of a viral infection may greatly reduce the severity of the illness (Weil, 1995). A sauna or steam bath produces the most effective sweating. Because that option may not be immediately available for most people, instruct them to prewarm their bed with an electric blanket or other means and fill the bath tub with comfortably hot water between 102 and 104 degrees Fahrenheit. They should submerge their body as much as possible for 15 minutes. The bath is followed by toweling off, jumping into the prewarmed bed, covering up to stay warm, and resting for at least one hour. This sequence can be done as often as two or three times a day to treat a cold or the flu.

A number of detoxifying baths can be suggested to patients. Instruct them that someone else should be in the house in case they get dizzy or exhausted and need assistance. You should provide the following general instructions:

- Wash the body thoroughly in a shower before the bath; rinse thoroughly.
- Have the bath water as hot as tolerable without burning, 102–104°F.
- Begin with a 5-minute soak; gradually build up the time over a number of baths until you can soak for 30 minutes.
- Drink 8 ounces of water during the bath.
- After soaking, take a cleansing shower; scrub with soap and rinse well to remove the toxins that have been excreted on the skin.
- Follow this procedure three times a week until your health has improved, and then one or two times a week to maintain health.

A number of substances can be added to the bath to help detoxify the body. The sulfur component of Epsom salts helps to rid the body of toxins as well as to increase sweating and increase the blood supply to the skin's surface. Instruct people to begin with 1/4 cup of Epsom salts per bath and gradually increase until they are using 4 cups per bath. Apple-cider vinegar changes the pH of the skin, which aids in the detoxification process. Again, it is best to begin

TRY THIS: *Stress Reducing Bath*

When experiencing stress of mind, body, or spirit, try taking a salt bath. To a tub of warm water (102–104°F), add 1/2 cup Epsom salts, 1/2 cup sea salt, and 1/2 cup baking soda. Soak for at least 15 minutes, followed by a cleansing shower.

with 1/4 cup and gradually increase to 1 cup. Baking soda baths, 8 ounces per bath, are alkalinizing and good for cleansing and drying weeping open sores. Ginger root baths increase sweating and help draw toxins to the skin surface. Instruct people to cut a thumb size piece of ginger root in small pieces. These pieces should be put in a pot of water and brought to a boil. Turn off the heat and let steep for 30 minutes. Strain the solution and pour into the bath. Any number of herbs can be brewed as a cup of tea and then added to the bath, which should only include one herb at a time. The most popular herbal baths are catnip, yarrow, peppermint, boneset, blessed thistle, pleurisy root, chamomile, blue vervain, and horsetail (Krohn et al., 1996).

REFERENCES

Alternative Medicine: Expanding Medical Horizons. 1994. A report to the National Institutes of Health on Alternative Medical Systems and Practices in the United States. U.S. Government Printing Office. Washington, DC.

BERRY, L. 1997. *Internal Cleansing.* Rocklin, CA: Prima Pub.

CASSILETH, B. R. 1998. *The Alternative Medicine Handbook.* New York: W. W. Norton.

COLLINGE, W. 1996. *Complete Guide to Alternative Medicine.* New York: Warner Books.

CRANTON, E. 1996. *Bypassing Bypass,* 2d ed. Trout Dale, VA: Medex Pub.

KROHN, J., F. TAYLOR, and J. PROSSER. 1996. *The Whole Way to Natural Detoxification.* Point Roberts, WA: Hartley & Marks.

LEVITON, R. 1997. Detoxifying the heart. *Alternative Medicine Online.* Future Medicine Publishing.

OLSZEWER, E. and J. P. CARTER. 1989. EDTA chelation therapy: A retrospective study of 2,870 patients. *J Advancement in Med.* 2: 197.

OLSZEWER, E. et al. 1990. A pilot double-blind study of sodium-magnesium EDTA in peripheral vascular disease. *J Nat Med Assoc.* 82(3): 173–177.

WEIL, A. 1995. *Natural Health, Natural Medicine.* Boston: Houghton Mifflin Co.

RESOURCES

American Board of Chelation Therapy
1407-B North Wells
Chicago, IL 60610

American College for Advancement in Medicine
23121 Verdugo Drive, Suite 204
Laguna Hills, CA 92653
800-532-3688
714-583-7666
www.acam.org
email: acam@acam.com

International Association for Colon Therapy
2051 Hilltop Dr., Suite A 11
Redding, CA 96002
916-222-1498

International Association for Colon Hydrotherapy
P.O. Box 461285
San Antonio, TX 78246
210-366-2888
email: iact@health.net

25 Animal-Assisted Therapy

No one is immune to the uplifting effects of birdsong. We all savor those warm spring mornings when we step outside and hear the light, musical conversation of wild birds. Domesticated birds provide their owners with similar pleasures, and those pleasures are compounded by the gift of companionship.

William H. Thomas, Life Worth Living

Animal-Assisted Therapy (AAT) is defined as the use of specifically selected animals as a treatment modality in health and human service settings. AAT has been steadily gaining in popularity in the United States and has been shown to be a successful intervention for people with a variety of physical or psychological conditions. Despite reluctance and skepticism on the part of many administrators of health care facilities, nurses have often advocated the use of animals as a therapeutic intervention. One of the earliest recorded observations of a connection between animals and health was made by Florence Nightingale (1969, p. 103) in 1860 when she noted that "a small pet is often an excellent companion for the sick, for long chronic cases especially." She further suggested that whenever possible, patients should participate in the care of the animal because this activity was helpful to their recovery. Long banned from health care facilities, dogs, cats, and other pets are gradually being welcomed with open arms.

BACKGROUND

The York Retreat in England, founded in 1792 for the treatment of people with mental illness, used small animals such as rabbits and poultry in their treatment plan. The goal was to decrease the use of restraints and medications by helping residents learn self-control through animals that relied on them for care. Bethel, a residential treatment center for people with epilepsy, founded

388

in 1867 in Germany, utilized pets as an important part of the treatment program. This pet program is still in place today and has expanded to include farm animals and a wild game park (Perelle and Granville, 1998). In the United States in the 1940s, injured World War II soldiers were encouraged to work with the hogs, cattle, and horses on the farm of the Army Air Corps Convalescent Hospital in New York. Since that time, animals have been used in many U.S. clinical settings from pediatrics to geriatrics, acute-care facilities to chronic care homes, from group accommodations to private homes, from prevention to healing, and even from schools to correctional facilities nationwide (Jorgenson, 1997).

PREPARATION

In the 1990s, the Delta Society developed the first comprehensive standards of practice for animal-assisted therapy. Now in its second edition, *Standards of Practice for Animal-Assisted Activities and Animal-Assisted Therapy* (1996) defines the role of animals in therapeutic programs.

Therapy dogs and cats are specifically selected for temperament, companionability, and interaction. Temperament is the animal's natural or instinctive behavior and is important in terms of the way the animal will react when stressed. A good therapy pet is calm, tolerant, and friendly. The second major criterion is that the animal has a person who is willing to volunteer time and energy in order to share the pet with others. Dogs must be obedience trained prior to participating in the program. A dog or cat must be at least one year of age before enrolling in the training and visiting program to better ensure that the pet has been effectively socialized and is comfortable interacting with numerous people in a crowded setting. In addition, the animal's immune system is more stabilized by this age. The animal's health must be verified by a veterinarian and all inoculations must be current. AAT-registering organizations require that a dog and its handler pass several tests prior to registration. In general, dogs have to demonstrate basic obedience skills and must be indifferent to crowds and distractions and unfazed by exuberant or clumsy handling, including ear tugging and "bear hugging." In addition, they must have a high tolerance for unfamiliar or loud noises and peculiar smells. Therapeutic riding horses must have a gentle, tolerant temperament, be well balanced and well muscled, and move with even strides. In addition to the familiar dogs and cats in pet therapy, other animals may include parrots, cockatoos, guinea pigs, rabbits, pot-bellied pigs, dwarf goats, llamas, donkeys, and horses.

Animal handler volunteers are trained in workshops or through home study courses. The handlers must pass a written test and their animals must pass a skills test. Participation in continuing education is required. Nurses, physical

and occupational therapists, psychotherapists, and other health care professionals must receive training to direct animal-assisted therapy programs. This
educational process is still in the beginning stages and at this time is primarily
accomplished through in-service training, and seminars and workshops at national and international professional meetings (Hines and Fredrickson, 1998).

Twelve countries, including the United States, offer formalized educational programs for registration, certification, or licensure of therapists. These
programs have intermittent sessions which may span one to two years. Most
frequently this specialized training is offered to physical therapists, occupational therapists, psychotherapists, and special education teachers (Fitzpatrick
and Tebay, 1998).

CONCEPTS

Companion Animals

Many people think of their animals as surrogate children. But one big exception is that these are children who rarely, if ever, disappoint their parents. Pets,
especially dogs, often seem to understand what their owners are feeling. For
some people, a pet is a reason to get up in the morning. It is something to nurture, touch, and stroke. For stress relief, it apparently does not matter much
whether the pet is a Labrador, a tom cat, or a canary. What is most important
is the person's relationship with the pet.

The contributions companion animals make to the emotional well-being
of people include providing unconditional love and opportunities for affection;
functioning as a confidant, playmate, and companion; and assisting in the
achievement of trust, responsibility, and empathy toward others. Studies of
children with pets indicate that the unconditional love and acceptance conveyed
in the child-animal relationship may validate a child's sense of self-worth. In
addition, older school-age children often turn to companion animals in times
of stress for reassurance. Children often perceive their companion animals as
play partners, most often during middle childhood than during adolescence or
early childhood (Melson, 1998; Triebenbacher, 1998).

Children with interactive pets such as dogs and cats are more attached to
their companion animals than are children with other types of pets such as
hamsters, fish, and turtles. Emotional bonds are more likely to be formed with
animals that are able to respond in an outwardly loving and affectionate way.
Behaviors such as tail wagging, barking, and purring often elicit affectionate
responses in human caregivers. In North America and Europe, pets are found
in the majority of homes with children. Families with children, especially
school-age children, are more likely to own companion animals than are

families without children. Multiple-pet ownership is also common. Pet ownership remains higher in rural versus urban areas, and in houses versus apartments. Still, across a variety of settings, the majority of children in Western countries are living with companion animals (Melson, 1998; Triebenbacher, 1998).

Therapy Animals

The characteristics that make many pets cherished family members—unconditional affection, responsiveness, and companionability—also make pets effective in therapy. In this age of high technological health care, it is sometimes easy to forget the importance of unconditional affection. Animals pay little attention to age or physical ability, but accept people as they are. It is insignificant if the person has no hair, is in a wheelchair, or is hallucinating. The underlying concept that supports the use of animals for therapeutic reasons is the bonding experience it provides. Frail or depressed older adults often brighten up and adopt a more positive outlook when they are in the presence of an animal "therapist."

Many health care professionals are finding that loneliness may be as serious as cancer and heart disease for older adults. Older people who stay active, find substitutes for work, and build new relationships as partners and friends die have been found most satisfied with life. Not all older adults, however, have options for remaining active and forming new friendships. Visiting with animals can help people feel less lonely and less depressed. Animals can provide a welcome change from routine or a distraction from disability or pain. People often talk to the animals and share with them their thoughts, feelings, and memories. When people talk to people, their blood pressure tends to go up because of questions of how one is being evaluated or judged. With animals, who are always eager to please and unconditionally accepting, people's blood pressure tends to go down (Jennings et al., 1998; Keil, 1998).

Animals also make it easier for two strangers to talk. They give people a common interest, provide a focus for conversation, and broaden the circle of friends. When animals visit long-term care facilities, residents laugh and mingle more than when the animals are not around. Animals also help stimulate socialization by providing an opportunity to share stories of animals the residents may have had in the past. Many people like to stroke the animal while talking about the pets who shared their lives.

Three significant problems that manifest within traditional long-term care facilities are loneliness, helplessness, and boredom. They often have not served as homes for people, but rather as institutions in which to store them. Residents may be intensely lonely, with long stretches of empty time. The basic concept of the Eden Alternative, a new approach to long-term care, is quite simple: long-term care facilities are viewed as habitats for human beings rather than institutions for the frail and elderly. The Eden Alternative seeks to eliminate the problems of loneliness, helplessness, and boredom by providing interaction with companion animals, the opportunity to care for other living things, and a milieu of variety and spontaneity. "Edenized" facilities share a commitment to change the system, and not just through "fur and feathers." Quality of life is emphasized as much as the quality of care. Residents and employees alike are encouraged to play a role in making that quality atmosphere happen. Administrators recognize that the care a resident receives is usually completed in 3–4 hours of the day, leaving 20 hours to live a life. As the U.S. population ages, and with growing frustration with traditional systems, long-term care facilities will have to be managed far differently than they are today. The Eden Alternative is the most innovative reform effort to date (Thomas, 1996; Thomas, 1998).

TREATMENT

Animal-Assisted Therapy

Animal-Assisted Therapy is the use of specifically selected animals as a treatment modality in health and human service settings. In AAT, an accredited professional guides the human-animal interaction toward specific, individualized therapeutic goals. In one treatment session, a variety of goals can be addressed: physical goals such as range of motion, balance, and mobility; cognitive goals such as improved memory or verbal expression; emotional goals such as increased self-esteem and motivation; and social goals such as building rapport and improved socialization skills. Linda Hume, L.P.N., AAT specialist, has developed a program of animal facilitation in occupational and physical therapy at Northeast Rehabilitation Hospital in Salem, New Hampshire. The following are a few of the goals and activities she has identified for AAT in her clinical setting (Hume, 1996):

- Increased upper extremity range of motion: throw an object for dog to retrieve; use of leash to maneuver dog; pet, stroke, brush animal
- Mobility: ambulate with dog
- Improved coordination: throw an object for dog to retrieve (releasing); reaching for object dog has retrieved
- Improved memory: asked to recall dog's name, breed, age, etc.; commanding dog to sit and remembering to release dog from command
- Increased language production: use of commands with dog; simply conversing to or about animal

- Object identification: direct dog to retrieve specific familiar items by appropriate name—ball, spoon, pen, cup
- Attention/Concentration: attending to dog, task, and therapist

Therapeutic horseback riding, available in at least 21 countries, is defined as all rehabilitative uses of horses. In equine-assisted psychotherapy, the riding is designed to support the psychotherapeutic treatment plan. Goals include increased self-confidence, improved self-esteem, refined social competence, the experience of pleasure, and the ability to establish a relationship with the horse. Remedial educational riding is used to further the educational and behavioral goals for school-age children with learning problems. The horse is used as a strong motivator for accomplishing specific treatment goals. Hippotherapy is the use of the rhythmic movement of the horse to increase sensory processing and improve posture, balance, and mobility in people with movement dysfunctions. The term derives from the Greek word *hippo* meaning horse. The transfer of movement from the horse to the client is designed primarily to achieve physical goals but may also effect psychological, cognitive, behavioral, and communication outcomes. Clients benefiting from hippotherapy include, but are not limited to, adults and children with cerebral palsy, multiple sclerosis, orthopedic problems, posttraumatic spasticity, strokes, scoliosis, genetic syndromes, and developmental delays (Fitzpatrick and Tebay, 1998).

Animal-Assisted Activities

A less formal approach, Animal-Assisted Activities (AAA) are motivational, educational, and recreational. The goal is to provide "meeting and greeting" human-animal interactions to enhance the quality of life, rather than a specific treatment plan. AAA is used in many types of facilities with a wide variety of animals. AAA visits to sheltered homeless families has been effective. Most shelters do not allow families to bring their pets, and seeing the visiting animal can be therapeutic, especially for children. AAA visits give homeless children a chance to participate in everyday experiences they may not have had recently, such as walking a dog or playing fetch (Albert, 1996).

Pet Visits

A family pet visit is an arrangement for a pet to visit the owner in the health care setting. The concept of pet visits as therapy for hospitalized people is not new, especially in facilities with rehabilitation and mental health units. The pet that visits may belong to a pet therapy program or may be the client's own pet. The University of Utah Hospital in Salt Lake City has had a pet visitation policy for many years. They believe that allowing a pet to visit can be a heal-ing experience for patients, family members, and even the pet. Pets are even allowed to visit in ICU settings, with the approval of the nurses, provided no medical contraindications are present (Martin, 1993).

Resident Animals

A resident animal lives at the health care facility. The staff is responsible for the complete health and well-being of the animal and residents are included in providing routine daily care. Grooming and brushing, for example, are good therapies for the hands. Some staff report that full-time pets become so per-ceptive that they actually gravitate to the rooms of people who are the most iso-lated or depressed. Those residents who have regular visits are more receptive to treatment, have a greater incentive to recover, and have an increased will to live (Keil, 1998).

Eden Alternative

In the Eden Alternative, nursing homes are places where the residents give as well as receive care and where a diversity of species create a natural habitat. The approach uses animals, plants, and children to interact with residents of long-term care centers, creating a "human habitat" that makes the residents feel more at home—and not so much in one. Resident animals are part of the total environment. Children and teenagers from schools and youth volunteer programs frequently visit the home. They come in and interact and build rela-tionships with residents, as opposed to the usual pattern of coming in, putting on a program, and leaving.

The Eden Alternative empowers residents and the staff members who come into daily contact with them. Residents have more say in their activities, menus, and daily routines; caregivers, maintenance workers, and other em-ployees can set their own work schedules, within given parameters. Support-ers of the program believe that employees frequently seem happier in Eden homes as evidenced by fewer sick days and lower staff turnover. The Eden Al-ternative is really about liberating the spirit of the people who are living and working in long-term care.

The movement remains loosely organized, spreading largely by word of mouth. North Carolina has declared unofficially that it is an Eden Alterna-tive state and has assembled a special coalition giving financial aid grants to encourage facilities to adopt Eden techniques. The Lt. Governor of Missouri, Roger B. Wilson, has asked the state's Division of Aging to help promote Eden. About 60 facilities there are in the process of implementing programs. Eden programs are also popular in New York, where William Thomas, M.D., founded the approach. Eden Alternative got its start in nursing homes but has grown to include adult day care services and assisted-living facilities (Levine, 1997).

Service Dogs

Service dogs are individually trained to do work or perform tasks for a person with a physical or emotional disability. They may legally go anywhere that a person with disabilities goes. Most people are familiar with guide dogs for those with visual impairment. Other service dogs can be trained to pull a wheelchair, open doors, retrieve dropped objects as small as a dime, and turn light switches on and off. Hearing dogs alert owners to important sounds that need a response. Seizure response dogs recognize behaviors associated with their owner's seizures and can be trained to stay with the person or get help. When breathing machines malfunction, service dogs can be trained to nose the phone receiver out of its cradle and hit the speed-dial buttons, all of which are programmed to 911. Training service dogs is an expensive and time-consuming project. The dog spends the first year of life with a foster family who is responsible for socialization and basic obedience training. Next comes five to six months of intensive training followed by six months of in-home training with the new owner. The benefit, of course, is that people can lead more independent and fulfilling lives.

In correctional institutes all across Ohio, puppies and prisoners are teaming up in an unusual program. A nonprofit organization called Pilot Dogs, Inc., places service puppies under the care of prisoners until the pups are ready for formal training as service dogs. Since the inception of the program in 1992, some 250 dogs have been placed in prisons. Inmates are chosen based on their records of good behavior and experience with dogs. No violent offenders are permitted to raise the dogs. The puppies sleep in crates in the cells with their partners and accompany them on their daily activities, including trips to the dining hall where the puppies learn to be well-behaved around people and become accustomed to the noise and crowds they will be faced with later. The prisoner is responsible for the care and well-being of the dog, housebreaking them, leash-training them, and putting them through a basic obedience course. After spending about 12 months at the correctional facility, the puppies are removed and placed in an intensive training program. A major advantage for the dogs is having human contact 24 hours a day, which is less likely to occur in regular foster homes. The chosen prisoners have the pleasure and delight of having a puppy to give love to and get love from. They also have the satisfaction of seeing the benefits of their training as the puppies progress (New Leash on Life, 1998).

RESEARCH

To date, much of the literature on the therapeutic use of animals in health care is anecdotal, but scientific research is beginning to appear. Research projects have demonstrated the following:

- A link can be made between animal companionship and improved cardiovascular health: for patients who were hospitalized with a diagnosis of myocardial infarction or angina pectoris, one year later, 28 percent of nonpet owners had died compared to 6 percent of pet owners (Friedmann et al., 1980). This study was replicated with similar results by Friedmann and Thomas in 1995.
- A study of 5,741 healthy participants in a cardiovascular screening program demonstrated that pet owners had significantly lower systolic blood pressure and plasma triglycerides than nonowners. Many pet owners had significantly lower cholesterol values (Jennings et al., 1998).
- A 10-month prospective study indicated that those people who owned a dog or a cat reported a significant reduction in minor health problems and a significant improvement in psychological well-being (Serpell, 1990).
- The introduction of visiting animals into a nursing home environment resulted in an immediate significant improvement in residents' social and self-maintenance behaviors, an increase that was maintained for at least one month after termination of the study (Perelle and Granville, 1998).
- Research being conducted by Southwest Texas State University at six Eden facilities has demonstrated a 33 percent decrease in the use of antianxiety and antidepressant drugs, and a 44 percent decrease in employee absenteeism at five sites.
- Hippotherapy research studies have been published in Germany, Switzerland, Austria, Italy, Belgium, Finland, and France. The U.S. studies are pending publication. Brazil, England, and Israel have studies in progress (Fitzpatrick and Tebay, 1998).
- Heipertz-Hengst (1994) has developed a standard client assessment form to be used before and after a hippotherapeutic treatment.
- In a study of 153 people with paraplegia and spasticity, 105 experienced reduction in spasticity for 2–36 hours after hippotherapy (Engelmann, 1994).

One of the largest organizations devoted to animal-assisted therapy is the Delta Society, composed of 1,500 members, 20 percent of whom are health care professionals. The objectives of the Delta Society are to promote study and research relating to human-animal interactions, increase the awareness of the significance of these interactions among health care professionals, and assess the role of the effect of human-pet bonds on the mental and physical well-being of people. Pets and People, a nonprofit volunteer agency founded in 1994, supports the research endeavors of graduate nursing students from the University of Southern Mississippi and Louisiana State University.

INTEGRATED NURSING PRACTICE

An important nursing role is that of advocate. Nurse advocates serve as links between clients and other health care professionals of the community. It is in that role that nurses in a wide variety of clinical settings can explore and encourage the therapeutic use of animals. The benefits of human-animal interaction are many and include such things as attachment, bonding, caring, pain management, stress management, motivation, communication, improved self-esteem, cardiovascular benefits, and improved coordination and balance. Disinterest on the part of health care professionals has been the major obstacle to growth in the field of animal-assisted therapy. As Hines and Fredrickson (1998, p. 36) have said, "Even in the area of cardiac health, in which studies have clearly indicated pet ownership as a positive factor, the medical community does not routinely incorporate this information into patient care."

To set up an animal-assisted therapy program, you must begin by approaching the facility's administration with a well-organized plan. This plan should include the following aspects:

- Theory and research background
- Goals and outcomes
- Clearly written policy and procedures
- Staff education about the proposed program
- A plan for volunteer recruitment and training
- A plan for testing and training of potential therapy animals
- A plan for implementation of the program
- A plan for evaluation of the program

You can anticipate some opposition to the initiation of an animal-assisted therapy program. One of the biggest concerns is the potential for transmission of infectious diseases. Although the risk is low, several zoonoses, or animal-transmitted infections, can occur. Seek the assistance of a veterinarian to identify the risks for specific types of infections and measures to prevent them. Infection risk can be reduced by making sure each animal is clean, vaccinated, and healthy;

keeping the animal out of the areas where food is prepared and served; and having residents wash their hands after the animal visits. Products can be sprayed on the animal's fur to reduce the risk of an allergic reaction. Huntington Memorial Hospital (1992) in Pasadena, California, has been host to more than 3,000 dog visits in five years. In that time, no zoonotic infection has been reported.

The Rehabilitation Unit at Duke University Medical Center, North Carolina, has begun a pilot program for therapeutic animals. The goals are to provide clients with the following opportunities (Jorgenson, 1997):

- Use recreational, animal-assisted activities to improve stress management
- Provide diversional activities
- Provide reminiscence therapy
- Increase gross and fine motor skills
- Improve cognitive skills
- Increase social interaction

If you are a pet owner, you can consider becoming a pet therapy volunteer. Many long-term care facilities encourage regular visits from people with trained and screened animals. Increasingly, these pets are also welcome at hospitals, cancer clinics, and hospices. This type of personal involvement in animal-assisted therapy can be wonderfully rewarding.

As a nurse you have wonderful opportunities to incorporate AAT in your work with people infected with human immunodeficiency virus (HIV) and those with Acquired Immune Deficiency Syndrome (AIDS). In the past, these individuals have been told to give up their pets for fear that their compromised immune system would place them at high risk for zoonotic infections. The reality is that people are more likely to contract zoonotic infections from contaminated food, water, soil, or even other people than from pets. You may need to explain to some clients that the HIV virus only infects humans and other primates and, therefore, cannot be spread from or to dogs, cats, birds, or even fish. With this understanding, you can become an advocate for the physical, emotional, and psychological benefits of pet companionship for those with HIV/AIDS.

With proper care and understanding and a healthy pet, the potential health risks of pet companionship are minimal and the benefits may far outweigh the risks. People living with HIV often deal with feelings of isolation, rejection, and lack of purpose. For such people, companion animals offer purpose, a feeling of being needed, a way to increase socialization, and a constant source of unconditional affection. If clients are selecting a new pet, they should consider one whose temperament, energy level, and environmental needs match their own. An older pet may be more appropriate than a young one. Box 25.1 describes the client teaching you should do with HIV/AIDS clients. The pre-

Box 25.1: Client Teaching: Pet Owners with HIV/AIDS

Veterinary Care

- Have your veterinarian examine your pet initially and then at least once a year.
- Keep your pet up to date on annual shots and rabies vaccination.
- Seek veterinary care immediately for sick pets.
- Street animals that are "adopted" should first be checked by a veterinarian before being brought into your home.

Pet Care

- Keep your pet clean and well groomed with short, blunt toenails.
- Keep the pet's living and feeding areas clean.
- Keep your cat's litter box out of the kitchen, use a litter box liner and change it daily.
- Always walk your pet on a leash and minimize the pet's contact with other animals and garbage.
- Cats should be kept indoors and be prevented from hunting birds and rodents.
- Feed your pet only commercially prepared pet foods; never feed raw meat or unpasteurized milk.
- Do not allow birds to fly free in your home; you must avoid their droppings.

General Hygiene

- Wash your hands frequently, especially before eating, smoking, or attending to open wounds.
- Keep your cat off all kitchen surfaces. If not possible, be sure to wipe down, with a gentle disinfectant, any surface on which food may be placed.
- Do not allow your dog to drink out of the toilet because it is a place of many germs.
- Try to avoid contact with your pet's bodily fluids. Gloves and a face mask should be worn for clean up including cleaning a litter box, aquarium, or bird cage.

Sources: POWARS—New York, NY; PAWS—San Francisco, CA; The Delta Society—Renton, WA; Action AIDS—Philadelphia, PA.

cautions are designed to protect the immunocompromised person from acquiring secondary infections.

A number of communities provide services to enable people with AIDS to keep their pets. Volunteers provide dog-walking service for people physically unable to walk their dogs, deliver pet food and supplies, clean litter boxes and bird cages, provide in-home care for cats whose owners must go to the hospital, and foster care for dogs in the same situation. You could volunteer your time and energy to this type of program, or if your community has no such program, you could establish one.

The Eden Alternative is a new way of thinking about long-term care facilities. Nurses are in an extraordinary position to teach others about what the Eden Alternative is and how they can use it to transform the facilities in which they practice. Before you can educate others, it is important that you become familiar with the concepts and the Ten Principles of the Eden Alternative. The principles, developed by Eden Alternative founder, William Thomas, M.D., and his wife, Judith, and are as follows:

1. Understand that loneliness, helplessness, and boredom account for the bulk of suffering among our frail elders.

2. Surrender the institutional point of view and adopt the Human Habitat model that makes pets, plants, and children the axis around which daily life turns.

3. Provide easy access to companionship by promoting close and continuing contact between the elements of the Human Habitat and the people who live and work within it.

4. Create opportunities to give as well as receive care by promoting our elders' participation in the daily round of activities that are necessary to maintain the Human Habitat.

5. Imbue daily life with variety and spontaneity by creating an environment in which unexpected and unpredictable interactions and happenings can take place.

6. Deemphasize the programmed activities approach to life and devote these resources to the maintenance and growth of the Human Habitat.

7. Deemphasize the role of prescription drugs in our elders' daily life and commit these resources to the maintenance and growth of the Human Habitat.

8. Deemphasize top-down bureaucratic authority in the facility and seek instead to place the maximum possible decision-making authority in the hands of those closest to those for whom we care.

TRY THIS: *Interacting with Your Pet*

When you are feeling tense or anxious and if you have a dog or a cat to whom you are attached, try this:

- Note your physical and emotional signs of tension: are your hands clenched? body trembling? restlessness? unable to relax? mouth dry? stomach upset? breathing more rapid? unable to concentrate? worrying?
- Do something with your pet for at least 20 minutes: play, groom, or talk.
- Conduct another self-assessment. What, if anything, has changed?

If you have a dog or a cat to whom you are attached, try this:

- Have a friend take your pulse and blood pressure.
- Gently play with your pet, stroke, pet, and talk to your animal for 15 minutes.
- Have your friend take your pulse and blood pressure again and compare the results to those taken prior to the interaction.

9. Understand that Edenizing is a never-ending process, NOT a program and that the Human Habitat, once created, should be helped to grow and develop like any other living thing.

10. Appoint leadership that places the need to improve resident quality of life over and above the inevitable objections to change. Leadership is the lifeblood of the Edenizing process and for it there is no substitute.

Miriam Stermer, a Certified Eden Associate from Charlotte, North Carolina, has further expanded these principles to enable you to evaluate the environment in which you practice or the environment in which your family elder may be living and what changes you might advocate to move in the direction of Edenizing the long-term care facility.

- What kind of companionship is provided for residents?
- How many and what kinds of animal live in the facility?
- What are the gardening opportunities?

- What opportunities do residents have to provide care rather than just receive care? Are residents encouraged to provide care for their plants and animals?
- Are children part of everyday life? Are there opportunities for one-to-one relationships?
- Are chemical restraints recognized as such? Does the facility pursue a restraint-free environment? Are problem behaviors approached in a holistic manner?
- Are planning teams consisting of residents, family members, staff, and community members in place?
- Has the facility committed time, money, and energy to make the approach an ongoing, continuing process?
- Does the administrator understand the Eden alternative philosophy and is she or he a leader in this process?

As the number of elderly persons increases in the United States, not only will the demand for more assisted living and long-term care facilities increase, but so too will the demand for alternatives to the traditional systems. As Thomas (1996, p. 14) describes it:

> As it stands now, nursing homes deliver a low perceived value at a high cost. To make matters worse, this situation is compounded by social trends that are weakening the sense of obligation across the generations. Ultimately, the elderly must depend on this sense of obligation for protection and sustenance.

Animal contact contributes to self-concept, social interaction, a decrease in loneliness and anxiety, and in general contributes to physical, psychological, and spiritual well-being. Nurses can and should be at the forefront of designing and supporting more humane approaches to those in our care.

REFERENCES

ALBERT, T. 1996. Visiting families who are homeless. *Pet Partners Newsletter.* 6(1): 1–2.

ENGELMANN, A. 1994. Hippotherapy results in paraplegic patients. In *Proceedings of the 8th International Therapeutic Riding Congress* (pp. 242–244). Levin, New Zealand: National Training Resource Center.

FITZPATRICK, J. C. and J. M. Tebay. 1998. Hippotherapy and therapeutic riding. In C. C. WILSON, D. C. TURNER, eds. *Companion Animals in Human Health.* Thousand Oaks, CA: Sage Pub., 41–58.

FRIEDMANN, E., A. H. KATCHER, J. J. LYNCH, and S. A. THOMAS. 1980. Animal companions and one-year survival of patients after discharge from a coronary care unit. *Public Health Reports.* 95(4): 307–312.

FRIEDMANN, E. and S. A. THOMAS. 1995. Pet ownership, social support, and one-year survival after acute myocardial infarction in the cardiac arrhythmia suppression trial CAST. *Am J Cardiology.* 76: 1213–1217.

HEIPERTZ-HENGST, C. 1994. Evaluation of outcome in hippotherapy. In *Proceedings of the 8th International Therapeutic Riding Congress* (pp. 217–221). Levin, New Zealand: National Training Resource Center.

HINES, L. and M. FREDRICKSON. 1998. Perspectives on animal-assisted activities and therapy. In C. C. WILSON and D. C. TURNER, eds. *Companion Animals in Human Health.* Thousand Oaks, CA: Sage Pub., 23–39.

Huntington Memorial Hospital. December 1992. Patients best friend? Hospital dogs raise spirits, not infection rates. *Hospital Infection Control.* Interagency Communication.

HUME, L. 1996. Animal facilitation in occupational and physical therapy sessions. www.rehabnet.com/aft/cdaft.html

JENNINGS, G. L. R et al. 1998. Animals and cardiovascular health. In C. C. WILSON and D. C. TURNER, eds. *Companion Animals in Human Health.* Thousand Oaks, CA: Sage Pub., 161–171.

JORGENSON, J. 1997. Therapeutic use of companion animals in health care. *Image.* 29(3): 249–254.

KEIL, C. P. 1998. In C. C. WILSON and D. C. TURNER, eds. *Companion Animals in Human Health.* Thousand Oaks, CA: Sage Pub., 123–134.

LEVINE, S. November 21, 1997. Creating an Eden for seniors. *Washington Post,* A01. washingtonpost.com/wp-srv/local/longterm/library/eden.html

MARTIN, S. 1993. Ask the experts. *Critical Care Nurse.* 13(2): 74, 79.

MELSON, G. F. 1998. The role of companion animals in human development. In C. C. WILSON and D. C. TURNER, eds. *Companion Animals in Human Health.* Thousand Oaks, CA: Sage Pub., 219–236.

New Leash on Life, 1998. *You and Your Dog.* 4(3): 12–13.

NIGHTINGALE, F. 1969. *Notes on Nursing.* New York: Dover Pub.

PERELLE, I. B. and D. A. GRANVILLE. 1998. Assessment of the effectiveness of a pet-facilitated therapy program in a nursing home setting. www.arrs.envirolink.org/psyeta/sa/sal.1/perelle.html

SERPELL, J. A. 1990. Evidence for long-term effects of pet ownership on human health. *Waltham Symposium 20: Pets, Benefits, & Practice.* First European Congress of the British Small Animal Veterinary Assoc. Cheltenham, England: BVA Pub.

Standards of Practice for Animal-Assisted Activities and Animal-Assisted Therapy, 2d ed. 1996. Renton, WA: Delta Society.

THOMAS, W. H. 1998. *Open Hearts, Open Minds.* Acton, MA: VanderWyk & Burnham.

THOMAS, W. H. 1996. *Life Worth Living.* Acton, MA: VanderWyk & Burnham.

TRIEBENBACHER, S. L. 1998. The relationship between attachment to companion animals and self-esteem. In C. C. WILSON and D. C. TURNER, eds. *Companion Animals in Human Health.* Thousand Oaks, CA: Sage Pub., 135–148.

RESOURCES

American Hippotherapy Association,
North American Riding for the Handicapped Association
P.O. Box 33150
Denver, CO 80233

The Delta Society
289 Perimeter Road E.
Renton, WA 98055-1329
800-869-6898
206-226-7357
www2.deltasociety.org/deltasociety/
email: deltasociety@cis.compuserve.com

The Eden Alternative
742 Turnpike Rd.
Sherburne, NY 13460
607-674-5232
607-674-6723 fax
www.edenalt.com

Federation of Riding for the Disabled International
Am Zaarshauschen 22
51427 Bergisch Gladbach, Germany

Pet Owners with HIV/AIDS Resource Service, Inc. (POWARS)
1674 Broadway, Suite 7A
New York, NY 10019
212-246-6307
212-246-6523 fax

Pets and People
Pat Gonser Ph.D., R.N.
P.O. Box 4266
West Station
Meridian MS 39307
601-483-8970
601-484-0402

Pilot Dogs Program
625 West Town St.
Columbus, OH 43215

St. John Ambulance Therapy Dog Program
1199 Deyell 3rd Line
Milbrook, Ontario LOA 1GO Canada

Therapy Dog International
719 Darla Lane
Fallbrook, CA 92028-1505
973-252-9800
973-252-7171 fax
email: tdi@gti.net

Therapy Dogs Incorporated
P.O. Box 2786
Cheyenne, WY 82003
307-638-3223

Therapet
P.O. Box 1696
Whitehouse, TX 75791
Shari Bernard, OTR
email: therapet@juno.com

Alternative Therapies for Common Health Problems

This appendix is meant to provide education relating to the management of minor health problems. These types of problems often respond well to alternative therapies and lifestyle modification. If in doubt of the seriousness of symptoms, see your health care practitioner. A number of suggestions are given for various problems. Select one that seems to be the most appropriate for your situation and keep notes on what seems to work and what does not. Modify these suggestions according to your individual needs.

Abrasions, scrapes

- Aromatherapy: after washing with soap and water, apply 1–3 drops of lavender or tea tree to wound; reapply oil 2 times a day until healed
- To disinfect, pour 3% hydrogen peroxide into the wound and let it foam up
- Apply the skin of a freshly peeled banana to the affected area, or cut a thin slice of raw potato and tape it over the affected area
- Herbs: sprinkle goldenseal powder in wound, crushed garlic mixed with honey makes a soothing salve—spread on a piece of clean gauze and cover the injured area

Acne

- Aromatherapy: bergamot, cedarwood, chamomile, clary sage, lemon grass, melissa, patchouli, rosemary, sandalwood, tea tree, thyme, ylang-ylang—can be made into a facial mask, compress, or topical cream; tea tree oil and lavender can be applied directly to blemishes

- Herbs: arnica, calendula skin products
- Drink plenty of water to flush out the system
- Supplements: 500 units of vitamin A, 5 mg zinc, or 1500 mg evening primrose oil

AIDS

- Acupuncture
- Herbs: curcumin, extract of boxwood plant
- Massage
- Supplements: Iron, vitamins C, E, and Bs; beta carotene, glutamine, selenium

Allergies

- Applied Kinesiology
- Herbs: stinging nettles to lessen runny nose and sneezing; teas made from chamomile, elder, or yarrow flowers can reduce reactions
- Homeopathy: allium cepa (onion); windflower, for swelling in the face— 1 tablet of apis every 15 minutes—maximum 6 doses
- Supplements: vitamin C to decrease histamine production

Alzheimer's disease (dementia)

- Herbs: ginkgo 120–240 mg daily
- Supplements: zinc, selenium, evening primrose oil

Alcohol abuse

- Acupuncture
- Herbs: milk thistle, kudzu
- Meditation
- Yoga

Amputations: phantom pain

- Magnets: improve blood flow to stump and cause phantom pain to disappear
- Massage

Anxiety

- Acupressure: press center of inside wrist 1 inch above crease toward elbow
- Animal-assisted therapy
- Aromatherapy: basil, bergamot, chamomile, frankincense deepens breathing to induce calmness, green apple, juniper, lemon balm, orange, neroli for panic attacks
- Biofeedback
- Healing Touch
- Herbs: valerian, passion flower, kava kava
- Homeopathy: St. Ignatius bean, arsenic
- Massage
- Meditation
- Reiki
- Relaxation techniques
- Therapeutic Touch
- Performance anxiety—hypnosis, guided imagery, Alexander Technique

Arthritis

- Aromatherapy: cedarwood, coriander, cypress massage or cold compress, compress of rosemary to swollen joints
- Exercise in water (nonweight-bearing) or moderate exercise as tolerated
- Feldenkrais Method
- Herbs: devil's claw, boswellia, evening primrose oil; ginger; capsaicin cream applied topically, glucosamine (1500 mg) and chondroitin (1200 mg) to help restore joint integrity; natural anti-inflammatories like willowbark, turmeric, and ginger
- Homeopathy: poison ivy
- Ice joints and then rub in analgesic oils
- Magnets placed over an inflamed area on regular basis
- Reflexology: all joints of the hands and feet should be worked for pain relief and mobility of corresponding body joints
- Supplements: thiamine, vitamins B_6, B_{12}
- Therapeutic Touch
- Yoga: practice slowly, seeing how far the affected joints can be moved without pain; do not exercise joints when they are inflamed

Asthma

- Acupuncture
- Alexander Technique: teaches a more relaxed way of breathing and enables you to manage yourself better during an asthma attack
- Aromatherapy: put several drops of cypress on a handkerchief and inhale deeply; put frankincense on a pillow at night to slow and deepen the breathing
- Biofeedback
- Breathing exercises
- Hypnosis
- Herbs: holy basil, elecampine, country mallow, malabar nut, bayberry; mix 3 parts tincture of lobelia with 1 part tincture of capsicum—take 20 drops in water at the start of an asthmatic attack—repeat every 30 minutes for a total of 3 or 4 doses
- Homeopathy: Arsenicum album, 1 tablet 3 times daily; maximum 1 week
- Meditation
- Reflexology: during an asthma attack, work the reflexes for the diaphragm and lungs on the balls of the feet
- Water—drink plenty of water to keep the respiratory tract secretions fluid
- Yoga: focus on expansive postures and breathing practices designed to increase the length of the exhalation

Athlete's foot

- Acupressure: do full foot or hand acupressure massage session twice a week to stimulate the immune and endocrine systems; do not press on broken, sore, or cracked skin areas
- Aromatherapy: cedarwood, lemon balm, rosemary; mix 2 drops lavender oil and 1 drop tea tree oil and apply between toes
- Herbs: black walnut tincture—apply directly to fungus patches and drink a tea of green crushed walnut hulls for fungus anywhere in body
- Naturopathy: take 2 Kyolic garlic tablets TID, decrease to BID when all infections are healed; dust your feet and shoes with garlic powder
- Supplements: take B-complex vitamins, 50–100 TID with meals; dust vitamin C powder directly onto affected area; zinc may help clear the skin and boost the immune system

Attention Deficit Disorder

- Biofeedback
- Supplements: B vitamins

Back pain

- Acupuncture
- Alexander Technique: teaches a more balanced used of body since muscular imbalance often contributes to back pain
- Applied kinesiology
- Biofeedback
- Chiropractic manipulation
- Herbs: valerian, nutmeg, gotu kola; to ease local discomfort soak a compress in 1/2 cup hot water containing 1 tbsp. camp bark and 1 tsp. cinnamon tinctures
- Homeopathy: 4 tablets of arnica as soon as possible after an injury and repeat every hour for the first day while awake, second day—4 tablets every 2 hours; third day—4 tablets four times
- Hydrotherapy: for acute back pain, use an ice pack on affected area for 20 minutes every 1–2 hours
- Magnets: place small magnets over area of muscle spasm in back
- Massage with warm oil
- Reflexology: work the spinal reflexes, especially the tender points, on the medial longitudinal arches of the feet (the bony ridges on the inside)
- Sleep on back with pillows under knees or on side with pillow between bent knees
- Yoga: lie down with legs bent, feet flat on floor, exhale fully and slowly for at least 12 breaths; long-term yoga practice can strengthen back muscles

Balance problems

- Qigong
- T'ai Chi
- Hippotherapy

Bee stings/insect bites

- Aromatherapy: tea tree, basil, bergamot, lavender, thyme, ylang-ylang
- Add enough water to baking soda or meat tenderizer to make a paste and apply it to the sting
- Cover affected area with a small amount of mashed fresh papaya.
- Herbs: apply fresh aloe vera sap directly to the bite; if bite becomes infected, bathe with marigold or echinacea tea; apply a fresh slice of onion to both bee and wasp stings; a mixture of honey and crushed garlic makes a soothing ointment
- Homeopathy: Apis, 1 tablet every 30 minutes, maximum 6 doses for burning and swelling

Bones (broken)

- Aromatherapy: massage in elemi oil prior to casting
- Bioelectromagnetics: place magnets into the dressings over fractures
- Healing Touch
- Reiki
- Therapeutic Touch

Bruises

- Aromatherapy: cypress, combine 1 drop of chamomile with 2 tsp. of ice cold water—soak a cotton pad and apply to affected area
- Herbs: witch hazel (topical), arnica tablets or massage tincture of arnica into bruised area; 200–400 mg 3 times a day of bromelain on an empty stomach
- Homeopathy: aconite, 1 or 2 doses only over 15 minutes immediately for the "shock" of the injury
- Hydrotherapy: cold compresses for first 12 hours with occasional breaks to prevent excessive chilling
- Supplements: 2,000 mg vitamin C 3 times a day for people who bruise easily; pineapple juice—enzymes speed the rate at which the blood causing the bruise dissolves

Burns (minor)

- Aromatherapy: for pain relief—chamomile, eucalyptus, geranium, lavender; to reduce inflammation—chamomile, clary sage, geranium, lavender,

myrrh, tea tree; to regenerate skin—chamomile, clary sage, eucalyptus, geranium, myrrh, rose, tea tree
- Herbs: aloe vera sap, calendula lotion, or raw honey
- Hydrotherapy: immediately immerse the affected part in ice water for 5–10 minutes with brief break during the first 20 minutes after the injury
- Magnets: place over site of injury to control pain and speed healing

Cancer

- Antioxidants: vitamins A, C, and E; Co-enzyme 10
- Imagery
- Massage
- Meditation
- Qigong
- Yoga

Canker sores

- Herbs: mix 1 cup of warm water with 1/4 teaspoon of salt and 1/2 teaspoon of goldenseal powder; licorice root gel, echinacea tincture, butternut, comfrey
- Supplements: vitamin A (25,000–50,000 IU daily) prevents infection from spreading; B-complex (50–100 IU TID); vitamin E (400–800 IU daily); selenium (200 mcg daily); acidophilus, 4 capsules, 4–6 times per day

Carpal tunnel syndrome

- Chiropractic manipulation
- Herbs: ginger compress
- Magnets placed over the front and back of the wrist to control symptoms
- Massage
- Pressure point therapies

Chest congestion

- Aromatherapy: cedarwood, steam inhalation of eucalyptus, frankincense; massage chest with lavender, inhale marjoram, peppermint, eucalyptus, or rosemary, drops of tea tree on handkerchief

- Herbs: tea made with peppermint and yarrow (1/2 tsp. each); sage or eucalyptus leaves in a bowl of steaming water—inhale with a towel draped over the head
- Magnets: wear on chest over bronchial tubes and at equal level on the back; sleeping on a magnetic mattress pad can be helpful

Cholesterol (high)

- Herbs: garlic, Indian gooseberry
- Meditation
- Supplements: Profibe (grapefruit fiber)
- Yoga

Circulation (poor)

- Aromatherapy: rosemary (increases circulation to skin), vetiver
- Biofeedback
- Exercise
- Healing Touch
- Herbs: ginkgo, garlic, cayenne, hawthorn, bilberry
- Hypnosis
- Imagery
- Magnets
- Massage
- Therapeutic Touch
- Yoga

Common cold

- Acupressure: if sinuses become blocked or painful
- Aromatherapy: inhale lavender, eucalyptus, or peppermint oil in steam vaporizer to speed recovery and lessens stuffiness; add 3 drops lemon oil, 2 drops thyme and tea tree oil, and 1 drop eucalyptus into hot bath
- Herbs: tea from fresh ginger and brown sugar, echinacea at the first sign of a cold, astragalus, garlic, goldenseal
- Homeopathy: allium cepa (onion), monkshood, aconite, or natrum muriaticum: 1 tablet up to every 4 hours, as needed—maximum 3–4 days.

- Reflexology: work the fingers and thumbs, the webs between the fingers, the pads beneath the fingers, and the spaces on the back of the hands for the reflexes of the head, lungs, and upper lymphatics
- Supplements: vitamin C, zinc lozenges

Cold sores

- Aromatherapy: apply tea tree oil at onset and continue until cleared
- Herbs: lemon-balm tea shows significant antiviral activity against herpes simplex; echinacea (600 mg daily) or goldenseal (100 mg daily)

Colic

- Aromatherapy: chamomile (rubbed on abdomen), coriander, orange, peppermint
- Massage abdomen; massage bottom of feet with warmed sesame oil

Constipation

- Aromatherapy: massage abdomen in a clockwise direction with orange, black pepper, ginger, or marjoram mixed in a carrier oil
- Exercise: especially activities that work the abdominal muscles such as rowing, swimming, walking, or sit-ups
- Herbs: dandelion root, chicory root, angelica root (20–30 drops of extract in a small glass of water 3 times a day), cascara sagrada, senna; psyllium—only use for several days, long-term use can be damaging
- Homeopathy: bryonia (wild hops) or nux vomica—1 tablet 3 times daily—maximum 1 week
- Drink 6–8 glasses of water daily
- Yoga: twisting postures and forward bends are often helpful

Corns

- Aromatherapy: mix 2 drops each of orange, lemon, and lavender oils in a basin of warm water and soak feet for at least 15 minutes per day

Cough

- Aromatherapy: cedarwood; several drops of cypress or tea tree on handkerchief and inhale deeply; add 3 drops eucalyptus and 2 drops thyme oil

to 2 tsp. vegetable oil—massage into neck and chest; steam inhalation using sandalwood, benzoin, eucalyptus, or frankincense
- Herbs: licorice, wild cherry bark, thyme; tincture of mullein in warm water 3 times a day
- Homeopathy: bryonia (wild hops), monkshood, rumex, stannum— 1 tablet 3 times daily until improved—maximum 2 weeks
- Reflexology: work the lung and diaphragm reflexes on and beneath balls of feet and webs between big toes and second toes

Depression

- Acupuncture
- Animal-assisted therapy
- Aromatherapy: bergamot, geranium, jasmine, lemon balm, rose, ylang-ylang; to bath add 15 drops geranium, 10 drops of bergamot, and 5 drops of lavender
- Exercise
- Flower essences: gentian, hornbeam, mustard, gorse, sweet chestnut
- Healing Touch
- Herbs: St. John's wort, valerian
- Meditation
- Reiki
- Supplements: B vitamins
- T'ai Chi
- Therapeutic Touch
- Transcranial magnetic stimulation

Diabetes

- Biofeedback
- Exercise
- Herbs: blueberry leaf tea, 2 cups a day on a regular basis; 100–200 mg of co-enzyme Q every day for a least 3 months to stabilize blood sugar
- Yoga

Diarrhea

- Aromatherapy: coriander, chamomile, neroli, lavender, or peppermint in carrier oil—gentle abdominal massage

- Herbs: 2 tsp. per cup of boiling water to make tea of black pepper, chamomile, coriander, rosemary, sandalwood, or thyme
- Homeopathy: podophyllum—1 tablet hourly until improved, then every 4 hours—maximum 5 days
- Supplements: zinc
- Replace lost fluids

Ear Infections

- Acupressure: massage just behind the tip of the mastoid bone at the bottom of the back of the ear to relieve pain
- Aromatherapy: put a drop of lavender on cotton and put it in the ear; use a chamomile tea bag that has been infused for a few minutes and place it on the side of the face or over the ear while it is still warm
- Craniosacral manipulation
- Herbs: warm mullein oil drops in ear
- Homeopathy: pulsatilla, belladonna, or aconite—1 tablet every 4 hours for 2–3 days
- Reflexology: work all fingers and toes paying close attention to the webs between the fingers and toes, especially between the 3rd, 4th, and 5th digits

Emotional distress

- Aromatherapy: chamomile, frankincense (deepens breathing to induce calmness), marjoram
- Breathing exercises
- Gratitude exercises
- Positive affirmations

Energy imbalance

- Applied Kinesiology
- Healing Touch
- Magnets
- Polarity Therapy
- Pressure point therapies
- Reiki
- Shiatsu massage

- Thai massage
- Therapeutic Touch

Fatigue

- Aromatherapy: peppermint, rose, rosemary, and basil stimulate the brain; lemon grass and rosemary are best for physical fatigue; use these oils in the bath, in massage oils, in vaporizers, or on a handkerchief; do not use peppermint or rosemary at night because they are too stimulating; rosemary should not be used by people with hypertension or epilepsy
- Herbs: ginseng (600 mg daily) especially for people over the age of 40
- Qigong
- Reflexology: a brisk complete foot treatment for more energy or a slow complete foot treatment to induce sleep
- Supplements: zinc, co-enzyme Q
- Yoga: start with relaxation and gentle movements on your back, progressing to kneeling, standing, and/or seated postures

Feet (tired)

- Aromatherapy: foot bath of 2 drops each of rosemary, sage, and peppermint oils in basin of hot water; soak for at least 15 minutes; rosemary (20 drops), sage (15 drops), and peppermint (10 drops) mixed in oil base can be applied directly to feet
- Massage
- Reflexology

Fever

- Aromatherapy: tea tree and juniper encourage the body to sweat; lavender and peppermint are cooling; chamomile is soothing and calming; use either in a bath or in cool water to sponge the body
- Herbs: to a large mug of boiling water add juice of 1 lemon, 2 tsp. honey, 1 tsp. grated ginger, 1/2 tsp. cinnamon, 1/2 tsp. nutmeg, and 1 tbsp. brandy or whisky
- Homeopathy: belladonna, aconite, ferrum phosphoricum, gelsemium—1 tablet every 30 minutes for six doses, then every 4 hours—maximum 3 days

Fibromyalgia

- Acupuncture
- Biofeedback
- Herbs: topical capsaicin
- Magnets: sleep on a magnetic mattress and use a magnetic pillow; magnets can also be placed over painful areas during the day
- Supplements: magnesium, malic acid

Fluid retention

- Massage feet and ankles
- Elevate legs

Headache (tension)

- Acupressure: press pressure points between eyebrows or at bottom of web between thumb and first finger
- Alexander Technique: helps improve posture to avoid buildup of tension in neck and shoulders
- Aromatherapy: basil, chamomile, massage lavender, peppermint, or eucalyptus around temples; rose compress to eyes
- Chiropractic manipulation
- Herbs: 1/2 tsp. each of betony and skullcap made into tea; ginseng (200 mg daily)
- Homeopathy: bryonia (wild hops), windflower, yellow jasmine, nux vomica—1 tablet every 4 hours as needed—maximum 6 doses
- Pulsating electromagnetic fields
- Relaxation techniques
- Therapeutic Touch
- Yoga

Heart disease

- Animal-assisted therapy
- Biofeedback
- Chelation therapy
- Herbs: 1–2 capsules of hawthorn four times a day for mild angina
- Meditation

- Supplements: vitamin E, L-carnitine (1,000 mg two times a day); coenzyme Q (30–100 mg per day) to improve utilization of oxygen at cellular level

Heat rash

- Herbs: sprinkle arrowroot powder on affected area; 1/2 cup of freshly grated ginger into a quart of boiling water—remove from heat immediately and steep for 5 minutes—cool and sponge ginger water onto affected areas and let it dry

Hemorrhoids

- Aromatherapy: massage geranium, chamomile, or lavender oil, mixed with a carrier oil, into the rectal area as needed
- Herbs: apply aloe vera gel to relieve itching; use compresses of witch hazel to clean area after bowel movement
- Homeopathy: aesculus, aloe, or hamamelis—1 tablet 2 times daily—maximum 2 weeks
- Hydrotherapy: sit in warm bath for 15 minutes several times a day

Hypertension

- Animal-assisted therapy
- Aromatherapy: ylang-ylang, clary sage, lavender, marjoram
- Biofeedback
- Herbs: garlic, hawthorn
- Massage
- Meditation
- Qigong
- Supplements: vitamin C; calcium for pregnancy-induced hypertension
- T'ai Chi
- Yoga

Immune enhancement

- Aromatherapy: elemi, eucalyptus
- Herbs: echinacea
- Massage

- Qigong
- Supplements: vitamin E, vitamin C, beta-carotene, garlic

Indigestion

- Aromatherapy: basil, chamomile, coriander, ginger, peppermint—use as a tea or in massage oil or warm compress over stomach area
- Herbs: chamomile, peppermint, ginger as a tea; for heaviness after a meal chew on cardamom or fennel seeds
- Homeopathy: windflower; nux vomica—1 tablet hourly for six doses, then three times daily—maximum 1 week

Infection (bacterial)

- Aromatherapy: calendula, geranium, rosemary, tea tree, lavender, eucalyptus, thyme, niaouli, bergamot—these oils work by attacking the organisms themselves, by killing airborne germs, and by strengthening the immune system
- Herbs: echinacea (600 mg three times a day) at first sign of infection; echinacea may be combined with goldenseal; garlic (2 g daily) in capsules

Infection (fungal)

- Aromatherapy: calendula, lemon balm, rosemary, tea tree
- Herbs: garlic

Infection (viral)

- Aromatherapy: eucalyptus, lemon balm, tea tree
- Herbs: goldenseal, echinacea, garlic
- Supplements: zinc, selenium

Infertility

- Meditation for unexplained infertility
- Supplements: zinc for men

Inflammation

- Aromatherapy: benzoin, birch, chamomile, clary sage, elemi, fennel, geranium, helichrysum, jasmine, myrrh, patchouli, rose, sandalwood
- Bee venom may slow down the body's inflammatory response by inhibiting the amount of free radicals or by stimulating the adrenal glands to release cortisol
- Homeopathy: belladonna
- Hydrotherapy: applications of heat and cold
- Magnets

Insomnia

- Aromatherapy: chamomile, which can also be used with children; clary sage, lavender, marjoram, neroli, or vetiver in bath or a pillow or as a room fragrance
- Exercise: not later than early evening
- Herbs: valerian, lemon balm, catnip, hops, passion flower, skullcap teas (if taste is unpleasant, add sugar, honey, or lemon)
- Homeopathy: windflower, nux vomica, arsenicum album—1 tablet before bed for 10 days or until improved
- Hydrotherapy: warm baths
- Magnets: use magnetic pillow or pad for sedating effect
- Meditation

Jet Lag

- Herbs: melatonin
- Drink fluids and avoid alcohol; do in-flight stretches

Labor pain

- Aromatherapy: blend of clary sage, rose, and ylang-ylang for massage—deep massage of lower back and hips during contractions, between contractions massage shoulders, back, hands, and feet; if contractions are lagging, a light massage of the breasts may stimulate activity
- Herbs: red raspberry tea, black cohosh tea
- Hypnosis

Liver disease

- Herbs: milk thistle, dandelion root tea
- Hydrotherapy: take steam baths or saunas frequently to help body eliminate toxins

Memory loss

- Aromatherapy: basil, black pepper, coriander, ginger, rosemary, thyme
- Exercise
- Herbs: 2 capsules twice a day of ginkgo
- Supplements: vitamin B_6

Menopause

- Aromatherapy: geranium, rose, fennel in bath or in body creams
- Herbs: black cohosh (4 tablets daily), vitex, agnue castii, rehmannia, ginseng, wild yam as tea; Chinese tonic of He Shou Wu, dong quai
- Meditation
- Supplements: vitamin E (200–800 IU daily), soy protein (50 g daily)

Menstrual discomfort

- Aromatherapy: basil; clary sage massage or warm compress; massage abdomen and lower back with jasmine, marjoram
- Herbs: tea of agnus castus with rosemary for premenstrual water retention; black haw for cramps—4 tsp. in glass of warm water, repeat after 4 hours if necessary; Chinese tonic of dong quai
- Homeopathy: viburnum, magnesium phosphate, sepia—1 tablet every 2–4 hours—maximum 12 doses
- Hydrotherapy: warm compresses
- Reflexology: massage uterine reflexes below inside ankle bones and ovarian reflexes beneath outside ankle bones
- Supplements: calcium and manganese, fish oil, parsley, celery, and dandelion leaves are all mild diuretics
- Yoga stretches and more relaxation and breathing exercises

Migraine headaches

- Aromatherapy: green apple (inhalant), lavender, mellissa, or peppermint put on a facecloth with cool water and used as a compress on the forehead or back of the neck
- Biofeedback
- Herbs: feverfew (prophylaxis)
- Homeopathy: iris, sanguinaria, glonoine—1 tablet every 30 minutes until improved—maximum 6 doses
- Hypnosis
- Pressure point therapies
- Pulsating electromagnetic fields

Morning sickness

- Acupressure: wristband—small weights that exerts pressure on a specific pressure point on the wrist
- Herbs: peppermint, catnip, ginger, chamomile teas

Muscle soreness

- Aromatherapy: chamomile, juniper
- Herbs: rub in wintergreen oil or capsicum cream
- Hydrotherapy: spa
- Massage
- Yoga

Nausea

- Acupressure: wristband—small weights that exert pressure on a specific pressure point on the wrist
- Aromatherapy: ginger, lavender, peppermint used as a compress and as teas
- Healing Touch
- Homeopathy: ipecacuanha, sepia, clossypium—1 tablet every half-hour—maximum 12 doses
- Imagery
- Reiki
- Therapeutic Touch

Osteoarthritis

- Acupuncture
- Alexander Technique: to relieve muscular tension and uneven weight-bearing
- Bioelectromagnetics
- Herbs: glucosamine and chondroitin to help restore joint integrity; natural anti-inflammatories like willowbark, turmeric, and ginger
- Hydrotherapy: soak in hot water or spa frequently; use ice packs on inflamed joints
- Pressure point therapies
- Relaxation exercises
- Supplements: vitamin B_6 (100 mg 2 times a day)
- Yoga: practice slowly, seeing how far you can move affected joints without pain; do not exercise when joints are inflamed

Osteoporosis

- Exercise: weight bearing unless advanced stage of disease
- Herbs: a tea of stinging nettles, alfalfa, or sage
- Supplements: calcium, vitamins D and C, hormone replacement therapy

Pain

- Alexander Technique
- Chiropractic manipulation
- Healing Touch
- Herbs: feverfew
- Hydrotherapy: hot water packs
- Hypnosis
- Imagery
- Magnets
- Pressure point therapies
- Reiki
- Sports massage
- Therapeutic Touch
- Trager Approach
- Trigger point massage

Physical disabilities

- Balance difficulties—T'ai Chi, yoga, hippotherapy

Poison ivy and poison oak

- Rinse the exposed area with soap and cold water; mix baking soda with water to form a paste and apply it to skin; once the paste has hardened, remove with cool water and apply a thin layer of honey to the area.
- For itching and discomfort, grind 1 cup raw, whole oats to a fine powder and add to tepid bath—soak for 20–30 minutes

Premenstrual syndrome

- Acupuncture
- Aromatherapy: massage or warm bath with rose oil, clary sage, ylang-ylang, lavender, lemon grass, sandalwood, jasmine, bergamot—you will have to decide, by trial and error, which one of these oils best suits you
- Deep breathing exercises for a least 20 minutes a day
- Herbs: vitex, black cohosh extract, agnus-castus (10–20 drops each morning); Helonias; Chinese tonic of dong quai
- Homeopathy: windflower, pulsatilla, lachesis—1 tablet 2 times daily—maximum 1 week; may be repeated next period
- Meditation
- Reflexology: massage uterine reflexes below inside ankle bones and ovarian reflexes beneath outside ankle bones
- Supplements: vitamin B_6, 2–3 g capsule of combined fish oil and evening primrose oil

Prostate enlargement (benign)

- Herbs: Saw palmetto (160 mg 2 times a day) pygeum africanum, stinging nettle root tea
- Supplements: 30 mg of zinc picolinate daily; add soy foods to diet

Psoriasis

- Diet: include foods with zinc, beta-carotene, vitamin D, and omega-3 fatty acids; avoid liver and other organ meats, foods that aggravate psoriasis

- Herbs: aloe vera extract in topical application—apply 3 times a day—do not cover
- Homeopathy: sepai, arsenicum iodatum, petroleum—1 tablet 2 times daily—maximum 2 weeks
- Sunshine on the skin is helpful

Sciatica

- Acupuncture
- Applied Kinesiology
- Chiropractic manipulation
- Hydrotherapy: warm water jets
- Reflexology

Sexual dysfunction

- Herbs: ginkgo (180 to 240 mg daily) for erectile problems; ashwaganda
- Hypnotherapy and imagery

Shingles

- Aromatherapy: eucalyptus, tea tree, lavender, chamomile, bergamot—smooth the oil gently over the affected areas and down either side of the spine; if body is too painful to touch, add oils to a water spray or use in a bath
- Herbs: echinacea (up to 2 g daily); St. John's wort tea, aloe vera gel to blistering area

Sinus problems

- Aromatherapy: basil, marjoram or eucalyptus—put on handkerchief or use with a vaporizer
- Herbs: ephedra, goldenseal, yarrow, coltsfoot—make a tea using 2 tsp. of herb per cup; use herbs in cream or oil and massage the sinus areas
- Homeopathy: hydrastis, kali bichromicum—1 tablet 3 times daily—maximum 10 days
- Hydrotherapy: hot and cold compresses, steam inhalation, nasal lavage
- Reflexology: massage the sinus reflexes on the tips of the fingers and toes

Skin (dry)

- Aromatherapy: mix 2 drops each of sandalwood, rose, and geranium oil with a tablespoon of almond oil—use as a topical evening moisturizer; other oils good for dry skin include jasmine, orange, and ylang-ylang used in a moisturizer or in a bath

Sore throat

- Aromatherapy: several drops of sandalwood on handkerchief or mix with carrier oil and massage into throat area and then wrap something warm around the throat
- Herbs: mix 1 cup of warm water with 1/4 teaspoon of salt and 1/2 teaspoon of goldenseal powder
- Homeopathy: monkshood, poison ivy, belladonna—1 tablet every 2 hours for 6 doses, then every 4 hours—maximum 3 days
- Reflexology: massage the throat reflexes around the "neck" of the big toes and thumbs

Sprain and strains

- Aromatherapy: chamomile, ginger, lavender as massage to area
- Healing Touch
- Herbs: 1/4 cup each of dry mustard powder and flour with warm water to make a thick paste, spread the paste onto cheesecloth or gauze, roll it up, and apply to the strained area
- Homeopathy: poison ivy—1 tablet 3 times daily—maximum 2 weeks
- Hydrotherapy: cold compresses to reduce swelling first 24 hours; then warm compresses to increase circulation
- Magnets: cover area with magnetic pad and secure with an Ace bandage—12 hours on and 12 hours off
- Myofascial release
- Pressure point therapies
- Reiki
- Therapeutic Touch

Surgery

- Hypnotherapy and visualization before surgery
- Magnets: place magnets over the incision site for 24 to 48 hours before surgery to improve postoperative recovery, place magnets over wound after surgery
- Meditation before and after surgery

Stress

- Aromatherapy: juniper, lavender, vetiver, ylang ylang, jasmine—use in massage oil or put in bath
- Breathing exercises; alternate nostril breathing (pranayama)
- Exercise
- Meditation
- Yoga: focus on slow movements and long exhalations

Sunburn

- Herbs: soak a soft cloth in cooled black or green tea and spread over the burned area—leave on 15–30 minutes; apply aloe vera sap to area
- Hydrotherapy: soak in a bath of tepid water and baking soda (1 pound) for 20–30 minutes; later that day or next take take a tepid bath with 1 or 2 cups of milk added
- Grated potato applied directly to the skin will decrease pain and prevent blistering; wrap in place with a clean cloth

Tension

- Aromatherapy: hot bath or massage using one of the following oils—bergamot, rose, cedarwood, chamomile, geranium, lavender, melissa, orange, or sandalwood
- Feldenkrais Method
- Healing Touch
- Herbs: valerian, passion flower, kava kava, ginseng as teas
- Massage
- Meditation
- Reiki
- Therapeutic Touch

Tinnitus

- Supplements: vitamin B_{12}

Urinary tract infection

- Aromatherapy: bergamot, sandalwood, lavender, or juniper in bath water
- Herbs: 2 capsules 3 times a day of uva ursi until symptoms disappear
- Supplements: unsweetened cranberry juice (300 ml daily) and vitamin C
- Urinate after sexual activity
- Drink plenty of water

Warts

- Aromatherapy: 1 drop each of lemon, thyme, and tea tree oil mixed in a base oil and swabbed 2 times a day
- Hypnosis
- Imagery

Weight control

- Aromatherapy: green apple
- Exercise
- Herbs: evening primrose oil
- Supplements: 2.5 g of vitamin B_5, 4 times a day

Wounds

- Aromatherapy: to disinfect—bergamot, chamomile, clary sage, jasmine, juniper, lavender, rose, tea tree; to relieve pain—bergamot, chamomile, geranium, jasmine, lavender, rosemary; to stop bleeding—cypress, geranium, rose; to reduce inflammation—chamomile, geranium, helichrysum, jasmine, patchouli; to promote formation of scar tissue—bergamot, chamomile, helichrysum, jasmine
- Bioelectromagnetics
- Herbs: echinacea, goldenseal
- Hydrotherapy: warm water irrigation

INDEX